Athletic Training Exam Review Third Edition

Lynn Van Ost, MEd, RN, PT, ATC
Hunterdon Medical Center
Flemington, New Jersey

Karen Manfré, MA, ATR
Hunterdon Central High School
Flemington, New Jersey

Karen Lew, MEd, ATC, LAT
Southeastern Louisiana University
Hammond, Louisiana

SLACK
INCORPORATED

Delivering the best in health care information and education worldwide
6900 Grove Road • Thorofare, NJ 08086

www.slackbooks.com

ISBN: 978-1-55642-764-0

The procedures and practices described in this book should be implemented in a manner consistent with the professional standards set for the circumstances that apply in each specific situation. Every effort has been made to confirm the accuracy of the information presented and to correctly relate generally accepted practices. The authors, editor, and publisher cannot accept responsibility for errors or exclusions or for the outcome of the material presented herein. There is no expressed or implied warranty of this book or information imparted by it. Care has been taken to ensure that drug selection and dosages are in accordance with currently accepted/recommended practice. Due to continuing research, changes in government policy and regulations, and various effects of drug reactions and interactions, it is recommended that the reader carefully review all materials and literature provided for each drug, especially those that are new or not frequently used. Any review or mention of specific companies or products is not intended as an endorsement by the author or publisher.

SLACK Incorporated uses a review process to evaluate submitted material. Prior to publication, educators or clinicians provide important feedback on the content that we publish. We welcome feedback on this work.

Published by: SLACK Incorporated
               6900 Grove Road
               Thorofare, NJ 08086 USA
               Telephone: 856-848-1000
               Fax: 856-853-5991
               www.slackbooks.com

Contact SLACK Incorporated for more information about other books in this field or about the availability of our books from distributors outside the United States.

Library of Congress Cataloging-in-Publication Data

Van Ost, Lynn.
   Athletic training exam review : a student guide to success / Lynn Van Ost, Karen Manfré, Karen Lew.-- 3rd ed.
      p. ; cm.
   Includes bibliographical references and index.
   ISBN-13: 978-1-55642-764-0 (alk. paper)
   ISBN-10: 1-55642-764-6 (alk. paper)
   1. Physical education and training--Examinations, questions, etc. 2. Athletic trainers--Examinations, questions, etc.
   [DNLM: 1. Physical Education and Training--Examination Questions. 2. Physical Fitness--Examination Questions.
   3. Exercise--Examination Questions. QT 18.2 V217a 2006] I. Manfré, Karen, 1952- II. Lew, Karen. III. Title.

RC1210.V36 2006
617.1'027076--dc22
                                                   2006004885

For permission to reprint material in another publication, contact SLACK Incorporated. Authorization to photocopy items for internal, personal, or academic use is granted by SLACK Incorporated provided that the appropriate fee is paid directly to Copyright Clearance Center. Prior to photocopying items, please contact the Copyright Clearance Center at 222 Rosewood Drive, Danvers, MA 01923 USA; phone: 978-750-8400; website: www.copyright.com; email: info@copyright.com

Printed in the United States of America.

Last digit is print number: 10 9 8 7 6 5 4 3 2

DEDICATION

We dedicate the third edition of this text to our families and friends. We could not have accomplished this pinnacle without your ongoing enthusiasm and encouragement. You have always been the light at the end of our journeys. We are very fortunate and blessed to have each of you in our lives.

Lynn Van Ost, MEd, RN, PT, ATC and Karen Manfré, MA, ATR

As we were completing the final portion of this text, Hurricane Katrina was bearing down on New Orleans and the Gulf Coast. I would not have been able to complete this text without the help of my family and friends. Lynn, Karen, Carrie, Lauren and everyone at SLACK Incorporated, thank you for your continued support of this important project. Mom, Dad, and Steven; you are my inspiration. There are so many people that have helped me along my journey in athletic training and without your guidance; I would not be where I am today. Greg, when I worry about things I cannot control, or fail to listen to the voice of reason, you are always available to put things in perspective. Thank you.

Karen Lew, MEd, ATC, LAT

CONTENTS

ACKNOWLEDGMENTS

We would like to extend a sincere thank you to many individuals who have helped us complete the third edition of this text. Carrie Kotlar, Lauren Plummer and everyone at SLACK Incorporated for once again taking us by the hand and being so kind and understanding throughout this process. Andy Wetstein, ATC for your inspiration from the beginning of this endeavor. Karen Lew, you are always such a positive member of this "team". When disaster struck you stood your ground and weathered the STORM till the end. We are grateful that you stuck it out with us.

Lynn Van Ost, Med, RN, ATC and Karen Manfré MA, ATR

I would like to thank the following people for their help with questions, constant feedback, and ideas. Your help is truly appreciated. I promise no more questions for at least another year. Gerard White, Cary Berthelot, and Cat Stemmans I appreciate the many questions you answered and the suggestions you offered for this book. Dr. Reiss Plauche, thank you for being there to answer questions and support me in all of my endeavors. Your encouragement means so much to me.

Karen Lew, MEd, ATC, LAT

ABOUT THE AUTHORS

Lynn Van Ost, MEd, RN, PT, ATC, graduated in 1982 with a Bachelor's in nursing from West Chester State College, West Chester, Pa; in 1987 from Temple University, Philadelphia, Pa, with a Master's in sports medicine/athletic training; and in 1988 from Temple University with a second Bachelor's in physical therapy. In addition to treating the general orthopedic population as a physical therapist, she has worked with both amateur and professional athletes and has over 11 years experience as an athletic trainer working with Olympic-level elite athletes at numerous international events, including the 1992 and 1996 Summer Olympic games. She currently works as a clinical specialist in sports medicine at Hunterdon Medical Center in Flemington, NJ.

Karen Manfré, MA, ATR, graduated from State University of New York at Brockport in 1977 with a Bachelor's in physical education/athletic training and from Rider University with a Master's in educational administration in 1999. She has been in education for over 20 years and has worked as an athletic trainer at many levels of competition, including professional, elite, and intercollegiate. She currently serves as the head athletic trainer for Hunterdon Central Regional High School in Flemington, NJ.

Karen Lew, MEd, ATC, LAT, graduated from the University of New Orleans in 1996 with a Bachelor's in health and physical education and from the University of Louisiana at Monroe with a Master's in education in 1997. She is involved with the athletic training education program at Southeastern Louisiana University where she currently serves as the program director of athletic training education. In addition to her duties at Southeastern Louisiana University, she has been involved with the Universal Cheerleaders' Association since 1993. During that time, she has served as an athletic trainer at a variety of camps, the Macy's Thanksgiving Day Parade, and the annual New Year's Day Parade in London, England.

FOREWORD

The profession of athletic training has gone through many changes since its creation in the 1950s, and today it continues to be a dynamic and vibrant health care profession. As part of this continuing metamorphosis, athletic training must continually respond to the changing needs of our patients/athletes, as well as the ever-expanding body of knowledge that undergirds our professional practice. The Board of Certification (BOC) certification examination is developed to address this changing professional practice, as well as the wealth of knowledge and skills required of certified athletic trainers. The intention of the BOC certification examination is to protect the public by ensuring that all those individuals who carry the title are able to demonstrate a minimum level of competence which has been determined to protect the public. This professional competence is defined by the BOC Role Delineation Study, as well as the *Professional Standards of Practice* (www.bocatc.org).

While many texts are developed by Certified Athletic Trainers who are involved in education, this text book is developed by highly qualified and experienced practitioners. Not only have Ms. Van Ost, Manfré, and Lew used their knowledge of the BOC certification examination and the Role Delineation Study in their development of this study guide, it is obvious that they also have brought their expansive clinical expertise to the development of clinically-relevant scenarios and questions. This exam review guide is developed in a very comprehensive and helpful format. In addition to its utilization as a study guide, it also can be used by educators to create simulated patient scenarios that are appropriate for clinical proficiency evaluations when no "real life" patients are available. While a text such as this can never replace the valuable experiences that students are able to gain with real patients, under the guidance and mentorship of qualified and experienced clinical educators, it can serve as a tool that can be used as an adjunct to their clinical teaching.

Paula Sammarone Turocy, EdD, ATC
Department Chair and Associate Professor
Rangos Rizakus Endowed Chair for Health Sciences and Ethics
Duquesne University
Pittsburgh, PA

INTRODUCTION

This study guide for the Board of Certification (BOC) certification examination was inspired and developed as a result of a strong passion for our profession. Athletic training is a unique health care profession in that the athletic trainer is often in the position of experiencing the results of his or her efforts. The athletes' victories are our victories, and their losses, our losses. We become friends, mentors, counselors, teachers, guardians, protectors, and healers. It takes a special individual to become a proficient and dedicated professional athletic trainer. Long hours are spent in the athletic training room, classroom, and on courts and fields preparing for the final examination that will allow you to place the letters ATC behind your name.

Our intent in writing this study guide is to assist you in accomplishing that final goal of passing the BOC certification examination. It is an accumulation of dedicated research and past experience. We have included a section on study techniques to assist you in your preparation for the examination and a general overview of the examination format to help you organize your thoughts.

This guide has been divided into six major areas: study techniques, general information and the examination format, sample written questions, sample written simulation questions, sample questions for the practical examination, and practical tips and advice for those who do not pass the first time.

The written questions have been organized according to related athletic training subject matter and the BOC's Role Delineation Study (5th Edition) Educational Domains and the Related Athletic Training Subject Matter to allow you to assess subjects in which you may be weak and subjects in which your strengths lie. Although this study guide will assist you in preparing for the certification examination, it should not be used in place of your textbooks or other sources of study from your academic program. It is not intended to be a "practice" examination; it is meant only to be used as an adjunct source of information and to tie everything you have learned in the classroom and during your fieldwork together.

In Chapters 1 and 2, we have provided some specific tools to help you organize yourself up to 6 months prior to the examination. Chapter 3 consists of over 1000 study questions. Over 800 of the questions are a "mixed bag" of subjects derived from the BOC's Role Delineation Study Educational Domains and the Related Athletic Training Subject Matter. The final 250 questions cover most of the related subject matter of athletic training. Chapter 4 includes 27 written simulation problems, testing your ability to make appropriate judgment calls and improve your problem-solving skills. Each problem presents a specific scenario with several possible options that you can choose to follow. Chapter 5 is a simulation for the practical examination. This section is comprised of 26 problems that are designed to test your manual athletic training skills.

The final chapter is directed at helping you if your test results are not favorable. We have included some suggestions on how to deal with the immediate difficulties not passing may cause and how to begin the process of developing a new approach for your next attempt. Provided you have applied the information you have learned in the classroom and on the field to the study strategies we have offered in this manual, you will not need to read this final chapter.

Unique to this third edition are all-new testing capabilities featuring an online component with written examination (multiple choice) questions. You can test your knowledge with three separate exams and receive the results for each when completed. Also, at the end of each sample exam, you will be able to review the questions along with the correct answers for a complete and comprehensive review. We wish you luck and look forward to welcoming you as a colleague.

STUDY TECHNIQUES AND TEST-TAKING STRATEGIES

The most obvious question that comes to mind when preparing for the Board of Certification (BOC) athletic trainer certification exam is "Where do I start?" Just the thought of studying for this examination can be overwhelming. There seems to be so much information and so little time to absorb it all. The good news is that none of this information should be new to you.

The purpose of this text is to provide you with a comprehensive review of previously learned material. In using this as a review tool, you can assess your strengths as well as your weaknesses. As you progress through this book, you should document areas that you need to review and research more information. The information contained throughout this book should serve as an excellent guide in your preparation for the BOC certification examination.

The best way to prevent you from feeling overwhelmed and to develop the motivation to study is to begin by taking small steps toward your goal. The first step is to learn new study strategies or improve the ones you currently find effective. Learning how to concentrate and organize your time in an efficient manner is the basis of good study skills. Remember, it is not necessarily the quantity of time you spend but the quality of time that counts.

IMPROVING CONCENTRATION

Concentration may be defined as the ability to focus on the task at hand. Here are some suggestions to improve your ability to concentrate while studying.

Eliminate Environmental Distractions

- Select one or two special study areas, preferably a place that is quiet and secluded (such as a library or park).
- Agree with those with whom you live (eg, roommates, spouses/relatives, and children) on a time you will be free to socialize and at what times you will study.
- Hang a "Do Not Disturb" sign on your door, wear a specific item of clothing, or tie a brightly colored ribbon to the door as your signal to others that you do not wish to be interrupted.
- Inform those who find it necessary to interrupt you during your study time on a regular basis that it is important they do not talk to you until you are ready to do so. Make sure you send a clear but tactful message, because they might not be aware that they are interfering with your ability to concentrate.
- Ignore distracting sights and sounds, such as the telephone, television, or loud music. Although some students state that they study better with music in the background, a silent room will provide no distractions at all. It is best to use your answering machine or voicemail so you are not tempted to answer the phone. While studying, make sure that your computer and cell phone are turned off.

Reduce Mind Wandering

- Stand up and walk away from your material when you find your mind wandering. Then come back, and try again.
- Concentrate only on the material you are reviewing. If you have errands or something suddenly pops into your mind, write it down on a note pad and tackle it at a later time.
- Make sure you stay in good shape, both physically and mentally. It is important to eat, sleep, and exercise routinely. You cannot concentrate or perform adequately if you are hungry or are a victim of sleep deprivation. Get out and exercise; it will relax you and clear your mind.
- If you have other major concerns about which you are currently worrying, such as personal problems at home or at work, make sure you attend to them when you are not studying. Try to find a way to resolve the problems as soon as possible so they do not distract you from the goal at hand.
- Remember to reward your studying with a social event or some quiet time alone doing an enjoyable activity that requires little focused concentration. Set a goal for your reward, such as reviewing a particular subject completely and to your satisfaction. Be careful not to set up your "time off" as your goal.

Improve Your Concentration

- Develop a good attitude toward the subject you are studying. Have an inquisitive mind; ask yourself additional questions, and search your books and notes for the answers. Skim through the textbook before reviewing a subject or create games for yourself. Try to make your study time as exciting and challenging as you can. The power of positive thinking will help you "ride the tide."
- Break down major areas into smaller components for study (eg, instead of tackling anatomy try a smaller subject, like the muscles of the lower extremity).
- When you get tired, take a break. Get something to drink or eat or take a stroll around the neighborhood. Try to become more aware of the amount of time you are able to adequately concentrate. It is probably best to study for only 2 to 3 hours at a time before taking a 10-minute break.
- Make sure you do not vary your study spots. The areas you have chosen for studying should be utilized only to study. Try to select a specific time to study, and do not get involved in any other activity in that area until you are done. Being consistent with both the time and place you choose to study will train you to be more efficient.

ADDITIONAL STUDY SUGGESTIONS

- *Form or attend a study group.* Make sure the individuals you ask to join the group are eager learners and are willing to participate on a regular basis. This will assure everyone that each person is contributing his or her fair share of work. Make sure the goals of the group are clearly defined so time is not wasted and that everyone has an equal role in accomplishing those goals.
- *Textbook review.* Only refer to your textbooks when it is necessary to review areas on which you are weak or to study a topic in more detail. Trying to read any of your textbooks from beginning to end is completely ineffective and will only cause you to panic. Use "subject focused books" (eg, a book on modalities or anatomy) rather than "general" athletic training books (eg, sports injury management or sports medicine).
- *Examination review courses.* Some schools will offer review courses for the examination. These courses are often given in the summer, when the school curriculum is less intense. It might be wise to contact a school that offers a Commission on Accreditation of Athletic Training Education (CAATE)-accredited curriculum to see if a review course is offered.
- *Class notes.* Your notes from your classes should comprise the majority of your study materials. The subjects outlined by the BOC as requirements for candidates planning to take the certification examination should have been sufficiently covered in your curriculum. If you are unsure of anything that was covered in a particular class, contact the professor so that he or she might help clear up your questions.
- *Audiovisual aids.* Audiovisual aids may help to clarify a confusing topic. It sometimes helps to be able to see or hear how a task is performed and have the ability to rerun the task several times to fully understand how it is done. If you learn better by hearing and seeing, ask your instructor or supervisor where you might obtain tapes or instructional videos (eg, handling an unconscious athlete, strength training techniques). You may also want to create your own video with friends or an instructor.
- *Practice with a buddy.* If you find you do not work well in groups but need to practice specific skills, enlist the assistance of a friend, especially another candidate whose needs are similar to yours. Feedback is important for accuracy and timing, and only someone familiar with what you are trying to accomplish can give you helpful insight. Working with someone in the same "boat" can also help

alleviate your anxieties. You may also recruit a certified athletic trainer that you are comfortable with to help you practice a skill in which you may be particularly weak.

- *Flash cards*. Make up flash cards with questions and answers, and carry them with you. This technique works especially well when studying factual information, such as anatomy, kinesiology, or therapeutic modalities. They are easy to carry and allow you to study in bits and pieces anytime, anywhere.
- *Multimedia*. Use CD-ROMs (eg, anatomy, goniometry, or manual muscle testing) to study from and clarify questions, or utilize the internet and explore helpful websites.

TIME MANAGEMENT

It is essential that you learn to organize your time and develop some specific test-taking techniques. Careful planning of your time will allow you to work more efficiently. Developing a purposeful calendar of events will allow you to prioritize your tasks and accomplish them step by step. Preparation is the key to success. Time spent organizing and planning will reduce your anxiety and allow you to think straight under pressure. The following ideas might be of help if you find either one or both of the above-mentioned areas to be a source of frustration.

- Plan a schedule for studying by creating a chart dividing the months into weeks and weeks into days and hours (see Appendix A). You may also try using a day planner or personal digital assistant (PDA).
- Fill in this chart with your planned study times, activities, and "down time." Keep a record of your study pattern, and review it on a weekly basis. If you are not spending enough time studying, where are you spending the time?
- When scheduling study times, be sure to allow yourself additional time for your harder topics. This will help you to avoid cramming, which is ineffective.
- Concentrate your study efforts on clinical situations, diseases, or areas with which you are not as familiar. For example, if you have never dealt with an athlete with a thoracic injury or a life-threatening allergic reaction, focus a bit more on those topics. Get more information until you are satisfied that the topic is well covered.
- Know the date of your examination, and make sure all the preliminaries are taken care of ahead of time (eg, you have turned in your application materials, your CPR card is current). This will help you organize your calendar.
- Think about the following questions and answer them to identify how you manage your time:

⇒ When are you most alert: in the morning, afternoon, or evening? What time is optimal for you to study?

⇒ How much sleep do you require to be most alert and able to concentrate?

⇒ When do you prefer to have your meals?

⇒ How much time do you like to exercise? What time is optimal for exercising?

⇒ How much time do you allow for relaxation or fun activities when you study?

⇒ What other priorities do you have in your life, and when are the best times to address them?

SPECIFIC TEST-TAKING STRATEGIES

By following a few simple guidelines when you actually sit down to take the test, you may eliminate a number of silly mistakes that can easily be made as a result of being too anxious.

- Preview your test, and look over the types and number of questions given.
- Read all the test instructions thoroughly before starting.
- Budget your time; note how many questions you must answer for each section and how much each question is worth. Estimate how much time you have to answer each question.
- Make sure you read the entire question and all the answers to the question before deciding which choice is best.
- If you are unsure of an answer, go with your first choice.
- Keep track of your time during the examination with your watch or a wall clock.
- Rephrase difficult questions in your own words, but be sure not to change the meaning of the question.
- Answer all the questions even if you have to guess. Do not leave any question unanswered.
- For multiple choice questions, if you have a question that has "all of the above" or "none of the above" as possible answers, go through each of the other answers and place a true or false next to it. If all or none of the answers are true or false, then all or none of the above applies.
- As you are reviewing the questions, mark them according to the level of difficulty. If you do not have any doubt about the answer, mark with a $, if you have some doubt about the content/answer, mark with a ?, and if there is a question you are not familiar with, identify it with an *. By coding the

questions, it will give you a basis of what you need to review.

- Write notes in the margin, or underline vocabulary you may need to review.
- Once you complete your review for the study period, make a comprehensive list of the materials that you need to review in your textbooks or with your instructor.

DECREASING YOUR TEST ANXIETY

Everyone feels some level of anxiety before taking a test; it is a normal response to feeling challenged. However, it is important to take control of your feelings so they do not overwhelm you and paralyze your thought process. Here are some ideas that you might try to make you more comfortable.

- Prepare early, approximately 6 months prior to the exam. Check to make sure you have everything in order to apply to take the test. If you are well prepared before the actual examination, it will be one less thing about which to worry. Assuming you have met all the requirements, this is the time to start organizing your study plan.
- Know the location of the test site, and leave enough time to get there early. Make sure to check the weather reports the night before to allow any changes in planning. If you live a good distance away, stay at a hotel the night before. If you are staying in the city or town in which the examination is being given, take the time to drive the route from your hotel to the examination site to avoid increasing your anxiety about specific directions or timing the next morning.
- Try to relax the night before the examination. Go out to dinner, or take in a fun movie with friends. This will help you to sleep well the night before the examination. Just be sure not to stay up late! You will want to be very alert the next morning.
- Eat a good breakfast the morning of the examination. You will not be able to concentrate if you are hungry, and you need fuel to stay alert.
- Make sure to dress comfortably. Wear clothing that is loose but neat, and wear layers of clothing so you can make adjustments if the room temperature is not to your liking. It is best to appear professional and avoid wearing athletic apparel, such as a sweatsuit. Do not wear a hat or bandanna on your head because this may attract attention, and under no circumstances should you wear clothing with a school or clinic logo.

- Do not cram the morning of the examination; this will only cause further stress. It might help to scan through one or two small topics prior to the test, but in general, you will know all you are going to know by that time anyway.
- While waiting for the test, try stretching a bit or running in place. If you know how to do progressive relaxation (ie, progressively tensing and relaxing your muscles from head to toe), feel free to try it. Find the bathroom and water fountain so you know where they are located.
- Close your eyes, and take some deep breaths; try to think positively and confidently. Remember, you have prepared yourself for this! If you go "blank" or find yourself panicking during the test, put your pencil down, close your eyes, and take a deep breath. Count to 10 or until you can focus again.
- Do not rehash your performance after the examination. What is done is done. Try to forget it for a couple of days. Plan to do something fun and stress-free after it is over.
- Do not compare yourself to your friends. You did the best you could, and every candidate's test scores will vary. Do not allow your score to be a measure of your self-worth.

WHAT TO BRING TO THE EXAMINATION

Be sure to bring the following items with you on the day of the examination:

- A map to the test site with written directions (or use Mapquest [www.mapquest.com]).
- Telephone numbers for the test site and BOC.
- Your test admission ticket.
- A photo ID (driver's license or passport).
- Your confirmation notice from the BOC.
- Change for a pay phone and snacks, if necessary.
- A watch (stop watch capabilities may be useful).
- Tissues.
- Reading glasses, if necessary.
- Money for lunch (or pack a lunch, and bring it with you).
- Proof of change of address or name change, if applicable.

GENERAL INFORMATION AND THE EXAMINATION FORMAT

Chapter 2

ELIGIBILITY AND APPLYING FOR THE BOC CERTIFICATION EXAMINATION

The NATA Professional Education Committee (NATA-PEC) was originally formed by the BOC to monitor the curriculum and field experiences provided by those schools offering athletic training programs. It was this committee's responsibility to ensure that all programs designed to prepare students to become certified athletic trainers met and maintained the academic and clinical standards set by the BOC. The NATA-PEC has since been replaced by the NATA Education Council (NATA-EC). This council is charged with setting the guidelines for the academic and clinical education of those students enrolled in accredited athletic training education programs.

Since it is not within the scope of this manual to include all the current policy changes being made by the NATA-EC regarding athletic training education, nor is it the intent of the authors to have this manual used as a complete source of these changes, it is best to obtain information pertaining to these developments directly from the NATA-EC if you have specific questions or concerns.

Those candidates who are eligible to take the BOC certification examination must have completed a program of study in athletic training that has been accredited by the Commission on Accreditation of Athletic Training Education (CAATE) beginning in 2006.

Candidates who have entered an accredited athletic training curriculum must have successfully completed the athletic training program in no less than 2 academic years and must have received their bachelor's degree from the college or university at which they completed their coursework. All eligible candidates may take the examination on the test date prior to graduation provided all the prerequisites have been met. For those candidates applying from an accredited athletic training program the endorsing athletic trainer is the program director. All endorsements should be in writing and notarized on the appropriate forms provided by the BOC in the application packet.

A CAATE-accredited athletic training program is divided into two components: didactic education and clinical experience. The didactic education component incorporates academic courses or academic credit that meets the requirements of the CAATE guidelines. These courses are designed to teach the athletic training student the clinical skills of the profession and provide a venue in which he or she may practice those skills. It has been recommended by the NATA-EC that these courses provide an academic syllabus and/or a clinical instruction manual that outlines the educational objectives and clinical skill outcomes. These outcomes are derived from the entry-level athletic training clinical proficiencies. The individual university or college determines the amount of academic credit assigned to a given course according to the institution's individual guidelines. Clinical academic coursework may include an internship, externship, or clinical laboratory class in addition to, but not in lieu of, formal academic clinical courses. Athletic training students are assigned to a designated approved clinical instructor (ACI) who is responsible for on-site daily supervision and the evaluation of the student's global performance.

The accredited athletic training program no longer requires a minimum number of hours. A student graduating from an accredited program will have had to successfully complete all of the athletic training education competencies and clinical proficiencies, which must be performed under the supervision of a BOC-certified athletic trainer. If a student is also preparing to take a state licensure examination, he or she must check with the specific state to ensure that he or she will meet all of the requirements of the state's governing board. These competencies and proficiencies will be fulfilled throughout the student's progression through the athletic training education program under the direct supervision of a certified athletic trainer. Many of these competencies and proficiencies will be done in the athletic training room, which should be located within an educational institution or professional sports venue and provide comprehensive athletic health care services (such as pre-practice and pre-game preparation, emergency and rehabilitative services, etc) to a competitive athletic population. Athletic training students may also experience a variety of secondary settings, such as a sports medicine center, emergency room, high school, or physician's office.

A current candidate must fulfill the requirements for eligibility to take the BOC certification examination, the following basic requirements must be met in order to apply:

- Proof of graduation from an accredited college or university.
- Proof of current cardiopulmonary resuscitation (CPR) certification.
- An approved curriculum candidate may apply to take the certification examination prior to graduation as long as he or she has completed all the required academic and clinical requirements outlined by the BOC. The examination may be taken on the test date that is the closest date to the candidate's anticipated date of graduation.

Candidates are required to register online utilizing the RegX option. RegX allows the user to register and submit the information needed to determine a candidate's eligibility. Once the BOC office in Omaha, NE receives the information from the candidate, they will notify the candidate of approval. After the candidate receives the approval notification, he or she may continue with the registration process. The application, once approved, is good for only 1 year. All applications will be processed by the BOC in Omaha, NE. This feature allows the candidate to register for the BOC certification examination online, as well as choose the test site and date of testing. You can access the RegX option by going to the BOC website at www.bocatc.org. All registration must now be completed electronically.

One of the benefits of using RegX will be that a candidate is no longer required to take all three parts of the exam on the same test date. A candidate may elect to take one, two, or all three parts on a specific date. Another advantage is the ability to see what sites are available and what sections are open. Having the ability to choose your own site, based on availability, will be a huge benefit.

It is advisable to register for the certification examination 5 months prior to the test so that you have plenty of time to make sure you have all your requirements completed and that any necessary forms are properly filled out and submitted in a timely fashion. Your test date and site will be assigned on a first-come, first-serve basis. We also suggest that you become an NATA member if you have not done so, as it will impact your application fee. The fee must be paid by check or money order and will cost less if you are an NATA member. Be sure to check with the BOC for current application fees. Be sure to complete your online application prior to the published deadline for the test date for which you are intending to sit. Applying early will help to ensure that it is accepted by the deadline. If you must postpone or cancel your test for any reason, you must request this in writing at least 30 days prior to your exam date. If you wish to reschedule your test date to a date later than your originally scheduled date, a $100 fee will be charged.

DEVELOPMENT OF THE BOC CERTIFICATION EXAMINATION

The development and administration of the BOC certification examination is the sole responsibility of the BOC. This private, nonprofit organization is governed by an eight-member board of directors consisting of five certified athletic trainers, a physician director, a public director, and a corporate/educational director. Within the organizational structure of the BOC are seven committees, each responsible for addressing various areas that are pertinent to the function of the BOC. Two of these committees—the Examination Administration Committee and the Examination Development Committee—are directly involved in the procedural aspects and design/validation of the examination. The questions for the test are developed, validated, and edited by certified athletic trainers. These questions are scrutinized to meet the specifications of the Role Delineation Study that were validated by the BOC. The Fifth Role Delineation Study began being implemented with the April 2006 test and will remain in use through 2011. All test questions developed for all three sections of the examination are based on the six domains of athletic training (prevention; recognition, evaluation, and assessment; immediate care; treatment, rehabilitation, and reconditioning; organization and administration; and professional development and responsibility).

THE BOC CERTIFICATION EXAMINATION FORMAT

The first certification examination given by the NATA in 1967 included 150 written questions and a practical section consisting of five questions. The original test was administered and manually scored by three athletic trainers. The certification examination has come a long way since that time and has experienced numerous changes. Currently, the test consists of three separate sections: the written section, the written simulation section, and the practical section. The examination is scored by computer, although additional precautions are taken by the testing center to ensure the test scores are accurate (eg, hand-scoring random tests and rescanning tests).

The Written Section

This section of the certification examination is a standard, 150 multiple-choice question examination based on the six domains of athletic training as identified by the Fifth Role Delineation Study validated in 2005. The questions randomly represent each domain and are worth one point each. Since there will only be one correct answer for each question, if you are unsure of an answer, we advise that you make an educated guess because your answer may be correct. You will not be penalized in this section for guessing. If you leave an answer unmarked or you choose an incorrect answer, a point will be deducted from your score.

Five different question formats have been used:
1. The basic A-type question with five possible correct answer choices.
2. "Not" type questions in which all the answers are correct except for one (eg, "Which of the following muscles is not located in the upper extremity?").
3. "Except" type questions in which all the answers are correct except for one (eg, "All of the following are good sources of vitamin A except:").
4. Completion questions in which a blank word or words must be filled into the stem statement to make it correct (eg, "The two primary movements of the knee joint are _____ and _____.").

5. Multiple-correct type questions in which you must pick all of the available correct choices of those presented and equate them to the list of correct answers.

An example of a multiple-correct type question might look like this:

Which of the following are included in the classification of drugs known as NSAIDs?
- I.   Motrin
- II. Proventil
- III. Dilantin
- IV. Indocin
- V.   Naprosyn

- A.   I, II, III
- B.   I, III, IV, V
- C.   I, IV, V
- D.   III, IV, V
- E.   I, II, V

In this case, C would be the correct answer because Motrin, Indocin, and Naprosyn are all NSAIDs.

Many of the questions will require you to recall information (eg, a specific fact), know a definition, or apply what you know about a particular subject to a situation or condition. For example, a sample question could be:

An athlete has weak shoulder flexors. Which of the following upper extremity proprioceptive neuromuscular facilitation (PNF) patterns would be appropriate to strengthen this muscle group?
- A.   D1 flexion
- B.   D2 extension
- C.   D3 flexion
- D.   Contract-relax
- E.   Slow Reversal

The answer would be A because a D1 flexion PNF pattern incorporates shoulder flexion.

For others you will have to analyze information presented in a question and come to a conclusion based on how the parts of the question relate to each other (eg, an athlete presents with a certain problem or condition and you must assess the situation).

The questions in this manual are reflective of each area of study; they are not meant to represent the full scope of the questions that will be covered in the examination. There are five possible choices for answers in the multiple choice section. Please carefully read each answer before identifying the correct answer as the choices may be similar in nature.

This section of the examination has a 3-hour time limit, which means you cannot spend more than 1 minute per question. Work at a steady pace, but do not rush.

Sometime during the written test, your name will be called and you will be escorted to the practical portion of the examination by a certified athletic trainer. Once you have completed the practical section, you will be escorted back to the testing area to finish the written examination.

When you feel satisfied that you have completed the written examination to the best of your ability, quickly scan your answer sheet to make sure you did not miss anything. Check that your answers correlate with the right questions. One missed answer can throw off your whole answer sheet. We also suggest you erase any unintentional marks you may have made on your answer sheet, as they may affect your score. You may leave the testing area once you are done or if the proctor announces the end of the examination period.

The Written Simulation Section

The written simulation section is a unique section of the certification examination in that it requires you to become more interactive and challenges your professional judgment and problem-solving skills. This section presents realistic scenarios in which you will have to make critical decisions regarding your care plan for the athlete. As you go through each scenario, you will have to make decisions regarding which actions are of immediate priority to ensure the athlete is provided proper care. As you continue through the sections of each scenario, additional information will be revealed to you, allowing you to process what is happening and make a decision on what steps you should follow next.

You will be provided with a problem booklet, an answer booklet, and a latent-image pen for this examination. The problem booklet contains the scenario with which you will be faced and a selection of possible actions from which to choose. You will decide on your answers and mark them with the latent-image pen in your answer booklet. Each answer is revealed as you make your response with the pen. A double asterisk designates the end of each answer. The answer booklet will be blank except for a list of numbers. To highlight your answers, you must highlight your response from the number toward the right until you reach the double asterisk. Do not scrub the pen against the page of the booklet, as you may mismark an answer by accident and highlight an answer you did not intend to highlight. You might also put a hole in your booklet if you rub too hard. Once an answer is marked it cannot be changed, so keep the latent-image pen away from your answer booklet when it is not in use. When answering questions in this part of the examination, keep in mind there is a process involved here, so only select answers that you believe are an immediate priority in solving the dilemma at hand. Follow any directions given if applicable. Make sure you carefully read through all of the possible actions first before you begin to prioritize them. This will help to minimize the chance of your making a mistake by missing an appropriate treatment option.

The written simulation is scored in a different fashion than any other part of the certification examination. Unlike the written examination, there is a penalty if you select an answer that is not appropriate for that situation or if all the correct answers are not selected. Each answer is assigned a positive point, no point (or zero), or a negative point value. There are a possible 50 points that may be scored for those answers that are correct and a possible 50 points that could be deducted from your total score for those answers that are incorrect. Neutral actions result in a zero point score and have no effect on your total score. It is not necessary to actually highlight the answers in the correct order for you to score points, but it is best if you approach your responses exactly how you would in a real-life situation, as it will increase your chances of being right. If you have specific questions concerning how the written simulation is scored, it is advised that you contact the BOC. You will be given 2.5 hours to finish the eight questions presented for the written simulation examination. To help you prepare for this section of the exam, there is an online component included with the text that you should utilize. This format will allow you to utilize a computer and receive immediate feedback regarding your answer selections.

The Practical Section

The practical section of the certification examination is designed to test your ability to apply your manual skills in an environment in which time and accuracy are significant factors in successfully completing the task. The room captain will ask you questions and you will be required to perform a specific task in reference to that question. You will be called during your written examination to take the practical portion and escorted to the test room by the model. This individual has been instructed not to talk about any portion of the examination as you are being escorted, so do not be offended if he or she does not answer you if you ask a question that might relate to the examination. You will bring your answer sheets with you and give them to the room captain. There will be a table in the room that will have various materials/supplies you can use during the examination. You will be instructed to examine these supplies so you know what is available for your use. You will be given a booklet that contains the questions that you will answer and be asked to read them to yourself as the examiners read the questions out loud. Your test will be tape-recorded by the room captain so you and the BOC will have a record of the test.

The time allotted per task begins immediately following the room captain's completion of reading the question. If you do not understand a question, you may ask to have it reread to you. The model has been instructed not to talk to you or help you in any way. He or she is only there for you to demonstrate on, so it will not be helpful to ask him or her what the question means. It is wise to stop and take a second to gather your thoughts (take a deep breath!) and think of what you are doing. You will be graded on the first thing that you perform. If you finish before the allotted time is up, recheck your performance to be sure you covered everything you wanted to cover. It is not necessary to explain what you are doing as you demonstrate each task. If explaining it aloud helps you, feel free to do so but you will not being graded on any of your verbal explanations.

In general, you may be asked questions regarding taping/splinting or wrapping techniques, athletic training evaluation skills (such as special tests, sensory testing, checking for vital signs, goniometric measurements, manual muscle testing, etc), rehabilitation techniques (such as PNF, mobilization techniques, etc), and treatment procedures. It is best to practice these techniques not only on other candidates, but also on certified athletic trainers who can give you constructive feedback. Use a stopwatch or clock to time yourself, since you will be under a time limit during the exam. You will be given 3 to 5 minutes to perform a taping/wrapping technique. Time varies for the rest of the tasks. You are usually given 1 minute for other tasks, especially those requiring you to perform special tests.

Points are scored as you perform the question and demonstrate all the necessary steps. You will lose a point if you do not perform the task in the allotted time, and you will not be given additional credit for completing a specific task before your time is up. Make sure you demonstrate your technique thoroughly, but only do what is necessary to perform the task. When evaluating and testing on the model, be sure to perform all your evaluations in a sequence. It is not necessary to demonstrate your special tests bilaterally. Make sure that you pay special attention to the side or location that you are instructed to test.

Written Examination Sample Questions

ATHLETIC TRAINING DOMAINS

Prevention

1. A sphygmomanometer is a device that measures which of the following?
   A. Grip strength
   B. Body fat percentage
   C. Intra-abdominal pressure
   D. Blood pressure
   E. None of the above

2. A Q-angle of >25 degrees may predispose an athlete to what postural deviation?
   A. Excessive genu varus
   B. Excessive genu valgus
   C. Genu recurvatum
   D. Coxa valgus
   E. Coxa vara

3. All of the following are factors in lower extremity overuse syndromes in runners except:
   A. Poor footwear
   B. Poor posture
   C. Change in surface
   D. Short strides
   E. A and B

4. All of the following questions are significant when screening a young athlete for an underlying cardiac abnormality except:
   A. Does the athlete have chest pain with activity?
   B. Does the athlete have a family history of sudden cardiac death in a family member under age 50?
   C. Does the athlete have numbness or tingling in either or both hands in cold weather?
   D. Does the athlete have a history of a "racing heart?"
   E. Does the athlete have a previous history of heart problem?

5. During a preparticipation physical, the team physician comes across a basketball player with the following profile: The athlete is tall with an arm span greater than his height, pectus carinatum or excavatum, high-arched palate, and myopia. What is the probable diagnosis?
   A. Paget's disease
   B. Milch disease
   C. Addison's disease
   D. Gigantism
   E. Marfan Syndrome

6. An athlete's pulmonary function is tested via spirometry. Several measurements are taken during this test. What is the maximum amount of air that can be expired after a maximum inspiration called?
   A. Maximum expiratory flow rate
   B. Forced expiratory volume
   C. Vital capacity
   D. Tidal volume
   E. Residual volume

7. During a preparticipation physical, an athlete is diagnosed with myopia. What is this athlete's problem?
   A. Double vision
   B. Farsightedness
   C. Blindness in one eye
   D. Nearsightedness
   E. None of the above

8. All of the following are functions of the liver except:
   A. Carbohydrate metabolism
   B. Detoxification of blood
   C. Protein synthesis
   D. Detoxification of urine
   E. Bile production

9. All of the following functions contribute to the athlete's ability to maintain a steady state during periods of increased metabolic needs while exercising except:
   A. Pulmonary diffusion
   B. Vascular adaptation
   C. Physical condition of the involved muscles
   D. A high-protein, pre-event meal
   E. A and C

10. One method of estimating body fat has been through the use of skin-fold measurements at four sites. These four sites include all of the following except:
    A. Biceps
    B. Triceps
    C. Suprailiac
    D. Suprascapular
    E. None of the above

11. In hot, wet environments, the athlete's ability to adjust to a significantly increased cardiovascular workload is limited by which factor?
    A. Hypoxia
    B. Hypervolemia
    C. Dehydration
    D. Hypernatremia
    E. Inability to dissipate heat by evaporation

12. When testing the physical conditioning of an athlete, the coach asks the athlete to sprint 50 yards. What does this test?
    A. Aerobic endurance
    B. Vital capacity
    C. Lower extremity power
    D. Power
    E. Anaerobic capacity

13. What is the definition of power?
    A. Power = work x force
    B. Power = speed x distance
    C. Power = force x distance
    D. Power = work x velocity
    E. Power = work x distance

14. During prolonged, intense training and conditioning of an athlete, what cardiac change may occur over a period of time?
    A. Development of heart murmurs
    B. Development of premature ventricular contractions (PVCs)
    C. Increase in heart size
    D. Decrease in heart size
    E. Mitral valve prolapse

15. If it was determined that a 25-year-old athlete should work at 80% of his maximal heart rate, what would be his target heart rate?
    A. 170 beats per minute (BPM)
    B. 156 BPM
    C. 145 BPM
    D. 140 BPM
    E. 130 BPM

16. How long (generally) should a "warm-up" be to adequately prepare the body for athletic performance?
    A. 5 to 10 minutes
    B. 35 to 45 minutes
    C. 60 minutes
    D. 15 to 30 minutes
    E. 45 to 60 minutes

17. On the average, an athlete expends between _____ to _____ calories per day.
    A. 4000 to 5000
    B. 2000 to 3000
    C. 2500 to 3000
    D. 2200 to 4400
    E. 1000 to 1800

18. An athlete's diet should consist of approximately _____ protein, _____ fat, and _____ carbohydrate.
    A. 12% to 15%, 40% to 50%, 55% to 70%
    B. 10% to 20%, 30% to 40%, 50% to 70%
    C. 5% to 10%, 30% to 45%, 60% to 80%
    D. 25% to 35%, 55% to 65%, 70% to 90%
    E. 45% to 55%, 10% to 20%, 45% to 55%

19. The pre-event meal should be planned by whom?
    A. The coach
    B. The athlete
    C. The athletic trainer
    D. A & B
    E. All of the above

20. The pre-event meal should be eaten _____ to _____ hours before competition to ensure proper digestion.
    A. 2 to 3 hours
    B. 3 to 4 hours
    C. 5 to 6 hours
    D. 6 to 8 hours
    E. 1 to 2 hours

21. How many glasses of water should an athlete consume on a daily basis?
    A. No more than 8
    B. 2 to 3
    C. 8 or more
    D. 5 to 7
    E. 4 to 6

22. Adequate calcium intake is essential in female athletes with inconsistent menstrual cycles. How much calcium should the female athlete consume a day?
    A. 500 to 700 mg
    B. 750 mg
    C. 1000 mg
    D. 1500 mg
    E. 1200 mg

23. When monitoring a carbohydrate-loading program for an endurance athlete, what should the athlete do the day prior to competition?
    A. Eat a high-carbohydrate meal and perform little or no exercise
    B. Eat a low-carbohydrate meal and participate in a regular amount of exercise
    C. Eat a high-carbohydrate meal and participate in a regular amount of exercise
    D. Hyperhydrate and rest the day before competition
    E. Eat a low protein diet and participate in a regular amount of exercise

24. When working on a bleeding athlete, what should the athletic trainer always do?
    A. Avoid touching the bloody areas
    B. Wash hands before treatment
    C. Wear gloves
    D. Wear eye protection
    E. Elevate the body part

25. Alpine skiing world championships are scheduled in Japan. Jet lag is bound to occur as a result of crossing several time zones. What should the athletic trainer recommend to the team members prior to their flight to combat the jet lag effect?
    A. Upon arrival, adjust all training, eating, and sleeping schedules to the local time of the country in which they are competing
    B. Consume caffeine only when traveling east
    C. Reset watches to the new time zone 3 days in advance to get used to the time change
    D. When traveling west, it is important to have a large breakfast in the morning to carry the athlete through the day
    E. None of the above

26. During a football practice in early September, the temperature is measured and found to be between 90°F to 100°F, but the humidity is under 70%. What should the athletic trainer recommend to the football staff?
    A. Suspend practice for the day
    B. Keep a careful watch on any athlete who is grossly overweight
    C. Have the athletes take a 10-minute rest every hour and change t-shirts when wet
    D. Limit practice to 30 minutes
    E. Schedule practice during the warmest part of the day

27. How is pediculosis spread between individuals?
    A. Coughing and sneezing
    B. Poor hand washing/hygiene
    C. Close sexual contact
    D. Contact with open sores
    E. Sharing eating utensils

28. When fitting the athlete with protective equipment, what factors should be considered?
    A. Athlete's skill level
    B. Athlete's height
    C. Athlete's weight
    D. Sport position
    E. All of the above

29. Which of the steps below are correct when fitting a football helmet?
    I.   Place the helmet over the head, tilt it backward, rotate it forward into position
    II. Try to turn the helmet side to side with the head in a stationary position
    III. Check to make sure the helmet sits three finger-breadths above the eyebrows
    IV. Press straight down on the crown of the helmet to see if the pressure is at the crown of the head
    V.   Check to see if the jaw pads fit snugly against the jaw
    VI. Check the chin strap adjustment for a tight fit

    A. I, II, IV, V, VI
    B. I, II, III, VI
    C. I, III, IV, V
    D. I, III, IV, VI
    E. I, III, IV, VI

30. All of the following conditions would disqualify an athlete from athletic competition except:
    A. Renal disease
    B. Uncontrolled hypertension
    C. Acute mononucleosis
    D. The absence of one testicle
    E. Human Immunodeficiency Virus

31. The _____ and _____ should be involved with the athlete and athletic trainer in selecting and maintaining the athlete's protective equipment.
    A. Coach, team physician
    B. Coach, equipment manager
    C. Equipment manager, team manager
    D. Team physician, coach
    E. Team physician, school nurse

32. Which of the following organizations certifies football helmets to make sure they are able to withstand repeated blows of high mass and low velocity?
    A. FDA
    B. NSA
    C. NATA
    D. NFL
    E. NOCSAE

33. Football helmets may fall into one or two categories. These two types are known as _____ or _____.
    A. Air- or fluid-filled, padded
    B. Gel-filled, padded
    C. Plastic, fiberglass
    D. Standard, adjustable
    E. Molded, non-molded

34. When is maximum protection provided by a properly fitting mouthguard?
    A. When it is made of a flexible, resilient material and is form-fitted to the teeth and upper jaw
    B. When it is made of a rigid, plastic material that is fitted to both the upper and lower jaw
    C. When it is certified by the NOCSAE
    D. When it is certified by the National Collegiate Athletic Association (NCAA)
    E. When it contains titanium fibers

35. Properly fitting shoulder pads should adequately cover the shoulder complex. Which structure should the epaulets and cups completely cover?
    A. The scapula
    B. The deltoids
    C. The pectoralis major
    D. The trapezius
    E. The pectoralis minor

36. A flak jacket is a piece of equipment designed to protect the athlete after what type of injury?
    A. Scapular injury
    B. Hip pointer injury
    C. Abdominal injury
    D. Rib injury
    E. Clavicle injury

37. Which of the following organizations sets the standards for eye protection for racquet sports?
    A. American College of Sports Medicine (ACSM)
    B. NATA
    C. FDA
    D. American Society for Testing and Materials (ASTM)
    E. NOCSAE

38. Of the following pieces of equipment, which is not an NCAA-mandated piece of equipment?
    A. Wrestling—ear guards
    B. Men's lacrosse—protective gloves
    C. Baseball—double ear flap helmet for batting
    D. Gymnastics—palm protectors for the uneven parallel bars
    E. Women's lacrosse—protective eyewear

39. A female gymnast is complaining of symptoms of premenstrual syndrome (PMS), such as irritability, anxiety, depression, and bloating. Which of the following vitamins might be helpful in alleviating these symptoms?
    A. Vitamin B_6
    B. Vitamin B_{12}
    C. Vitamin K
    D. Vitamin A
    E. Vitamin C

40. While discussing general nutrition principles with a female swimmer who is a strict vegetarian, the athletic trainer should be aware that her diet might lack what mineral?
    A. Choline
    B. Iron
    C. Niacin
    D. Folate
    E. Potassium

41. Which type of drink would not be appropriate prior to a long-distance run?
    A. Water
    B. Regular soda
    C. Gatorade
    D. Water with lemon juice added
    E. Any drink containing sodium

42. A megadose of which of the following vitamins is potentially very dangerous?
    A. Thiamin
    B. Vitamin B_6
    C. Vitamin C
    D. Vitamin B_{12}
    E. Vitamin A

43. Under what condition(s) is an athlete likely to experience a stress fracture of a bone?
    A. After a few high loads or many small loads are applied to the bone
    B. After a large traumatic insult to the bone
    C. After a traumatic incident that is quickly followed by a few small loads to the bone
    D. After one or two small loads are applied to the bone
    E. None of the above

44. Which of the following should be included in a preparticipation physical examination?
    I. Height and weight
    II. Orthopedic screening
    III. Vital signs
    IV. Ear/nose/throat exam
    V. Blood work

    A. I, II, V
    B. II, IV, V
    C. I, II III, IV
    D. I, III, V
    E. All of the above

45. Which of the following can cause an indirect sports fatality?
    A. Contact sports
    B. A blow to the head
    C. Blunt chest trauma
    D. Rodeo riding
    E. Heat stroke

46. One of your athletes has just purchased a bicycle helmet and found a crack in the shell. To which organization should the manufacturer of the helmet report this defect?
    A. NATA
    B. Consumer Product Safety Commission
    C. NOCSAE
    D. United States Olympic Committee (USOC)
    E. National Academy of Sports Medicine (NASM)

47. During a preparticipation physical examination, what type of assessment should be utilized to document the maturity of an athlete's secondary sexual characteristics?
    A. Tanner's five stages of assessment
    B. HOPS assessment scale
    C. Glasgow scale
    D. Erickson's hierarchy
    E. Maslow's maturity scale

48. During a preparticipation physical examination, what should the team physician and athletic trainer do jointly?
    A. Perform blood tests
    B. Perform Sentinel's test
    C. Review each examination for the final approval to participate
    D. Perform an orthopedic screening
    E. Perform psychological fitness assessments

49. According to the Americans with Disabilities Act, who should make the final decision regarding a disabled athlete's participation in a sport?
    A. Athletic trainer
    B. Team physician and school nurse
    C. Individual athlete
    D. Parents
    E. Team physician

50. Which of the following individuals is most susceptible to heat stroke and, therefore, must be carefully educated regarding the importance of adequate fluid intake during activity in hot, humid weather?
    A. Basketball guard
    B. A wrestler
    C. Female gymnast
    D. Swimmer
    E. A defensive lineman in football

51. When using an ice pack at home to decrease pain and swelling of an injured limb, what should the athletic trainer recommend to the athlete to prevent a cryotherapy injury?
    A. Add acetone to the ice at a 3:1 ratio
    B. Keep the injured limb elevated while using ice
    C. Place a damp towel between the athlete's skin and the ice pack
    D. Leave the ice pack on the body part between 20 to 40 minutes at a time
    E. All of the above

52. One of your athletes has been diagnosed with impetigo. What should the athletic trainer recommend to the athlete to prevent spread of the infection to other individuals?
    A. Clean his clothing daily with bleach
    B. Wear gloves
    C. Practice safe sex
    D. Prevent others from borrowing his clothing or using his towels
    E. Cover his mouth when coughing and avoid socializing in large crowds

53. A wrestler comes to the athletic training room inquiring about a "drug that will make him lose weight quickly." He mentions a diuretic. Which of the following drugs has been banned by the International Olympic Committee (IOC) and causes diuresis?
    A. Furosemide
    B. Salbutamol
    C. Caffeine (<12 mcg/mL)
    D. Salicylates
    E. None of the above

54. A baseball player complains of recurrent ingrown toenails. What might the athletic trainer suggest to prevent this problem?
    A. Have the athlete put a small amount of cotton under his nails
    B. Have the athlete wear shoes with a large toe-box
    C. Have the athlete trim his toenails in a rounded shape parallel to the border of the cuticle
    D. Have the athlete trim his toenails weekly and cut them straight across
    E. Have the athlete purchase larger shoes

55. When advising an athlete about the proper construction of a running shoe, which of the following criteria will help prevent foot and ankle injuries?
    I. The midsole should be somewhat soft, but should not easily flatten out with pressure
    II. The shoe should have good forefoot flexibility
    III. The heel counter should be shallow and firm
    IV. The heel counter should be strong and fit well around the foot
    V. The upper should be constructed of quality leather or rubber

    A. I, II, IV
    B. I, III, IV, V
    C. II, III, IV
    D. II, IV, V
    E. I, II, III

56. To prevent the feeling of sedation during the day while taking medications for allergic rhinitis, the athletic trainer should suggest the athlete not take which of the following medications until he or she is ready to go to bed?
    A. Expectorants
    B. Antihistamines
    C. Decongestants
    D. Nonsteroidal anti-inflammatory drugs (NSAIDs)
    E. Anti-pyretic agents

57. Why is it important for an athlete to follow a varied diet that reflects the food pyramid?
    A. The athlete will maintain a healthy appetite
    B. Vitamin toxicity will be avoided
    C. Strict vegetarians tend to become anemic
    D. All of the above
    E. None of the above

58. To prevent the possibility of an acute compartment syndrome, the athletic trainer should advise his or her field hockey players to wear which of the following pieces of equipment?
    A. Thigh pads
    B. Mouthguards
    C. Helmets
    D. Gloves
    E. Shin guards

59. The dangers of possible hypothermia during exercise in very cold weather are significantly pronounced by _____ and _____.
    A. Light clothing, low chill factor
    B. Wind, wet weather
    C. Layered clothing, dry weather
    D. Wind, dry weather
    E. Heavy clothing, wind

60. A female athlete should choose a sports bra that is supportive enough to prevent stretching of which structure?
    A. The skin
    B. The pectoralis major
    C. Cooper's ligaments
    D. The nipples
    E. Ligamentum pectoris

61. When instructing an athlete in the proper technique of applying an elastic wrap to control pain and edema of an extremity, the athletic trainer should instruct the athlete to remove the wrap if all except the following occurs at the distal end of the extremity:
    A. Numbness
    B. Coolness
    C. Tingling
    D. Cyanosis
    E. Pink hue to the skin

62. When counseling an athlete about the adverse effects of anabolic steroids on females, all of the following effects should be included except:
    A. Severe acne
    B. Increased libido
    C. Increased body fat
    D. Development of a deep voice
    E. Change in menstrual cycle

63. What should the athletic trainer advise his or her athletes to do to minimize the negative effects of jet lag?
    A. Drink an adequate amount of fluids, especially water, to avoid dehydration
    B. Keep watches set to their "home" time zone
    C. Get up and go to bed 2 to 3 hours earlier for each time zone crossed
    D. Wear warm clothing to avoid getting cold while on the plane
    E. Get at least eight hours of sleep at night the week before the flight

64. You are aware of the general use of smokeless tobacco among your high school baseball players. You decide to develop a seminar for the coaches and players to discourage its use. Which of the following are effects of the chronic use of chewing tobacco?
    I. Leukoplakia
    II. Mouth and throat cancer
    III. Increased aggression
    IV. Bad breath
    V. Mood swings
    VI. Gynecomastia

    A. I, II, IV
    B. III, V, VI
    C. I, II, III
    D. II, III, IV
    E. II, III, IV, V

65. One of your basketball players comes into the athletic training room insisting that his ankles need to be taped even though he has no known injury. The athlete should be advised of which of the following?
    A. To let the athletic trainer know if he starts developing any knee problems
    B. An elastic or neoprene ankle brace is more effective than taping in preventing an injury
    C. For the ankle taping to be effective, the athlete should rely on ankle-strengthening exercises rather than prophylactic taping if there is no injury present
    D. Advise the athlete to contact his family physician to evaluate his ankles
    E. None of the above

66. It is well-known that many athletes will utilize nutritional supplements in an effort to enhance performance. An athlete asks you to explain the action of an antioxidant. Which of the following best describes the role of an antioxidant?
    A. A nutrient that protects the cell from the detrimental effects of substances that may cause health problems, such as premature aging
    B. A mineral that is known to protect the body from cancer
    C. A vitamin that is known to protect the body from heart disease
    D. A substance that is found in vegetables and dairy products and prevents certain types of cancer and osteoporosis
    E. None of the above

67. In order to prevent medial epicondylitis, all of the following actions should be avoided via technique modification except:
    A. Too much wrist flexion at follow-through during a golf swing
    B. Excessive elbow valgus when throwing a javelin
    C. Hyperextension of the wrist when performing a backhand shot in tennis
    D. Excessive wrist flexion during a racquetball forehand shot
    E. A and B

68. Which of the following athletes should avoid high volume, high intensity plyometric exercises?
    A. Athletes who weigh more than 220 lbs
    B. Premenstrual female athletes
    C. Athletes who weigh less than 75 kg
    D. Diabetic athletes
    E. Asthmatic athletes

69. All of the following free-weight exercises require one or more spotters except:
    A. Free-weight exercise in which the bar passes over the face
    B. Free-weight exercise in which a bar moves over the head
    C. Free-weight exercise in which a bar curls up in front of the chest
    D. Free-weight exercise in which the bar is positioned on the back
    E. Free-weight exercise in which the bar moves over the chest

70. Keratoderma can be prevented by all of the following except:
    A. Wearing two pairs of socks
    B. Applying a lubricant to the skin to prevent friction
    C. Using an antifungal ointment
    D. Using a glove or moleskin
    E. Wearing properly fitting shoes

71. How may an urinary tract infection (UTI) be avoided in a female athlete?
    A. Drinking fluids that are acidic, such as orange juice
    B. Practicing sanitary bowel and bladder habits
    C. Avoiding food high in magnesium
    D. Avoid wearing colored underwear
    E. None of the above

72. According to NCAA guidelines, how long a period of time should be allowed for acclimatization to prevent heat illness?
    A. 7 to 10 days
    B. 24 to 72 hours
    C. 2 to 7 days
    D. 10 to 14 days
    E. One month

73. How many servings of fruit should an athlete have as a minimum daily requirement?
    A. 2 to 6 servings
    B. 5 to 7 servings
    C. 2 to 4 servings
    D. Number of servings are according to the athlete's age
    E. Number of servings are according to the athlete's height and weight

74. At the secondary school level, the athletic training student should be involved in the educational efforts involving blood-borne pathogens. These educational items should include all of the following except:
    A. Education on the availability of herpes testing
    B. Education/training in the use of universal precautions and wound care
    C. Education on access to hepatitis B virus (HBV) vaccinations and testing
    D. Education of parents and guardians regarding the students' risk of infection
    E. Education on the modes of infection and risk of infection from the athletes they care for

75. According to the ACSM, when performing flexibility exercises, how long should a stretch be held for optimal results?
    A. 5 to 10 seconds; after 10 seconds minimal/no results are achieved
    B. 10 to 30 seconds; only as long as it feels comfortable
    C. 45 to 60 seconds; no less than 45 seconds
    D. 60 to 90 seconds; until the athlete feels some mild discomfort
    E. A minimum of one and a half to two minutes

76. A diet that is very low in carbohydrates may result in all of the following except:
    A. Fatigue
    B. Hypoglycemia
    C. Ketosis
    D. Very high blood pH levels
    E. Headaches

77. Which of the following is not a neural effect of resistance training?
    A. Increased motor unit activation and recruitment
    B. Increased discharge frequency of motoneurons
    C. Increased muscle capillary density
    D. Decreased neural inhibitions
    E. Increased neuromuscular efficiency

78. General maintenance and cleaning tasks of the athletic training room and activities areas of an athletic facility should include all of the following except:
    A. Wood flooring should be kept free of splinters, holes, protruding nails, uneven boards, and screws
    B. All areas should be swept, vacuumed, and mopped according to designated cleaning schedules
    C. Check to make sure that athletic uniforms/equipment are properly stored and inventoried on a regular basis
    D. Lighting apparatuses should be checked and changed on a regular basis
    E. Check to see that ground fault interrupters are working and appropriately located

79. To prevent a hazardous electrical problem in the athletic training room, _____ and _____ should never be used.
    A. Multiple adapters, extension cords
    B. Ground fault interrupters, three-pronged wall outlets
    C. Ground fault interrupters, florescent lights
    D. Hanging lights, three-pronged wall outlets
    E. Equipment with electrical cords, equipment that conforms to National Electrical Code guidelines.

80. During a preparticipation physical examination that utilizes stations, which of the following personnel is able to perform an examination for adenopathy, abnormalities of the genitalia, and hernias in an athlete?
    A. Athletic training student
    B. Physician or physicians' assistant
    C. Physical therapist
    D. Certified athletic trainer
    E. School nurse

81. "Counting the number of seconds from lightning flash until the sound of thunder divided by five" describes the "flash-to-bang" method utilized by athletic trainers to roughly calculate which of the following?
    A. How far away thunder is occurring
    B. The amount of time before play is resumed
    C. How far away lightning is occurring
    D. The intensity of the thunder
    E. None of the above

82. When is it best to have athletes practice outdoors in an urban environment?
    A. Early in the morning
    B. In the middle of the afternoon
    C. Early afternoon
    D. Very late afternoon/early evening
    E. Never

83. There are two types of heel cups that are designed to help prevent heel bruises. Of these two heel cups, which has an elevated heel that can compress downward so that the heel never actually makes contact with the interior of the shoe?
    A. A rubberized padded cup
    B. A rigid plastic cup
    C. A jelly-filled cushion cup
    D. An air-filled cushion cup
    E. All of the above

84. What is the primary purpose of the Achilles' tendon tape job?
    A. To give support and help prevent inversion ankle sprains
    B. Used with acute ankle sprains to help prevent swelling if an elastic wrap is not available
    C. To prevent the medial foot from flattening
    D. To restrict the amount of dorsiflexion at the ankle
    E. A and C

85. Which of the following is not recommended for the prevention of heat-related illnesses?
    A. Check the humidity and temperature daily
    B. Drink 20 ounces of water every 15 minutes
    C. Wear layers of lightweight clothing
    D. Acclimatize
    E. All of the above

86. Which of the following is not a preventive measure for fungal skin infections?
    A. Use powders to absorb moisture
    B. Wear the same pair of shoes everyday
    C. Shower frequently
    D. Avoid contact with contaminated surfaces
    E. Toweling off completely following a shower

87. All of the following are measures for preventing infectious diseases except:
    A. Appropriate diet, recovery time between workouts, and sleep
    B. Use individual water bottles, towels, uniforms, and personal equipment
    C. Frequent laundering of uniforms
    D. Use water to clean contaminated surfaces or equipment
    E. B and C

88. Which of the following stages of disease prevention focuses on early detection and appropriate referral?
    A. Primary stage
    B. Secondary stage
    C. Initial stage
    D. Tertiary stage
    E. None of the above

89. All of the following are predisposing conditions to heat illness except:
    A. Medications
    B. Age
    C. Conditioning level
    D. Hydration status
    E. Small body mass

90. All of the following symptoms are considered "red flags," requiring urgent referral to a physician, except:
    A. Persistent headaches
    B. Constant pain
    C. Insomnia
    D. Malaise, fatigue
    E. Hunger

91. All of the following are effects of immobilization on muscle except:
    A. Increase in muscle contraction time
    B. Increase in muscle tension produced
    C. Decrease in muscle fiber size
    D. Decrease in total muscle weight
    E. Decrease in neuromuscular efficiency

92. All of the following types of infection are transmitted through the air except:
    A. Meningitis
    B. Pneumonia
    C. Tuberculosis
    D. Scarlet fever
    E. Malaria

93. Which of the following is a type of exercise that involves a muscle contraction in which the length of the muscle is changing while the contraction is performed at a constant velocity?
    A. Isokinetic
    B. Isotonic
    C. Isometric
    D. Progressive resistance
    E. Proprioceptive Neuromuscular Facilitation

94. A shoe with _____ and _____ cleats has been shown to reduce the risk of knee injuries.
    A. Longer, fewer
    B. Shorter, more
    C. Longer, more
    D. Shorter, fewer
    E. Longer, sharper

95. What type of stretching is not recommended because of the potential for causing muscle soreness and possible injury when done over a period of time?
    A. Ballistic
    B. PNF
    C. Static
    D. Concentric
    E. None of the above

96. When exercising in cold temperatures, what should be done by the athlete to prevent hypothermia?
    A. Keep his or her clothes dry
    B. Warm up exercises and remain active
    C. Wear warm clothing
    D. None of the above
    E. All of the above

97. Sixty-five percent of the heat produced by the body during exercise is lost through what?
    A. Convection
    B. Conduction
    C. Evaporation
    D. Radiation
    E. None of the above

98. Where is the most heat lost from the body in cold weather?
    A. Hands
    B. Feet
    C. Torso
    D. Head and neck
    E. A and B

99. What does a sunscreen sun protection factor (SPF) of 5 represent?
    A. An individual can be exposed to ultraviolet light five times longer than he or she could without having the sunscreen on before his or her skin turns red
    B. An individual will be protected from the sun 105%
    C. Nothing
    D. The sunscreen contains 5% of SPF
    E. The number of applications it takes for 100% protection

100. All of the following are signs and symptoms of dehydration except:
    A. Sunken, soft eyes
    B. High specific gravity of urine
    C. Weight loss
    D. Thirst
    E. Seizures

101. Athlete's foot (tinea pedis) may be prevented by all of the following except:
    A. Dusting the feet daily with powder
    B. Completely drying feet after getting them wet, including between toes
    C. Wearing sandals when showering in a public facility
    D. Washing the feet on a regular basis
    E. Sharing shoes with teammates

102. All of the following are items used to prevent internal ear damage from excessive noise except:
    A. Ear plugs
    B. Ear muffs
    C. Semi-aural devices
    D. A head band
    E. B and C

103. Which of the following is not a cause of a weight-training injury?
    A. The use of a "spotter"
    B. Barbell or platform defects
    C. Poor technique
    D. Not properly warming up before lifting weights
    E. C and D

104. All of the following are intrinsic factors of injury except:
    A. Flexibility
    B. Weather
    C. Age
    D. Weight
    E. C and D

105. A soccer player sustains a strain to the quadriceps muscle group. You are trying to prevent atrophy during rehabilitation. What method of treatment would you use?
    A. Ultrasound and transcutaneous electrical nerve stimulation (TENS)
    B. Interferential current (IFC)
    C. Stretching
    D. High volt galvanic stimulation
    E. Russian stimulation

106. Which of the following is a D2 pattern of an extremity?
    A. External rotation with flexion and abduction to internal rotation with extension and adduction
    B. External rotation with flexion and adduction to internal rotation with flexion and abduction
    C. External rotation with adduction and flexion to internal rotation with abduction and flexion
    D. External rotation with abduction and extension to internal rotation with adduction and flexion
    E. None of the above

107. An athlete reports to you that another member of the women's gymnastics team has a recognizable problem with eating. She reports that the athlete binge eats, followed by self-inducted vomiting. What is this athlete suffering from?
    A. Anorexia nervosa
    B. Amenorrhea
    C. Bulimia nervosa
    D. None of the above
    E. B and C

108. Which of the following is a condition that is associated with the enlargement of the spleen?
    A. Graves' disease
    B. Constipation
    C. Appendicitis
    D. Hepatitis
    E. Mononucleosis

109. All of the following are true when fitting shoulder pads except:
    A. Axillary straps should not be very tight but just enough to be snug around the chest to keep the shoulder pads in place
    B. Shoulder pads should stop at the midsternum
    C. Acromioclavicular (AC) joint should have a channel of foam padding
    D. Lateral flaps should cover down to the deltoid tuberosity
    E. The neck opening must allow the athlete to raise the arm overhead, but not allow the pad to shift

110. According to NATA guidelines, an athletic trainer who is suspected of being infected with HIV should do all of the following except:
    A. Seek medical care and ongoing evaluation
    B. Take procedures to ensure health of patients and self
    C. Wait until it is convenient to be tested because it is not immediately life threatening
    D. Inform appropriate medical personnel
    E. Disclose condition to school administration

111. Which of the following minerals decreases the risk of osteoporosis and increases the density of the bone?
    A. Zinc
    B. Folate
    C. Molybdenum
    D. Iron
    E. Calcium

112. All of the following are signs of anorexia nervosa except:
    A. Dramatic weight loss
    B. Obsession with weight gain
    C. Social isolation
    D. Reaching competitive weight and continuing to lose weight in off-season
    E. Significant weight gain during the off-season

113. When trying to decrease the chance of injury during activity, one should stretch thoroughly. Which one of these stretches represents bouncing type movement to achieve a stretch?
    A. Ballistic
    B. Dynamic
    C. Static
    D. Active
    E. PNF-slow-reverse hold

114. While assisting an athlete in stretching exercises, the athletic trainer should follow some guidelines. Which one of the following is not true?
    A. The athlete should be relaxed
    B. The stretch should be stopped when the athlete reports mild discomfort
    C. The stretch should be unilaterally administered
    D. The body part should be stretched for up to 30 seconds
    E. All of the above

115. Athletes can prevent lower leg injuries by all of the following except:
    A. Stretching
    B. Proper footwear
    C. Proprioceptive training
    D. Strength training
    E. All of the above

116. Which of the following is not a way for a throwing athlete to prevent injuries while training?
    A. Minimizing the effects of microtrauma during training
    B. Maintaining cardiovascular and lower extremity conditioning
    C. Good communication between the athlete, athletic trainer, coach, and physician during training
    D. All of the above
    E. B and C

117. Prevention of a chronic or debilitating illness or injury through appropriate care and rehabilitation is called what?
    A. Primary prevention
    B. Secondary prevention
    C. Tertiary prevention
    D. All of the above
    E. None of the above

118. _____ refers to the concept of dividing the annual training plan into smaller segments, phases, or cycles.
    A. Specificity
    B. Frequency
    C. Duration
    D. Segmental division
    E. Periodization

119. Extrinsic risk factors of athletic injury include which of the following?
    A. Training errors
    B. Poor or inappropriate coaching
    C. Improper technique
    D. All of the above
    E. None of the above

120. _____ states that muscle strength, power, endurance, and hypertrophy increase only when muscles perform workloads greater than those loads previously encountered.
    A. P.R.E. principle
    B. The DAPRE principle
    C. The strength-duration curve
    D. The power training principle
    E. The overload principle

121. An athlete with mononucleosis should not play sports until the symptoms subside because of which of the following problems?
    A. Enlarged spleen
    B. Stress on the liver
    C. Possible kidney complications
    D. Because of malaise and fatigue
    E. Possible gallbladder rupture

122. An athlete with a concussion should be held out of play for which of the following reasons despite the severity of the concussion?
    A. Tingling in hands and feet
    B. Possibility of second impact syndrome
    C. Possibility of compartment syndrome
    D. Possibility of brachial plexus problems
    E. None of the above

123. When a football player has a possible cervical injury, which of the following should you do first?
    A. Remove the shoulder pads (only)
    B. Remove the helmet (only)
    C. Remove the shoulder pads then the helmet
    D. Place the athlete on a spine board
    E. None of the above

124. A player presents to you with a suspected shoulder dislocation. What should you do?
    A. Evaluate the injury then reduce the dislocation as soon as possible
    B. Evaluate the shoulder motion and send the athlete to the hospital
    C. Tell the athlete to sit and wait until you have time to deal with it
    D. Check the neurovascular status of the upper extremity, including dermatomes and myotomes
    E. Immediately immobilize the joint and refer the athlete to team physician

125. Shoulder pads provide protection for which type of injury?
    A. AC joint separation
    B. Glenohumeral joint separation
    C. Rotator cuff tendinitis
    D. Impingement
    E. Brachial plexus injuries

Recognition, Evaluation, and Assessment

1. A positive Thompson's sign is indicative of what problem?
    A. Tight hip flexor
    B. Tight iliotibial band
    C. Ruptured anterior tibialis tendon
    D. Ruptured posterior tibialis tendon
    E. Ruptured achilles' tendon

2. Which of the following is a simple movement to check the integrity of the radial nerve?
    A. Elbow flexion
    B. Wrist extension
    C. Forearm supination
    D. Thumb-to-little finger opposition
    E. Shoulder flexion

3. A grade I ankle inversion sprain involves which structure?
    A. Tibiofibular ligament
    B. Posterior talofibular ligament
    C. Calcaneofibular ligament
    D. Anterior talofibular ligament
    E. Spring ligament

4. You are covering a football game when two players collide. You notice that one player grabs his neck and shakes his arm. When you examine him, he complains of lateral neck discomfort and a feeling of "numbness" or "burning" down his arm. His arm is hanging limp by his side. In a few minutes, the symptoms subside. What do you suspect?
    A. Carpal tunnel syndrome
    B. Long thoracic nerve injury
    C. A "burner" or pinched nerve syndrome
    D. Dorsal scapular nerve injury
    E. Thoracic outlet syndrome

5. Which test, if positive, is indicative of a torn posterior cruciate ligament?
    A. Sag sign
    B. Anterior drawer sign
    C. McMurray's sign
    D. Ober's sign
    E. Lachman's sign

6. At what point should the athletic trainer's initial evaluation of an injury begin?
    A. At the moment the injury is witnessed
    B. Once the athlete has been stabilized in the athletic training room
    C. Once the athletic trainer receives a medical referral from a doctor
    D. After the athlete is seen by the team doctor
    E. B and D

7. Which scale is important in assessing the severity of a head injury?
    A. Beck's Orientation Scale
    B. Romberg's Cognition Scale
    C. Ranchos Los Amigos Amnesia Scale
    D. Intracranial Pressure Scale
    E. Glasgow Coma Scale

8. What quick test can be performed to check if nerve root L5 is intact?
    A. Have the athlete flex his or her hip while standing
    B. Have the athlete walk on his or her toes
    C. Have the athlete extend his or her great toe
    D. Have the athlete extend his or her hip
    E. Have the athlete flex his or her knee

9. A positive Phalen's sign is suspect of what problem?
    A. Tarsal tunnel syndrome
    B. Long thoracic nerve injury
    C. Thoracic outlet syndrome
    D. Suprascapular entrapment syndrome
    E. Carpal tunnel syndrome

10. Trendelenburg's test is a method used to evaluate the competence of what structures?
    A. Hip flexors
    B. Peroneal muscles
    C. Hip abductors
    D. Erector spinae
    E. Abdominals

11. What evaluative test is used to examine the integrity of the lateral collateral ligament of the knee?
    A. Pivot shift test
    B. Valgus stress test
    C. Lachman's test
    D. Varus stress test
    E. None of the above

12. What does a positive drop-arm sign indicate?
    A. Posterior shoulder subluxation
    B. Torn rotator cuff muscle
    C. Axillary nerve injury
    D. A labral tear
    E. Humeral head fracture

13. If there is inflammation at the site of the medial epicondyle of the elbow, which of the following would be positive?
    A. Tennis elbow test
    B. Golfer's elbow test
    C. Tinel's sign
    D. Finkelstein's test
    E. Allen's test

14. All of the following are signs of an injury except:
    A. Change in skin color or texture
    B. Change in body temperature
    C. Change in blood pressure
    D. Complaint of headaches
    E. Change in respiratory rate

15. Information gained during the palpation phase of the athletic trainer's initial assessment might include all of the following except:
    A. Presence of crepitus
    B. Sensory function
    C. Presence of a deformity
    D. Degree of functional movement
    E. A and B

16. During an upper quarter screen, checking the strength of thumb extension correlates to what nerve root?
    A. T1
    B. T3
    C. C5
    D. C4
    E. C8

17. A positive "clunk" test is indicative of what pathology?
    A. Unstable ankle
    B. Olecranon fracture
    C. Meniscus tear of the knee
    D. Glenoid labrum tear
    E. Anterior cruciate ligament tear

18. A baseball player comes to see the athletic trainer and is complaining of diffuse pain, clicking, and a sensation of "slipping" of his right shoulder when throwing. What pathology might the athletic trainer suspect with this type of presentation?
    A. Torn rotator cuff
    B. Thrower's exostosis
    C. AC joint pathology
    D. Labral pathology
    E. Bicipital tendinitis

19. Two major symptoms of a spontaneous pneumothorax include _____ and _____.
    A. Bradycardia, cyanosis
    B. Sudden chest pain, dyspnea
    C. Apnea with rales, rhonchi
    D. Left shoulder pain, cyanosis
    E. Diaphoresis, bradycardia

20. The _____ pulse and _____ pulse should be palpated after an acute traumatic injury to the knee area to make sure the peripheral circulation to the involved limb is adequate.
    A. Posterior tibial, dorsalis pedis
    B. Anterior tibial, plantar
    C. Saphenous, dorsalis pedis
    D. Femoral, posterior tibial
    E. Femoral, popliteal

21. Foot drop may be indicative of what pathology?
    A. Plantar nerve injury
    B. Shin splints
    C. Osteochondritis dissecans
    D. Achilles' tendonitis
    E. Peroneal nerve injury

22. A type V Salter-Harris fracture involves what kind of fracture through the physeal plate?
    A. The epiphysis and metaphysis separate without fragmentation
    B. A crush injury to the epiphysis
    C. The epiphysis and metaphysis separate with fragmentation
    D. The epiphysis, metaphysis, and physis all separate from each other
    E. None of the above

23. An athlete you have just evaluated for a possible head injury has a noticeable facial droop on the left side of his face. Which cranial nerve(s) is involved?
    A. I
    B. IV, V
    C. VII
    D. III, IX
    E. II, VI

24. During your examination of an athlete who has been complaining of weakness when using the rowing machine in the weight room, you notice his right latissimus dorsi muscle appears atrophied. Which nerve is affected?
    A. Trigeminal
    B. Thoracodorsal
    C. Dorsal scapular
    D. Thoracic spinal
    E. None of the above

25. A second-degree burn will have which of the following characteristics?
    A. A raised, reddened appearance
    B. A white, mottled appearance
    C. A blackened, hard appearance
    D. A reddened area with blisters
    E. Blanched, shiny appearance

26. The athlete may have difficulty performing what actions if the medial and lateral pectoral nerves are injured?
    A. Flexion, adduction, and internal rotation of the upper arm
    B. Shoulder shrugs
    C. Abduction and external rotation of the upper arm
    D. Extension, internal rotation, and adduction of the upper arm
    E. Flexion, abduction, and external rotation of the upper arm

27. A gymnast reports to the athletic trainer with a complaint of low back pain, which has been present for approximately 1 week. After being sent to the doctor for evaluation, a "Scottie dog" defect is seen on x-ray. This finding confirms which condition?
    A. Fractured transverse process of a vertebrae
    B. Fractured demifacet of a vertebrae
    C. Spondylolisthesis
    D. Spondylolysis
    E. A and B

28. An athlete is poked in the eye with a finger and comes to the athletic trainer for evaluation. He is having significant difficulty opening his eye. Which of the following muscles might have sustained an injury?
    A. Levator capitis inferioris
    B. Splenius capitis
    C. Levator palpebrae superioris
    D. Levator palpebrae orbitis
    E. Scalenes

29. An athlete is brought to the athletic training room after being struck in the back of the head with a bat by accident. He is complaining of blurred vision. Which lobe of the brain has been affected?
    A. Frontal
    B. Parietal
    C. Temporal
    D. Occipital
    E. None of the above

30. What internal organ is diseased if the athlete presents with jaundice?
    A. Spleen
    B. Pancreas
    C. Gallbladder
    D. Kidney
    E. Liver

31. Which two structures are injured with a Bankart lesion?
    A. Anterior capsule of the shoulder and the glenoid labrum
    B. The inferior capsule of the shoulder and glenoid fossa
    C. The articular surface of the humeral head and glenoid labrum
    D. The surgical neck of the humerus and the coracoacromial ligament
    E. The acromioclavicular joint and glenoid fossa

32. An athlete has a wrist injury that is limiting his ability to supinate his forearm. In what plane of motion does supination and pronation of the forearm take place (in the anatomical position)?
    A. Frontal
    B. Horizontal
    C. Sagittal
    D. Vertical
    E. A and C

33. What is the sensation that an athlete might experience just prior to an epileptic seizure called?
    A. An aura
    B. An hallucination
    C. A delusion
    D. Pre-epileptic vertigo
    E. A premonition

34. The inflammatory process includes all of the following signs and symptoms except:
    A. Redness
    B. Pain
    C. Warmth
    D. Swelling
    E. Numbness

35. Changes in blood pressure may occur as a result of many factors. Two of these factors may include _____ and _____.
    A. Exercise, change in posture
    B. Change in posture, respiratory rate
    C. Level of consciousness, body size
    D. Respiratory rate, pH levels of the blood
    E. Change in mood, respiratory rate

36. Type I diabetes is characterized by an impaired capacity to secrete insulin due to a beta cell defect. This type of diabetes is commonly seen in what type of individual?
    A. Obese, geriatric
    B. Lean, insulin dependent
    C. Noninsulin dependent, obese
    D. Noninsulin dependent, juvenile
    E. None of the above

37. All of the following are true about infectious mononucleosis except:
    A. The attack rate is highest between 15 to 25 years olds
    B. The virus is excreted in saliva
    C. The primary symptom is low back pain
    D. It is caused by transmission of the Epstein-Barr virus
    E. It causes splenomegaly in over half of all cases

38. Which of the following organisms is one of the most common causes of vaginitis in women?
    A. Acquired immunodeficiency syndrome (AIDS)
    B. Genital herpes
    C. Chlamydia trachomatis
    D. Candida
    E. All of the above

39. All of the following are risk factors for osteoporosis except:
    A. Early menopause
    B. High consumption of alcohol, cigarettes, and caffeine
    C. Sedentary lifestyle
    D. Obesity
    E. Lack of folic acid in the diet

40. An athlete with an infection or serious disease, such as leukemia, might demonstrate an abnormally raised white blood cell count. What is the normal leukocyte count?
    A. 200,000 to 400,000/cu mm
    B. 500 to 1500/cu mm
    C. 4000 to 10,000/cu mm
    D. 1000 to 40,000/cu mm
    E. 250 to 500 /cu mm

41. What is the primary target of the AIDS virus in the body?
    A. Neutrophils
    B. Basophils
    C. T-helper lymphocytes
    D. Phagocytes
    E. Red blood cells

42. EIA stands for what clinical entity?
    A. Exercise-induced arrhythmia
    B. Exercise-induced asthma
    C. Exercise-induced allergy
    D. Exercise-induced aneurysm
    E. None of the above

43. What type of gait deviation might the athletic trainer see with an athlete who has sustained an ankle injury and has decreased range of motion in dorsiflexion?
    A. Lateral trunk bending
    B. Trendelenburg gait
    C. Hip hiking
    D. Wide walking base
    E. Extension lag

44. A soccer player has fractured his right lower leg, been placed in a cast, and given crutches. The addition of crutches does what to his center of gravity?
    A. Moves it to the left
    B. Moves it to the midabdominal area
    C. Moves it to the right
    D. There is no effect on the center of gravity
    E. Enlarges the base of support

45. You notice one of your gymnasts has lost a significant amount of weight over the last month. She is always concerned about her image when she discusses her performance with you. What might you suspect as the problem?
    A. Drug dependence
    B. Depression
    C. Narcissism
    D. Bipolar disease
    E. Anorexia nervosa

46. An athlete who sustains a severe or career-ending injury may go through a progression of emotional reactions, which are frequently seen with an individual who has experienced a significant loss. All of the following are included in this series of reactions except:
    A. Bargaining
    B. Anger
    C. Acceptance
    D. Denial
    E. Guilt

47. All of the following are symptoms of an overtrained athlete except:
    A. Emotional liability
    B. Loss of appetite
    C. Reduced concentration
    D. Excessive motivation
    E. Fatigue

48. Which of the following signs/symptoms are present in a depressed athlete?
    A. Decreased appetite
    B. Insomnia
    C. Fatigue
    D. Feeling of hopelessness
    E. All of the above

49. The athletic trainer notices one of the baseball players routinely cleans his cleats after every game and practice so no dirt is visible and checks his equipment bag multiple times to assure himself his "lucky towel" is with him. This is an example of what type of behavior?
    A. Schizophrenic
    B. Anxiety
    C. Obsessive-compulsive
    D. Passive-aggressive
    E. A and B

50. All of the following are possible factors regarding why an athlete might be injury prone except:
    A. Bad luck
    B. Problems at home
    C. Joint hypermobility
    D. Poor endurance
    E. Poor coordination

51. Results of severe fluid restriction during weight loss attempts by a wrestler may include which of the following?
    A. Higher resting heart rate
    B. Increased renal flow
    C. Increased stroke volume
    D. Higher O_2 consumption
    E. Lower resting heart rate

52. What is wrong with an athlete eating a 12- to 16-ounce steak, baked potato, scrambled eggs, and coffee with sugar 4 hours prior to an event?
    A. Coffee with sugar may take as long as 3 hours to metabolize
    B. The intestinal tract will be full at the time of competition because it is a large meal
    C. The athlete may be hungry 8 hours later after he or she competes
    D. Nothing; the pre-event meal should be at least 500 calories or more
    E. Nothing; the athlete should eat whatever makes him or her feel comfortable

53. What happens when an athlete consumes a simple sugar prior to an event?
    A. May cause a sudden decrease in blood glucose because of a sudden increase in insulin production
    B. May lead to a sudden increase in blood glucose because of a decrease in insulin production
    C. May lead to increased blood levels of electrolytes
    D. May lead to hyperlipidemia
    E. May cause a sudden increase in bilirubin levels

54. Which of the following is not a good source of vitamin C?
    A. Broccoli
    B. Strawberries
    C. Oranges
    D. Nuts
    E. Spinach

55. An athlete informs the athletic trainer that he is taking tetracycline for a respiratory infection. Tetracycline will bind with which of the following two minerals to form a nonabsorbable complex (and therefore should not be taken before meals)?
    A. Potassium and zinc
    B. Sodium and magnesium
    C. Iron and calcium
    D. Iron and phosphorus
    E. Folic acid and niacin

56. In general, what is a healthy percent body fat range for a female athlete?
    A. 20% to 25%
    B. 15% to 30%
    C. 5% to 10%
    D. 13% to 18%
    E. 10% to 13%

57. A loss of water equaling what percent of body weight will begin to threaten athletic performances?
    A. 10% to 20%
    B. 0.5% to 1%
    C. 1% to 2%
    D. 1% to 1.5%
    E. 2% to 3%

58. Which of the following medications is not an NSAID?
    A. Aspirin
    B. Motrin
    C. Tylenol
    D. Orudis KT
    E. Aleve

59. Which of the following medications is not an antihistamine drug?
    A. Dimetapp
    B. Ultram
    C. Benadryl
    D. Claritin
    E. Tavist D

60. An athlete comes to your office complaining of intense itching and burning pain between his toes, and he cannot find anything to help alleviate the symptoms. The area is reddened with some white flakes. What might you recommend?
    A. Neosporin ointment
    B. Tinactin spray
    C. Silvadene cream
    D. Eucerin cream
    E. Hydrocortisone

61. An athlete collides with a teammate during an ice hockey game and sustains a blow to the jaw with a hockey stick. He is holding his lower face with his hands and is in intense pain. All of the following procedures will assist the athletic trainer in determining if there is a fracture of the jaw except:
    A. Have the athlete bite and observe for a malocclusion
    B. Palpate the jaw for a hematoma
    C. Ask the athlete to open and close his mouth, noting asymmetry with movement
    D. Palpate for jaw deformity when it is at rest, open, and closed
    E. See if the athlete can retract his jaw and observe for difficulty with movement

62. An athlete sustains a blunt trauma injury to the upper right quadrant of the abdomen. What structure might be injured in this area?
    A. Liver
    B. Gallbladder
    C. Spleen
    D. Pancreas
    E. Kidney

63. Which of the following symptoms represents a second-degree concussion?
    I. Blurring or loss of consciousness lasting from 20 seconds to 5 minutes
    II. Headache and amnesia are often present
    III. Athlete is often confused and disoriented
    IV. There are no positive signs on neurologic testing and examination
    V. There is no complaint of a headache
    VI. Altered level of consciousness lasts less than 10 to 20 seconds

    A. II, IV, VI
    B. I, IV, V
    C. I, II, III
    D. IV, V, VI
    E. All of the above

64. "Cauliflower ear" is an injury to which structure of the ear?
    A. Tympanic membrane
    B. External auditory canal
    C. Pinna
    D. Eustachian tube
    E. None of the above

65. What may proteinuria indicate?
    A. Pancreatitis
    B. Possible gallstones
    C. Renal or urinary tract pathology
    D. Diabetes
    E. Crohn's disease

66. What would be the most appropriate type of roentgenogram for a possible tibial stress fracture?
    A. X-ray
    B. Pet scan
    C. Magnetic resonance imaging (MRI)
    D. Computer tomography (CT) scan
    E. Bone scan

67. Which of the following is one of the most common eye injuries sustained in athletics?
    A. Detached iris
    B. Detached retina
    C. Zygomatic fracture
    D. Corneal abrasion
    E. None of the above

68. All of the following parameters should be assessed when checking the neurovascular status of an injured limb except:
    A. Sensation
    B. The pulse distal to the injury
    C. Motor function
    D. Joint range of motion
    E. Atrophic changes

69. A baseball player has been stung by a bee. This player has a history of a severe allergy to bee stings. A couple of minutes after being stung, the area becomes red and raised and begins to itch. The athlete begins to complain that his tongue feels thick, and he starts to have difficulty breathing. What type of shock is he beginning to develop?
    A. Neurogenic
    B. Metabolic
    C. Hypovolemic
    D. Respiratory
    E. Anaphylactic

70. After an acute musculoskeletal injury, such as a shoulder dislocation, the body releases a natural opiate-like substance that provides temporary pain relief. What is this substance called?
    A. Prostaglandins
    B. Substance P
    C. Endorphins
    D. Insulin
    E. None of the above

71. What is the typical mechanism of injury for an anterior shoulder dislocation?
    A. Shoulder abduction with internal rotation
    B. Maximal shoulder extension
    C. Shoulder abduction with external rotation
    D. Shoulder adduction with internal rotation
    E. Shoulder flexion with internal rotation

72. Which of the symptoms below are seen with acute mountain sickness?
    I. Insomnia
    II. Vomiting
    III. Shortness of breath with exertion
    IV. Headache
    V. Fatigue

    A. II, III, IV
    B. I, III, IV, V
    C. I, II, IV, V
    D. I, II, III, V
    E. II, III, IV

73. Which muscle grade denotes active muscle movement in a gravity-eliminated position?
    A. -3/5
    B. +3/5
    C. 5/5
    D. 1/5
    E. 2/5

74. All of the following are useful in evaluating low back pathology except:
    A. Valsalva's maneuver
    B. Bilateral straight leg test
    C. Scouring test
    D. Lasègue's test
    E. Slump test

75. What is the best position for the athlete to be in to muscle test the piriformis?
    A. Sitting
    B. Prone
    C. Supine
    D. Side lying
    E. Standing

76. What is the average range of motion of elbow flexion?
    A. 0 to 90 degrees
    B. 0 to 135 degrees
    C. 0 to 115 degrees
    D. 0 to 100 degrees
    E. 0 to 180 degrees

77. What is the proper method to manually muscle test the biceps femoris muscle?
    A. Sitting, resisting knee extension
    B. Lying prone, resisting knee flexion with the tibia in external rotation
    C. Sitting, resisting hip flexion
    D. Lying prone, resisting knee flexion with the tibia in internal rotation
    E. Sitting, resisting elbow flexion

78. What is a quick method of testing the motor ability of the S1 nerve root?
    A. Have the athlete walk on his or her toes
    B. Have the athlete manually resist ankle inversion
    C. Have the athlete manually resist great toe extension
    D. Assess the athlete's ability to squat
    E. Resisted ankle inversion

79. To test the function of the rhomboid major muscle, the athletic trainer should ask the athlete to perform what movement?
    A. Scapular retraction
    B. Shoulder internal rotation
    C. Scapular protraction
    D. Shoulder shrug
    E. Shoulder external rotation

80. Which muscle supinates the forearm and flexes the shoulder?
    A. Brachialis
    B. Coracobrachialis
    C. Biceps brachii
    D. Flexor pollicis longus
    E. Pronator quadratus

81. All of the following movements occur in the sagittal plane except:
    A. Hip abduction
    B. Shoulder flexion
    C. Knee extension
    D. Hip flexion
    E. Elbow flexion

82. Which muscle flexes both the foot and the knee?
    A. Biceps femoris
    B. Flexor digitorum
    C. Posterior tibialis
    D. Anterior tibialis
    E. Gastrocnemius

83. The flexor pollicis longus is responsible for which of the following action(s)?
    A. Great toe flexion
    B. Thumb flexion
    C. Thumb flexion and adduction
    D. Thumb flexion and abduction
    E. None of the above

84. Asking the athlete to move his or her eyes from side to side and up and down tests the integrity of which cranial nerve?
    A. II
    B. V
    C. I
    D. III
    E. None of the above

85. The rectus femoris muscle _____ and _____ when it contracts.
    A. Flexes the hip, externally rotates the hip
    B. Extends the hip, flexes the knee
    C. Flexes the knee, plantar flexes the ankle
    D. Flexes the hip, extends the knee
    E. Extends the hip, extends the knee

86. Which of the following muscles is not involved in internal rotation of the hip?
    A. Adductor magnus
    B. Gluteus maximus
    C. Gracilis
    D. Tensor fascia latae
    E. Gluteus minimus

87. Which of the following cervical nerve roots represent the sensory dermatomes of the hand?
    I. C5
    II. C6
    III. C7
    IV. C8
    V. T1

    A. I, II, III
    B. II, III IV
    C. III, IV, V
    D. I, III, IV
    E. I, III, V

88. Which of the following muscles does not adduct the shoulder?
    A. Pectoralis major
    B. Teres major
    C. Subscapularis
    D. Latissimus dorsi
    E. Serratus anterior

89. Which of the following muscles does not extend the trunk?
    A. Semispinalis (thoracic)
    B. Erector spinae
    C. Quadratus lumborum
    D. Multifidi
    E. Gluteus Maximus

90. The supinator muscle is innervated by which of the following nerves?
    A. Musculocutaneous nerve
    B. Axillary nerve
    C. Radial nerve
    D. Median nerve
    E. A and D

91. Following multiple ankle sprains over the course of the year, the athletic trainer detects some weakness of the invertors and evertors of an athlete's ankle. Which of the following muscles does not invert the ankle?
    A. Tibialis posterior
    B. Extensor digitorum longus
    C. Flexor digitorum longus
    D. Flexor hallucis longus
    E. C and D

92. During digestion, food passes through the small intestine as it is being broken down into smaller components. Which area of the small intestine does it pass through first?
    A. Ileum
    B. Esophagus
    C. Jejunum
    D. Cecum
    E. Duodenum

93. What nerve passes through the carpal tunnel?
    A. Musculocutaneous
    B. Radial
    C. Median
    D. Ulnar
    E. Cubital

94. Which of the following structures is not part of the pelvis?
    A. Coccyx
    B. Pubic symphysis
    C. Ileum
    D. Innominate bones
    E. Sacrum

95. Which nerves innervate the hip adductor musculature?
    A. Femoral, superior gluteal
    B. Femoral, tibial
    C. Femoral, obturator
    D. Femoral, obturator, inferior gluteal
    E. Tibial, obturator

96. Which of the following muscles abducts the little finger of the hand?
    A. Interossei
    B. Abductor digiti minimi
    C. Lumbricals
    D. Abductor digitorum brevis
    E. None of the above

97. Which of the following muscles does not extend and laterally flex the neck?
    A. Splenius capitis
    B. Splenius cervicis
    C. Levator scapulae
    D. Sternocleidomastoid
    E. Multifidus

98. Which of these muscles are innervated by the tibial nerve?
    I. Gastrocnemius
    II. Flexor hallucis longus
    III. Extensor hallucis longus
    IV. Tibialis anterior
    V. Biceps femoris

    A. I, II, III, IV
    B. II, III, V
    C. I, II, V
    D. I, III, IV, V
    E. I, II, III

99. All of the following are controlled by the cranial nerves except:
    A. Vision
    B. Smell
    C. Tongue movement
    D. Cervical flexion
    E. Hearing

100. What position is the "recommended" position for manually muscle testing the gluteus medius muscle?
    A. Side lying, with the affected limb on top
    B. Supine
    C. Prone
    D. Sitting
    E. Standing

101. What is the average range of motion of knee flexion?
    A. 0 to 180 degrees
    B. 0 to 120 degrees
    C. 0 to 100 degrees
    D. 0 to 155 degrees
    E. 0 to 135 degrees

102. True leg-length discrepancy is measured between which two points?
    A. The posterior inferior iliac spine to the medial malleolus
    B. The umbilicus to the midpatella
    C. The umbilicus to the lateral malleolus
    D. The anterior superior iliac spine to the medial malleolus
    E. The anterior superior iliac spine to Gerdy's tubercle

103. In what position should the athlete be to manually muscle test the hip flexors, and where should the athletic trainer's force be directed during testing?
    A. Prone, with the force directed down onto the posterior thigh
    B. Side lying, with the force directed down onto the side of the thigh
    C. Sitting, with the force directed down onto the anterior aspect of the thigh
    D. Sitting, with the force directed down onto the medial aspect of the thigh
    E. None of the above

104. What position should the athlete's shoulder be in to manually muscle test the deltoids?
    A. Abducted to 0 degrees and externally rotated to 45 degrees
    B. Abducted to 90 degrees
    C. Flexed with the palm down
    D. Extended with the palm up
    E. Extended with palm down

105. What is an excessive lateral curvature of the vertebral column called?
    A. Kyphosis
    B. Spondylolysis
    C. Scoliosis
    D. Lordosis
    E. None of the above

106. During your evaluation of an athlete's shoulder, you notice his left scapula is "winging." What does this indicate?
    A. Rhomboid weakness
    B. Deltoid weakness
    C. Serratus anterior weakness
    D. Upper trapezius weakness
    E. Long thoracic nerve entrapment

107. The maximal rate at which oxygen is consumed and utilized while exercising is known as the maximal oxygen consumption, or VO_2 max. What is the normal range of VO_2 max for an average college athlete?
    A. 80 to 100 mL/kg/min
    B. 45 to 60 mL/kg/min
    C. 70 to 80 mL/kg/min
    D. 45 to 60 dL/g/min
    E. 25 to 40 mL/kg/min

108. Which of the following is an indirect method of monitoring oxygen consumption?
    A. Measuring respiratory rate
    B. Measuring vital capacity
    C. Drawing blood gases during testing
    D. Measuring tidal volume
    E. Measuring heart rate

109. During exercise, the body's oxygen stores are greatly diminished. The recovery O_2 is used for all the following except:
    A. Replacing O_2 dissolved in tissue fluids
    B. Returning muscle myoglobin to resting values
    C. Increasing venous oxyhemoglobin to pre-exercise levels
    D. Returning the catecholamine level in the blood to normal
    E. A and B

110. Submaximal exercise tests, which evaluate physical working capacity (PWC) by measuring heart rate increases with exercise, include all of the following except:
    A. Progressive pulse rate test
    B. Harvard step test
    C. Cooper 12-minute run-walk test
    D. The Saltin-Astrand VO_2 debt test
    E. None of the above

111. A _____ is a device used to measure joint range of motion.
    A. Goniometer
    B. Dynamometer
    C. Caliper
    D. Flexometer
    E. Sphygmomanometer

112. Tenderness and pain with induration and swelling of the pretibial musculature following overexertion is indicative of which syndrome?
    A. Chondromalacia
    B. Pes anserinus bursitis
    C. Periostitis
    D. Nerve compression syndrome
    E. Tarsal tunnel syndrome

113. Speed's test is an evaluative test for which of the following problems?
    A. Thoracic outlet syndrome
    B. Supraspinatus tendinitis
    C. Bicipital tendinitis
    D. Ruptured biceps tendon
    E. Rupture of the brachialis muscle

114. Who is the only person who can legally diagnose a medical problem?
    A. The school nurse
    B. A physician
    C. The athletic trainer
    D. An emergency medical technician (EMT) or paramedic
    E. Physical therapist

115. If the calcaneofibular ligament of the ankle is torn, which of the following would be positive?
    A. Talar tilt test
    B. Anterior drawer sign
    C. Distraction test
    D. Clunk test
    E. Hawkins-Kennedy Test

116. When taking a history during a physical examination of an athlete, all of the following information is pertinent except:
    A. The mechanism of the injury
    B. If a "pop" or "snap" was heard or felt
    C. If the athlete is on medication
    D. Whether or not the athlete has medical insurance
    E. History of previous injury

117. What problem might the athletic trainer see if the L4 nerve root was compressed?
    A. Hip flexor weakness
    B. Plantar flexion weakness
    C. Knee extension weakness
    D. Dorsiflexion weakness
    E. Drop foot

118. With the athlete sitting, the scapula stabilized, and the shoulder maximally flexed, the athlete complains of pain and appears apprehensive. This is a positive _____ test.
    A. Yergason's
    B. Speed's
    C. Neer's
    D. Compression
    E. Hawkins-Kennedy

119. If a palpable "clunk" or shift at approximately 20 to 30 degrees of knee flexion is found during a pivot-shift test, this may be indicative of what?
    A. Anterolateral rotary instability of the knee
    B. Anteromedial rotary instability of the knee
    C. Posterolateral rotary instability of the knee
    D. Posteromedial rotary instability of the knee
    E. All of the above

120. "Spearing" in football is a dangerous technique. Football coaches have discontinued this practice when teaching tackling techniques because it may cause severe head and neck injuries. What is the resulting force on the cervical spine when a football player spears an opponent?
    A. Sudden neck extension
    B. Sudden neck hyperflexion with rotation
    C. Sudden neck lateral flexion
    D. Sudden neck rotation
    E. Sudden vertebral axial distraction

121. What is the most common mechanism of injury for an anterior shoulder dislocation?
    A. Adduction and external rotation
    B. Abduction and internal rotation
    C. Adduction and internal rotation
    D. Abduction and external rotation
    E. Abduction and extension

122. Which of the following conditions often contributes to shoulder impingement?
    A. Acute bicipital tendinitis
    B. Suprascapular nerve entrapment
    C. Adhesive capsulitis
    D. Glenohumeral instability
    E. Serratus anterior weakness

123. An athlete has just been diagnosed with plantar fasciitis. All of the following would be appropriate measures to provide support/relief to the affected area except:
    A. An orthotic for arch support
    B. Low dye taping
    C. Metatarsal pad
    D. A heel cup
    E. Stretching program

124. An athlete has been diagnosed with bulimia and has a known history of laxative abuse. Complications of chronic laxative use include which of the following?
    A. Electrolyte imbalance and dehydration
    B. Hyperactivity
    C. Hematemesis
    D. Chronic nasal congestion
    E. All of the above

125. An athlete comes to the athletic training room after being kicked in the lower leg by an opponent during a football game. He is complaining of decreased sensation in the L4 dermatome. What is this change in sensation called?
    A. Paresthesia
    B. Hypoesthesia
    C. Hyperesthesia
    D. Referred pain
    E. Anesthesia

126. _____ and _____ are two signs of diabetic coma.
    A. Drowsiness, acetone-smelling breath
    B. Seizures and pale, clammy skin
    C. Seizures, a bounding pulse
    D. Flushed skin, giddiness
    E. Pale skin, weak pulse

127. Which of the following tests is used to detect a possible meniscal tear in the knee?
    A. Faber's test
    B. Allen's test
    C. Jerk test
    D. Lachman's test
    E. McMurray's Test

128. An athlete reports to the athletic trainer with the presence of lesions on his upper lip and mouth area that look like blisters with a crusted yellow appearance and a red, weeping base. What is the probable cause of these lesions?
    A. Impetigo
    B. HIV
    C. Shingles
    D. A fungus infection
    E. Hives

129. An athlete is brought to the athletic training room after sustaining a hard kick to the abdominal area. Which of the following symptoms is not a sign of a significant abdominal injury?
    A. Slow, deep respirations
    B. Increased heart rate, decreased blood pressure
    C. Ashen colored skin
    D. Rapid, shallow respirations
    E. Rebound tenderness

130. A football quarterback is "sacked" during a game. He comes off the field holding his throwing arm and complains of chest and anterior shoulder pain. After evaluating the athlete, the athletic trainer suspects a torn pectoralis major muscle. Which of the following physical findings will be seen if the athletic trainer is correct?
    A. Ecchymosis around the xyphoid process
    B. Palpable defect in the posterior axilla
    C. Weakness in abduction and external rotation
    D. Weakness in adduction, flexion, and internal rotation of the affected arm
    E. All of the above

131. While training in a high-altitude climate (eg, 9000 to 10000 ft), a rock climber experiences acute dyspnea, cough, headache, and weakness. What is the probable cause of these symptoms?
    A. Asthma
    B. Pleurisy
    C. Bronchitis
    D. Pulmonary edema
    E. None of the above

132. A second-degree medial collateral ligament sprain is characterized by all of the following except:
    A. Pain along the medial joint line
    B. No gross knee instability, but mild ligamentous laxity is noted in full knee extension during valgus stress testing
    C. Difficulty in actively flexing and extending the knee
    D. Immediate, severe pain following the feeling of a "pop" in the knee; the pain quickly subsides and the athlete is left feeling a dull ache in the knee joint
    E. A and B

133. What is the usual mechanism of injury for a Colles' fracture?
    A. A fall on a closed fist
    B. A fall on a bent elbow
    C. A fall on an outstretched arm and hand
    D. A twisting movement of the knee when the lower leg is planted
    E. Direct trauma to the forearm

134. Allen's test is used to test what?
    A. The integrity of the vertebral arteries
    B. The integrity of the radial and ulnar arteries of the hand
    C. For carpal tunnel syndrome
    D. For tarsal tunnel nerve entrapment
    E. Integrity of the ulnar nerve

135. Which of the carpal bones is most commonly dislocated?
    A. Scaphoid
    B. Lunate
    C. Cuboid
    D. Hamate
    E. Triquitrum

136. What type of force typically causes injury to the medial collateral ligament, medial meniscus, and anterior cruciate ligament of the knee?
    A. A valgus force with the tibia in external rotation
    B. A varus force with the knee in full extension
    C. A valgus force with the femur in external rotation
    D. A valgus force with the knee in recurvatum
    E. None of the above

137. An athlete sustains a neck injury during an ice hockey game and is complaining of numbness and tingling along the ulnar border of his forearm and fourth and fifth fingers. Which of the following roentgenograms would be most appropriate in detecting nerve root compression?
    A. Electromyography or nerve root conduction velocity test
    B. CT scan or MRI
    C. Myelography
    D. Sonography
    E. Plain film radiograph

138. Which of the following is an example of a papule?
    A. A freckle
    B. A wart
    C. A hive
    D. A friction blister
    E. All of the above

139. When testing for paresthesia of the C5 nerve root, where should the athletic trainer perform pinprick testing?
    A. Base of the neck
    B. At the nipple line
    C. The medial aspect of the arm
    D. The lateral aspect of the forearm
    E. The lateral aspect of the upper arm over the middle deltoid

140. What is the proper position to manually muscle test the anterior deltoid?
    A. Shoulder in full internal rotation with the palm facing the floor, the force directed downward
    B. Shoulder at 90 degrees of abduction, full external rotation, and supination with the force directed downward
    C. Resistance to the first 30 degrees of abduction
    D. Arm at 90 degrees of flexion, palm facing downward, and the force is in the downward direction
    E. None of the above

141. What is one of the most common symptoms of a lumbar discogenic injury?
    A. Dull, localized backache
    B. Localized swelling with muscle guarding
    C. Inability to backward bend
    D. Sharp, radiating pain down the back of the leg
    E. All of the above

142. When an athlete reports to the athletic trainer complaining of lateral hip pain, all of the following conditions might be the source of pain except:
    A. Trochanteric bursitis
    B. Strain of the gluteus medius
    C. Lumbar discogenic disease
    D. Avulsion of the ischial tuberosity
    E. Strain of the tensor fasciae latae

143. All of the following injuries might be associated with a "popping" sensation of the knee joint except:
    A. Anterior cruciate ligament injury
    B. Torn meniscus
    C. Subluxed patella
    D. Iliotibial band friction syndrome
    E. B and C

144. The contact phase of the running gait is divided into which components?
    A. Forward swing and foot strike
    B. Foot strike, midsupport, and take-off
    C. Follow-through, forward swing, and foot descent
    D. Midsupport, take-off, and foot descent
    E. Foot strike, follow-through, foot descent

145. Foot pronation results in _____ of the tibia during midsupport in the running gait.
    A. External rotation
    B. Internal rotation
    C. Abduction
    D. Adduction
    E. None of the above

146. A wrestler comes into the athletic training room after sustaining a major elbow injury. There is intense pain, and the area is grossly swollen. The athlete is unable to straighten his elbow, and the forearm appears shortened. The athletic trainer suspects an acute dislocation. Which two areas would the athletic trainer check for possible vascular impairment?
    A. Ulnar and radial pulses
    B. Radial pulse and color of the nailbeds after compression
    C. Brachial and radial pulses
    D. Arterial and venous circulation
    E. Axilla and anticubital fossa

147. An athlete sustains a blow to the head with a temporary loss of consciousness. He appears to have a lucid period in which he seems to be normal for a period of a couple of hours and then becomes significantly lethargic. What type of medical emergency would the athletic trainer suspect?
    A. Ruptured intervertebral disc at level C3,4
    B. Extradural hemorrhage
    C. Basilar fracture
    D. Subdural hemorrhage
    E. None of the above

148. Concussions are usually graded on the _____ and _____ of neurologic impairment.
    A. Frequency, severity
    B. Frequency, duration
    C. Length, severity
    D. Duration, frequency
    E. Type, length

149. A tennis player comes to the athletic trainer complaining of medial thigh pain. He is limping and has pain with resisted hip adduction and hip flexion. There is diffuse tenderness and ecchymosis along the proximal aspect of the medial thigh. What is the probable cause of the pain?
    A. Hip flexor rupture
    B. Groin strain
    C. Medial hamstring strain
    D. Popliteal strain
    E. None of the above

150. A lacrosse player comes limping into the athletic training room with assistance from a coach. He is holding his leg in slight hip and knee flexion. There is a large bulge in the proximal thigh. During the exam, the athletic trainer requests the athlete to extend his knee as he sits on the edge of a taping table. He is able to partially straighten his leg, although there is pain down the anterior thigh area with the attempt to move it. What does the athletic trainer suspect is wrong?
    A. Biceps femoris rupture
    B. Femoral nerve injury
    C. Ruptured rectus femoris muscle
    D. Obturator nerve injury
    E. Iliopsoas rupture

151. A basketball player reports to the athletic training room complaining of a "burning" pain along the lateral aspect of his right knee during and after running. No edema or ecchymosis is found during the exam, but he is tender to palpation of the affected area. Which of the following special tests might be positive?
    A. Lachman's test
    B. Patellar apprehension test
    C. Ober's test
    D. Sag sign
    E. Faber's test

152. An athlete presents with loss of strength at the L3 and L4 nerve root levels. What muscle should the athletic trainer test to confirm an injury at this level?
    A. Gluteus minimus
    B. Flexor hallucis longus
    C. Gluteus maximus
    D. Adductor magnus
    E. Quadriceps

153. The athletic trainer asks an athlete to shrug his shoulders after a neck and shoulder injury. He has difficulty performing this movement, even though it is not painful. What nerve is injured?
    A. Spinal accessory
    B. Dorsal scapular
    C. Long thoracic
    D. Suprascapular
    E. None of the above

154. How is the strength of the pes anserinus musculature manually muscle tested?
    A. Resistance to knee flexion and internal rotation of the lower leg
    B. Resistance to knee extension and hip adduction
    C. Resistance to knee flexion and external rotation of the lower leg
    D. Resistance to knee extension and internal rotation of the lower leg
    E. Resistance to knee flexion and ankle inversion

155. During a track meet, you notice one of the runners appears somewhat disoriented. During your assessment of this athlete, you find he is complaining of being light-headed, his skin is cool and clammy, he is sweating profusely, and his radial pulse is rapid. You take a rectal temperature and find it is mildly elevated (102°F). You suspect the athlete is suffering from which of the following problems?
    A. Heat cramps
    B. Prickly heat
    C. Heat stroke
    D. Heat exhaustion
    E. None of the above

156. One of your female gymnasts has been complaining of feeling generally fatigued on a constant basis. After being examined by the team physician, he orders a complete blood count (CBC). This blood test assesses all of the following except:
    A. Red blood cell count
    B. White blood cell count
    C. Plasma volume
    D. Hemoglobin levels
    E. Platelet count

157. While elevating an athlete's shoulder, you note that the athlete is unable to abduct through the full range of motion against gravity. When performing a manual muscle test, this finding would be assigned which of the following muscle grades?
    A. +2/5
    B. 3/5
    C. -4/5
    D. 1/5
    E. -3/5

158. You evaluate a basketball player who has sustained a finger injury while attempting to catch a ball. During your examination, you observe that the athlete is unable to extend the distal phalanx and the tip of his finger is positioned in approximately 30 degrees of flexion. You determine the athlete has a mallet finger. This injury is caused by which of the following?
    A. Tenosynovitis of the abductor pollicis longus
    B. A subungual hematoma
    C. A sprain of the extensor pollicis brevis
    D. An avulsion of the extensor tendon from its insertion
    E. Dupuytren's contracture

159. During your examination of a football player who has sustained a low back injury during a tackle, you find that he is reporting dulled sensation along the dorsum of his right foot, he has difficulty walking on his heels, and his patellar tendon reflex is diminished. You suspect which of the following nerve root(s) is affected?
    A. L3
    B. L4
    C. L2
    D. S1 to S3
    E. L5

160. When evaluating the inert structures of a joint, passive range of motion is used to determine all of the following except:
    A. The athlete's willingness to move
    B. Limitations of joint motion
    C. Joint stability
    D. Muscle elasticity
    E. Soft tissue elasticity

Immediate Care

1. All of the following drugs may be used with phonophoresis during the acute phase of treatment except:
    A. Dexamethasone
    B. Hydrocortisone 1%
    C. Lidocaine
    D. Naproxen
    E. Hydrocortisone 10 %

2. One of your athletes has been diagnosed with psoriasis. All of the following medications are appropriate for treatment of this condition except:
    A. Aristocort
    B. Kenalog
    C. Topicort
    D. Betadine
    E. A and B

3. Which of the following is not a medication that is delivered via a metered-dose inhaler for exercise-induced asthma (EIA)?
    A. Proventil
    B. Alupent
    C. Atrovent
    D. Ventolin
    E. Butisol

4. What medication is often used for anxiety or panic attacks?
    A. Zantac
    B. Xanax
    C. Thorazine
    D. Prozac
    E. None of the above

5. What is the primary mode of action of penicillin?
    A. Increases the number of T-lymphocytes in the bloodstream
    B. Inhibits the metabolism of the bacteria
    C. Prevents bacterial reproduction
    D. Breaks down the cell wall of the bacteria
    E. Prevents viral reproduction

6. Which of the following is considered a medical emergency?
    A. Acute compartment syndrome
    B. Navicular fracture
    C. Bulimia
    D. Mitral valve prolapse
    E. Cellulitis

7. All of the following treatments would be inappropriate for an acute quadriceps contusion except:
    A. Light massage
    B. Pulsed ultrasound
    C. Ice massage followed by gentle stretch
    D. Ice pack with compression wrap with the knee in flexion
    E. Heat pack and massage

8. Deep frostbite is a medical emergency. What would the proper course of treatment be for this problem?
    A. Very slow, careful rewarming of the body part with warm water
    B. Firm, sustained pressure of the hand on the affected body part
    C. Rapid rewarming of the affected body part with warm water
    D. Quick friction in order to increase local circulation
    E. None of the above

9. During which of the circumstances below should an athlete be immediately referred to a dentist?
    I.   The tooth is knocked out
    II. When a tooth is displaced 2 mm or more
    III. When a crown is fractured and the tooth is still alive
    IV. When a filling is knocked out or fractured and the athlete is sensitive to hot or cold food
    V.   When an artificial plate is broken during competition

    A. I, II, III
    B. I, II, III, V
    C. I, V
    D. II, III, IV
    E. I, III, IV

10. A male athlete sustains a direct blow to the genital area. How can the athletic trainer immediately decrease the pain?
    A. Use an ice pack to the area with the athlete in supine, knees in extension
    B. Use direct pressure on the testes
    C. Have the athlete lie supine with his knees bent to his chest to decrease the strain on the scrotum and apply ice to the affected area
    D. Have the athlete lie on his side with his knees extended
    E. Place a moist heat pack over the area

11. When performing two-person CPR, what is the correct compression-to-breath ratio?
    A. 5:2
    B. 15:2
    C. 15:1
    D. 5:1
    E. 2:5

12. Shock after a severe injury can result from _____ or _____.
    A. Pain, increased blood pressure
    B. Decreased heart rate, infection
    C. Hemorrhage, hypothermia
    D. Hemorrhage, stagnation of blood
    E. Increased heart rate, pain

13. An athlete who had been diagnosed with infectious mononucleosis has just been cleared by the team doctor to return to full activity. How long should the athlete remain out of contact participation from the time of onset to the time of full recovery?
    A. 2 weeks
    B. At least 3 weeks
    C. 6 months
    D. A maximum of 6 weeks
    E. Minimum of 2 months

14. A rugby player sustains a confirmed head injury during a game and had been removed from the game. All of the following are symptoms/signs of increasing intracerebral pressure that the athletic trainer should monitor except:
    A. Nausea and vomiting
    B. Pupil irregularity
    C. Increase in systolic blood pressure with decrease in diastolic blood pressure
    D. Romberg's sign
    E. Changes in cognition

15. If an athlete is unconscious from a blow to the head, he or she should be assumed to have a neck injury in addition to a possible head injury. If the airway appears to be impaired, all of the following would be appropriate steps in management except:
    A. Cut the face mask with an appropriate tool and move it out of the way
    B. Leave the helmet on
    C. Stabilize the head and neck
    D. Do a finger sweep of the mouth to remove any debris and clear the airway
    E. Activate EMS

16. During the foreign body airway obstruction maneuver, the athletic trainer should grasp one fist with the other hand and place the thumb side of the fist where?
    A. On the abdomen between the xyphoid process and the umbilicus
    B. On the manubrium
    C. On the abdomen between the umbilicus and the symphysis pubis
    D. Between the scapula
    E. None of the above

17. An athlete is brought into the athletic training room with a 2.5-inch nail embedded in his foot. All of the following actions are appropriate in the treatment of this injury except:
    A. Immediately remove the nail from the foot
    B. Keep the athlete calm
    C. Pack the nail and foot as they are in a large dressing to help control the bleeding and stabilize the object
    D. Transport the athlete to the hospital with the nail still embedded in the foot
    E. Verify that the athlete's tetanus shot is current

18. Which of the measures below are appropriate steps in the management of an athlete who is experiencing a seizure?
    I. Keep spectators out of the way
    II. Protect the patient's head and body from injury
    III. Turn the patient on his or her side
    IV. If the athlete is in status epilepticus or it is a first seizure, immediately seek additional medical support
    V. Try to keep the athlete's mouth open by any means to prevent airway obstruction
    VI. Call the athlete's next of kin to inform him or her of the problem and of the care given

    A. II, IV, V, VI
    B. I, II, III, IV
    C. II, III, IV, VI
    D. I, II, IV, V
    E. III, IV, V, VI

19. It is critical that CPR be administered as soon as possible during a life-threatening situation. In what amount of time is brain damage likely to occur if the brain is deprived of oxygen?
    A. 2 to 4 minutes
    B. 10 to 12 minutes
    C. 4 to 6 minutes
    D. 10 minutes
    E. After 15 minutes

20. During CPR, it is most convenient and efficient to monitor the athlete's circulation by palpating the carotid artery. Where is the pulse located?
    A. In the groove between the larynx and the sternocleidomastoid muscle
    B. Between the mastoid process and pharynx
    C. At the base of the neck superior to the manubrium
    D. 2 inches below the base of the earlobe on the side of the neck
    E. Antecubital fossa of the elbow

21. During CPR, the adult sternum must be compressed to what depth for compression to be effective?
    A. 0.5 to 1 inch
    B. 1 to 1.5 inches
    C. 1.5 to 2 inches
    D. 2 to 2.5 inches
    E. 2.5 to 3 inches

22. Which type of heat injury is considered a medical emergency?
    A. Dehydration
    B. Heat cramps
    C. Heat stroke
    D. Heat exhaustion
    E. All of the above except A.

23. Which of the following signs and symptoms are characteristic of a tension pneumothorax?
    I. Tracheal deviation
    II. Distended neck veins
    III. Unilateral absence of breath sounds
    IV. Dizziness
    V. Cyanosis

    A. II, III, IV
    B. I, IV, V
    C. I, III, IV, V
    D. I, II, III, V
    E. I, III, IV

24. An athlete has been kicked in the low back area during a soccer game. He is complaining of significant flank pain, is having difficulty voiding, and there is blood in his urine. What should the athletic trainer suspect is injured?
    A. The spleen
    B. The large intestine
    C. The lumbar fascia
    D. The testicles
    E. The kidney

25. When evaluating an unconscious athlete, what should the athletic trainer do first?
    A. Check for sources of bleeding
    B. Take vital signs
    C. Check for normal extremity movement
    D. Take the athlete's pulse rate
    E. Check that the athlete's airway is open and he or she is breathing normally

26. What is the most common and devastating mechanism of injury seen in neck injuries sustained during football?
    A. Cervical hyperextension
    B. Forceful cervical lateral flexion
    C. Cervical hyperflexion and rotation
    D. Cervical hyperflexion and axial compression
    E. None of the above

27. Where would the athlete complain of pain with acute appendicitis?
    A. Lower right quadrant of the abdomen
    B. Right lateral hip area
    C. Inner right thigh
    D. Anterior right thigh area
    E. Lower back

28. What is the prudent method of transporting an athlete with a suspected spinal injury?
    A. Do not move the athlete until a doctor is present
    B. Use of a stretcher
    C. Fireman's carry
    D. Use a spine board with medical assistance
    E. Use a wheelchair

29. When fitting an athlete for crutches, the elbow should be bent to approximately what angle?
    A. 90 degrees
    B. 10 degrees
    C. 45 degrees
    D. 0 degrees
    E. 30 degrees

30. Under what condition can CPR be stopped?
    A. If a rib is fractured during the effort
    B. The athlete vomits
    C. The athlete aspirates
    D. Not until the athletic trainer is exhausted, spontaneous respirations and pulse have returned, or a physician or another party continues CPR in place of the athletic trainer
    E. A and C

31. After an athlete has suffered a ruptured spleen, he or she may experience pain that radiates down the left shoulder and approximately one third of the way down the upper left arm. What is this pain called?
    A. Visceral pain
    B. Radicular pain
    C. Kehr's sign
    D. Angina
    E. Radiation

32. What is the appropriate treatment for an athlete who has sustained a rib fracture?
    A. Use of a rib belt
    B. There is no specific treatment
    C. Total bedrest
    D. Use of a pillow to splint the ribs when coughing
    E. C and D

33. All of the following are basic functions of athletic taping and bandaging except:
    A. To support an injured body part
    B. To protect wounds from infection
    C. To enhance the athlete's skill
    D. To hold protective equipment in place
    E. B and D

34. Taping continuously around a limb may cause what problem?
    A. Ineffective support
    B. Difficulty in tape removal
    C. Compromised circulation
    D. There is no problem with this method
    E. Blisters

35. What is the compression-to-breath ratio during one-person adult CPR?
    A. 5:1
    B. 15:2
    C. 15:1
    D. 5:2
    E. 2:15

36. An athlete reports to the athletic trainer with a deep laceration to his thigh. The cut is approximately 1/8-inch deep, 1-inch long, and bleeding moderately. What would be the proper steps for the athletic trainer to take to treat this wound?
    A. Use a pressure bandage to control the bleeding, keep the wound clean and free of debris, use Steri-Strips for temporary closure, and apply ice and compression to the area
    B. Use a pressure bandage to control the bleeding, keep the wound clean, suture the laceration, and cover with a sterile dressing
    C. Wipe the area clean with soap and water, use an antibiotic ointment to minimize infection, suture the wound, and cover it with a sterile dressing
    D. Wipe the area clean with soap and water, apply a large adhesive bandage, and apply ice to the area
    E. None of the above

37. An athlete comes to the athletic trainer holding a tooth that has just been knocked out of his mouth. What would be the proper steps for the athletic trainer to take to allow for a successful reimplantation?
    A. Try to put it back in place and use a topical ointment for pain
    B. Put the tooth in a jar of water, tell the athlete to store it in a refrigerator until he can see a dentist
    C. There is nothing the athletic trainer can do because the tooth is dead
    D. Place the tooth in a cloth soaked with saline or water and get the athlete to a dentist within 30 minutes
    E. None of the above

38. During an emergency, all of the following information should be given over the telephone by the athletic trainer to emergency personnel except:
    A. The type of emergency
    B. The current status of the athlete
    C. Where the athlete is currently located
    D. The type of treatment currently being given to the athlete
    E. The name of the next of kin

39. An athlete has a suspected fracture involving the knee. Which of the following areas should be splinted?
    A. The ankle and lower leg areas
    B. The knee and thigh
    C. The ankle, knee, and thigh
    D. The lower limb joints and one side of the trunk
    E. The hip and ankle

40. Which of the following cells release histamine and serotonin during the cellular response phase of tissue healing?
    A. Macrophages
    B. Erythrocytes
    C. Granulocytes
    D. Leukocytes
    E. Mast cells and platelets

41. The acute phase of an injury lasts approximately 3 to 4 days. What occurs at the time of initial trauma?
    A. Phagocytosis, followed by vasoconstriction and diapedesis
    B. Transitory vasodilatation, inflammation, and phagocytosis
    C. Transitory vasoconstriction, followed by vaso-dilatation and increased permeability
    D. Vasoconstriction, increased permeability, and granulation
    E. All of the above

42. Where do primitive stem cells mature into mature red and white blood cells and platelets?
    A. Liver
    B. Spleen
    C. Gallbladder
    D. Bone marrow
    E. Epididymis

43. An athlete has just been injured on the basketball court, and the athletic trainer begins administering first aid. During the initial contact, the athletic trainer notices the athlete is hyperactive, argumentative, and sarcastic in his responses to questions. All of the following actions by the athletic trainer are inappropriate except:
    A. Telling the athlete he or she is a wimp and that it is "not that bad"
    B. Being abrupt and telling the athlete to snap out of it
    C. Allowing the athlete to express his emotions as they occur
    D. Calling the referee over to calm the athlete
    E. Walking away to prevent an argument

44. The athletic trainer notices an athlete is prone to abnormal bruising. After discussing the problem with the team doctor, he recommends which of the following vitamins?
    A. E
    B. D
    C. C
    D. Niacin
    E. K

45. An acronym used for the immediate care of an acute musculoskeletal injury is which of the following?
    A. RICE
    B. NSAID
    C. REST
    D. STAT
    E. HOPS

46. A drug that is used to increase the effect of another, such as aspirin when used in combination with codeine, is known as what?
    A. Synergistic
    B. Cumulative
    C. Paradoxical
    D. Potentiating
    E. Titrating

47. Which of the following is not the proper action for an athlete to take if lightning is observed during a game?
    A. Avoid standing near metal bleachers on the field
    B. Stand near a telephone pole
    C. Assume a crouched position in a ditch
    D. Take cover in an automobile if he or she cannot get indoors
    E. A and C

48. One of your cross-country runners has an ongoing problem with tinea pedis. Which of the following actions should you take to assist this athlete in mini-mizing the problem?
    A. Use talcum powder daily and keep his feet dry after showering
    B. Use Kwell shampoo twice a day or as directed by a physician
    C. Remove the infected toenail to prevent the infection from spreading
    D. Make sure the athlete uses sunblock with an SPF of 15 or higher
    E. None of the above

49. An athlete comes to the athletic training room with what appears to be a tick embedded in his lower leg. The athletic trainer should instruct the athlete not to do which of the following?
    A. Keep the area clean and free of other debris
    B. Pull the tick off with tweezers
    C. Cover the tick with mineral oil
    D. Put fingernail polish remover onto its body
    E. All of the above

50. What is a major side effect of the NSAID group?
    A. Vertigo
    B. Tinnitus
    C. Drowsiness
    D. Blurred vision
    E. Gastrointestinal upset

51. Your athlete is on a medication for a *Staphylococcus aureus* infection. Which of the following adverse reactions might you expect with antibiotic treatment?
    A. Palpitations
    B. Abdominal cramping
    C. Dry mouth
    D. Headache
    E. All of the above

52. What is the normal dosage for one tablet of aspirin?
    A. 200 mg
    B. 400 mg
    C. 500 mg
    D. 375 mg
    E. 325 mg

53. All of the following are possible side effects of oral contraceptives except:
    A. Nausea and vomiting
    B. Shortness of breath
    C. Fluid retention
    D. Amenorrhea
    E. Feeling "sluggish"

54. Anabolic steroids are often abused by athletes. Which of the following results may occur in the female athlete after ingesting testosterone?
    A. Decreased libido
    B. Gynecomastia
    C. Hirsutism
    D. Increased body fat
    E. All of the above

55. What is the best way to prevent otitis externa?
    A. Avoid contact activities for 7 to 10 days
    B. Use ear plugs during activity
    C. Dry the external auditory canal after swimming
    D. Wear adequate protective devices for the ear
    E. All of the above

56. Under which of the following conditions should an athletic helmet be removed after an injury?
    A. If the athlete requests it be removed
    B. If, after a reasonable period of time, the face mask cannot be removed to gain access to the airway
    C. The chief EMT requests that it be removed
    D. If the helmet causes immobilization of the head or jaw
    E. The helmet should never be removed

57. Which of the following tools has the interassociation task force recommended not be used as the primary tool for loop-strap removal on a football helmet after an injury?
    A. A box-cutter
    B. The "trainer's" angel
    C. A screwdriver
    D. The anvil pruner
    E. B and D

58. A predisposing condition such as spinal stenosis may mean an athlete is more likely to:
    A. Experience vertigo after an injury to the head
    B. Demonstrate nystagmus after an injury to the head
    C. Develop "glove and stocking" symptoms after a neck injury
    D. Develop paralysis after a fracture-dislocation
    E. Develop lower extremity neuropathies

59. Spinal immobilization is best achieved with the full-body splint. All of the following are examples of full-body immobilization equipment except:
    A. The standard rigid spine board
    B. Vacuum mattress
    C. A Stryker frame
    D. Scoop stretcher
    E. Miller full body splint

60. After an acute injury, chemical mediators are given off by various cells. Which of the following chemicals is the first to appear?
    A. Serotonin
    B. Heparin
    C. Prostaglandins
    D. Histamine
    E. Thrombin

61. Which of the following means "the abnormal development of tissue"?
    A. Atrophy
    B. Dysplasia
    C. Metaplasia
    D. Hyperplasia
    E. Hypertrophy

62. _____ and _____ are two conditions that will interfere with fracture healing.
    A. Poor blood supply, poor immobilization
    B. Infection, callus formation
    C. Granulation, callus formation
    D. Hematoma formation, the influx of endosteal cells
    E. Increased blood supply, callus formation

63. One of your athletes has just been stung by a bee. He appears to be showing signs of anaphylaxis. Which of the following medications would be appropriate to administer to stop the reaction?
    A. Epinephrine
    B. Heparin
    C. An antitussive
    D. A histamine-2 blocker
    E. None of the above

64. _____ and _____ are both examples of histamine-2 blockers.
    A. Xanax, Tegretol
    B. Benadryl, Seldane
    C. Proventil, Ventolin
    D. Tagamet, Zantac
    E. Benadryl, Tagamet

65. Which of the following drugs must the athletic trainer determine the athlete is not allergic to prior to administering a NSAID?
    A. Famotidine
    B. Acetaminophen
    C. Sulfa
    D. Sudafed
    E. Aspirin

66. When transporting an athlete off the field by manual conveyance, it is most convenient to do this with how many athletic trainers?
    A. 6
    B. 4
    C. 1
    D. 3
    E. 2

67. What is the average respiratory rate for an adult (18 years of age or older)?
    A. 30 to 80 breaths/min
    B. 20 to 30 breaths/min
    C. 12 to 15 breaths/min
    D. 5 to 10 breaths/min
    E. 40 to 50 breaths/min

68. Where should the bell of a stethoscope be placed when taking blood pressure?
    A. Over the brachial artery
    B. Over the brachial vein
    C. Over the popliteal fossa
    D. Over the radial artery
    E. Over the ulnar artery

69. Orthostatic syncope is caused by which of the following conditions?
    A. Increased intracranial pressure
    B. Sudden peripheral vasodilatation
    C. Poisoning
    D. An acute reduction in cardiac output
    E. All of the above

70. Which type of food should the athletic trainer recommend the athlete avoid if gallbladder pathology is suspected?
    A. Foods low in carbohydrates
    B. Foods high in protein
    C. Fatty foods
    D. Foods high in vitamin K
    E. All of the above

71. An athlete who has a seizure should be referred to a physician under which of the following conditions?
    A. After a seizure that lasts more than 5 min
    B. There is no history of previous seizures
    C. If the seizure does not fit into the person's pattern of previous seizures
    D. All of the above
    E. None of the above

72. Your team physician sends a prescription to you for your athlete that reads "whirlpool treatments TID." What does TID mean?
    A. Twice a day
    B. Every three hours
    C. Four times a day
    D. Three times a week
    E. Three times a day

73. If necessary, the removal of the helmet and shoulder pads from an athlete with a suspected spinal cord injury should be coordinated to avoid which of the following?
    A. Cervical hyperextension
    B. Airway obstruction
    C. Cervical hyperflexion
    D. Thoracic rotation
    E. Thoracic compression

74. The interassociation task force recommends that no fewer than _____ persons lift athletes suspected of having a spinal cord injury.
    A. Four plus
    B. Two plus
    C. Three plus
    D. Ten plus
    E. Eight plus

75. Which of the following instruments is used to visually examine the ear canal and tympanic membrane?
    A. Ophthalmoscope
    B. Laryngoscope
    C. Arthroscope
    D. Endoscope
    E. Otoscope

76. What is the primary reason an athletic trainer would perform pulmonary auscultation?
    A. To check for a systolic bruit
    B. To identify potential abnormal breath sounds
    C. To diagnose cardiothoracic pathology
    D. To diagnose pulmonary pathology
    E. All of the above

77. One of your female athletes presents with dysuria, a sense of urgency to urinate, decreased urine volume, nocturia, low back pain, and pyuria. What do you suspect this athlete has?
    A. Pyoperitonitis
    B. Dermatitis
    C. Prostatitis
    D. Vaginitis
    E. Cystitis

78. One of your athletes presents with rhinorrhea, rhinitis, a sore throat, nonproductive cough, low grade fever, headache, chills, and malaise. What action(s) should the athletic trainer take?
    A. Do not allow the athlete to work out for 10 to 14 days and refer him or her to a physician
    B. Transport the athlete to the nearest emergency room
    C. Limit the athlete's activities until the fever resolves and resume full activity as the symptoms resolve
    D. Begin the athlete on a course of antipyretics and analgesics
    E. Call the team physician for advice

79. All of the following symptoms should alert the athletic trainer to serious pathology that requires immediate referral to a physician except:
    A. Itchy skin, especially when it involves areas on the feet and toes
    B. Painful urination
    C. Unexpected weight loss
    D. Night pain
    E. Palpable lump in the breast or axilla

80. For which of the following injuries would the use of a hard-shell pad be appropriate?
    A. Cover a large skin infection
    B. A toe injury
    C. A painful contusion
    D. Plantar fasciitis
    E. None of the above

81. When choosing a prophylactic knee brace, the brace should meet all the following criteria except:
    A. It should always be custom-molded to avoid a poorly fitting brace
    B. It should not interfere with normal knee function
    C. It should not increase injuries to the lower extremity
    D. It should be cost-effective and durable
    E. B and D

82. When selecting a running shoe, the athletic trainer should recommend a sneaker with what type of sole?
    A. Polyurethane
    B. Rubber or polyurethane
    C. A hard rubber material infused with plastic
    D. Carbon-based materials
    E. None of the above

83. Of the following orthotic devices, which is the most difficult to fit and has the highest degree of complications?
    A. The semisoft orthotic device
    B. The soft orthotic device
    C. The semirigid orthotic device
    D. The rigid orthotic device
    E. None of the above

84. An AED is used for what purpose?
    A. To provide immobilization of the lumbar spine and pelvis after a spinal injury
    B. To treat arrythmias of the heart
    C. To treat hypovolemic shock
    D. To assess the athlete's level of consciousness after a head injury
    E. To defibrillate the heart when an unconscious victim has no pulse

85. When resolving a conflict, there are many approaches that an athletic trainer can take to successfully manage a difficult situation. Of the following conflict resolution methods, which one is least likely to successfully resolve a problem?
    A. Compromise
    B. Collaboration
    C. Negotiation
    D. Avoidance
    E. A and B

86. One of your athletes presents with abnormal pain that he describes as burning. He states that it becomes worse when he lies in supine or consumes caffeine, spicy foods, or alcohol. What might you suspect is the problem?
    A. Kidney stone
    B. Ruptured spleen
    C. Bowel obstruction
    D. Hernia
    E. Esophageal reflux or peptic ulcer

87. One of your athletes presents with a sudden onset of chest pain, dyspnea, hemoptysis, and cyanosis. What do you suspect is the problem?
    A. Pneumothorax
    B. Lung cancer
    C. Endocarditis
    D. Pulmonary infection
    E. Acute appendicitis

88. One of your athletes presents with diarrhea, vomiting, and abdominal cramping 1 to 6 hours after eating at a local restaurant. What do you suspect is the problem?
    A. Kidney stone
    B. Bowel obstruction
    C. Viral gastroenteritis
    D. Dysentery
    E. Food poisoning

89. How long should the abdomen be auscultated before the athletic trainer decides if the bowel sounds are absent?
    A. 30 to 60 seconds
    B. 2 to 3 minutes
    C. 60 to 90 seconds
    D. At least 5 minutes per region
    E. None of the above

90. One of your athletes begins to complain of intense itching of the skin under the cold pack that you applied to his shoulder 5 minutes ago. When you remove the pack you notice that hives have developed on the area that has been cooled. What is the athlete experiencing?
    A. Paroxysmal cold hemoglobinuria
    B. Hypothermia
    C. Cold urticaria
    D. Raynaud's disease
    E. Frostbite

91. When treating an athlete who presents with undifferentiated somatoform disorder, the athletic trainer should do all of the following except:
    A. Provide care for a bona fide injury
    B. Develop a sound relationship with the athlete to gain his or her trust
    C. Avoid doing more harm by dismissing the athlete as a "symptom magnifier"
    D. Provide the athlete with psychological counseling focused on having the athlete recognize and acknowledge the source of his or her anger
    E. All of the above

92. When using iontophoresis, the athletic trainer should be aware of possible _____ and _____ as a result of ion flux during treatment.
    A. Vertigo, light-headedness
    B. Sensation changes, increased swelling
    C. Skin irritation, chemical burns
    D. Vasodilatation, skin mottling
    E. Allergic reaction, increased swelling

93. Why is it important that an athlete with an abdominal injury never be given anything to eat or drink?
    A. It increases the risks of surgery if an operative procedure becomes necessary
    B. It will increase the athlete's blood glucose
    C. It will cause blood to be shunted to the viscera, causing hypovolemic shock
    D. It will cause metabolic acidosis
    E. None of the above

94. One of your diabetic athletes appears confused and is dizzy, apprehensive, and diaphoretic. How should this athlete be treated?
    A. This athlete is in diabetic ketoacidosis and should be given an immediate insulin injection
    B. This athlete should be treated for insulin shock and should be transported to the nearest hospital if he or she does not respond to sugar within 2 to 3 minutes
    C. This athlete is hyperthermic and needs to be placed in a cool, dark room until the symptoms pass
    D. The athletic trainer should monitor vital signs every 15 minutes, keep the athlete oriented, and administer insulin by mouth. If there is no change in 5 to 10 minutes, the athlete should be transported to the hospital
    E. None of the above

95. When taking a blood pressure with a sphygmomanometer, at what point is the systolic pressure noted?
    A. The point at which the pulse disappears
    B. The point at which the pulse is first heard
    C. At a point between 150 and 200 mmHg
    D. When the brachial pulse is first palpated as the cuff is deflated
    E. When the radial pulse is first heard as the cuff deflates

96. The ideal relationship between the athletic trainer and athlete is built on _____ and _____.
    A. Encouragement, effective listening
    B. A positive attitude, a sense of humor
    C. Luck, "good chemistry"
    D. Trust, mutual respect
    E. Trust, a good insurance policy

97. Which of the following is not a good reason to refer an athlete to a psychiatrist or psychologist?
    A. The athlete is showing undue concern over minor injuries, but the concern is brief
    B. His or her psychological stress is intense or persistent
    C. There is any suggestion of suicide
    D. There is a loss of contact with reality
    E. C and D

98. An athlete receives a head injury during a soccer game. While performing the on-field evaluation, the athletic trainer notices that the athlete has a hearing defect after testing for air and bone conduction using a tuning fork. Which cranial nerve is injured?
    A. IX (glossopharyngeal)
    B. VI (abducens)
    C. XII (hypoglossal)
    D. IV (trochlear)
    E. VIII (vestibulocochlear)

99. Which of the following is the proper protocol for administering Tylenol to an adult athlete (assuming the athlete is not allergic to acetaminophen)?
    A. Initial dose: two tablets, 200 mg each, repeat every 4 to 6 hours, PRN
    B. Initial dose: two tablets, 225 mg each, repeat every 4 to 6 hours, PRN
    C. Initial dose: two tablets, 325 mg each, repeat every 4 hours, PRN
    D. Initial dose: two tablets, 12.5 mg each, repeat every 6 hours, PRN
    E. Initial dose three tablets, 200 mg each, repeat every 8 to 12 hours, PRN

100. Which of the following is the proper protocol for administering Advil to an adult athlete (assuming he or she is not allergic to ibuprofen or aspirin and does not have renal or gastrointestinal pathology)?
    A. Initial dose: one to two tablets, 200 mg each, repeat every 6 hours, PRN. Do not exceed six tablets in a 24-hour period without consulting with a physician
    B. Initial dose: four tablets, 200 mg each, repeat every 6 hours, PRN
    C. Initial dose: one tablet, 400 mg, repeat in 4 to 6 hours with two tablets, 100 mg each, PRN
    D. Initial dose: one tablet, 600 mg, repeat in 4 to 6 hours, PRN. Do not exceed four tablets in a 24-hour period without consulting with a physician
    E. None of the above

101. Which of the following is the proper protocol for administering Pepcid AC to an adult athlete (assuming the athlete does not have difficulty swallowing or has persistent abdominal pain)?
    A. Initial dose: two tablets, 5 mg each with milk up to twice a day. Do not administer more than four tablets in a 24-hour period
    B. Initial dose: one tablet, 10 mg each with water up to twice a day. Do not administer more than two tablets in a 24-hour period
    C. Initial dose: one tablet, 75 mg with water up to twice a day. Do not administer more than two tablets in a 24-hour period
    D. Initial dose: one tablet, 5 mg with water up to four times a day
    E. None of the above

102. One of your athletes is complaining of constipation related to a dietary change. Which of the following would be the most appropriate recommendation for the athletic trainer to make?
    A. Recommend a diet high in fish oils
    B. Recommend increased fluid intake and increased intake of fruits, bulk vegetables, and cereal
    C. Recommend an increased diet of red meat and legumes
    D. Decrease the intake of green, leafy vegetables, and cereals to decrease bulk
    E. All of the above

103. Which of the following categories of drugs does not have a synergistic effect to cryotherapy?
    A. Nonsteroidal anti-inflammatory analgesics
    B. Skeletal muscle relaxants
    C. Systemic antibiotics
    D. Anti-inflammatory steroids (glucocorticoids)
    E. A and B

104. Which of the following categories of drugs has an antagonistic effect to superficial and deep heat therapy?
    A. Peripheral vasodilators
    B. Skeletal muscle relaxants
    C. Nonsteroidal anti-inflammatory analgesics
    D. Systemic vasoconstrictors
    E. All of the above

105. Which of the following are the three most common sites for avulsion fractures and apophysitis in the pelvic region?
    I. Ischial tuberosity and hamstring attachment
    II. Pubic symphysis and the adductor magnus attachment
    III. Anterior inferior iliac spine and the rectus femoris attachment
    IV. Iliac crest and quadratus lumborum attachment
    V. Anterior superior iliac spine where the sartorius attaches

    A. I, III, V
    B. III, IV, V
    C. I, II, IV
    D. I, III, IV
    E. I, II, III, IV

106. What is the possible consequence of a poorly managed shin contusion?
    A. Anterior tibialis tendinitis
    B. A fasciotomy
    C. Osteochondritis dissecans
    D. Osteomyelitis
    E. Extensor digitorum contracture

107. Which of the following is not part of the treatment for plantar fasciitis?
    A. Heel cups
    B. Soft orthotics
    C. Ultrasound
    D. Arch taping
    E. Use of a metatarsal bar

108. All of the following structures should be evaluated before and after a dislocated elbow is reduced except:
    A. The median nerve
    B. The radial nerve
    C. The neurovascular status of the brachial artery
    D. The ulnar nerve
    E. The axillary nerve

109. Which of the following is the appropriate treatment of a Bennett's fracture?
    A. RICE and analgesics followed by immobilization of the MTP joint for 3 weeks
    B. RICE and analgesics followed by immobilization of the CMC joint; it is structurally unstable and the athlete should be immediately referred to an orthopedic surgeon
    C. RICE and analgesics followed by immobilization of the wrist in slight flexion for 6 weeks
    D. RICE and analgesics followed by a protective splint of the PIP joint for 6 to 8 weeks
    E. None of the above

110. One of your athletes is experiencing an anxiety attack. He is hyperventilating. You talk to him to calm him down and have him slowly rebreathe into a paper bag. What process does rebreathing into a paper bag reverse?
    A. The release of adrenocorticotropic hormone (ACTH) from the pituitary gland
    B. Respiratory acidosis
    C. Metabolic alkalosis
    D. Metabolic acidosis
    E. Respiratory alkalosis

111. Which end feel is an abrupt, firm, springy resistance to motion?
    A. Tissue stretch
    B. Bony block
    C. Capsular restriction
    D. Muscle spasm
    E. Scar tissue adhesions

112. Which of the following is not a component of a primary survey?
    A. Check for sensations of numbness, tingling, or burning
    B. Check surroundings and environment
    C. Check athlete for ABC
    D. Check for severe bleeding
    E. B and D

113. Which of the following should be done for an unconscious athlete suffering from insulin shock?
    A. Immediately give the athlete an injection of epinephrine so his or her airway will open
    B. Immediately give the athlete a glass of orange juice or other high sugar drink
    C. Immediately transport the athlete to an emergency care facility
    D. Immediately give the athlete some sugar-free candy in order to counteract the high levels of sugar in his or her body
    E. All of the above

114. When symptoms are experienced distal to the pathology, this is known as what?
    A. Referred symptoms
    B. Physiological symptoms
    C. Radicular symptoms
    D. Psychosomatic symptoms
    E. Contrecoup symptoms

115. Which is not a sign/symptom of postconcussion syndrome?
    A. Dizziness
    B. Restlessness
    C. Behavioral changes
    D. Visual disturbances
    E. All of the above are signs or symptoms of postconcussion syndrome

116. What special test identifies ulnar nerve compression or transmission interference at the elbow?
    A. Finkelstein's test
    B. Tarsal tunnel test
    C. Elbow flexion test
    D. Tinel's sign
    E. Yergason's test

117. All of the following are signs/symptoms of anaphylactic shock except:
    A. Development of rash or hives
    B. Wheezing sounds coming from the chest
    C. An increase in blood pressure
    D. Rapid, weak pulse
    E. A and D

118. Which of the following is not a major type of open wound?
    A. Laceration
    B. Contusion
    C. Abrasion
    D. Avulsion
    E. Incision

119. Which of the following is a condition of rapidly rising internal body temperature that occurs when the body's mechanisms for the release of heat are overwhelmed?
    A. Hyperthermia
    B. Heat exhaustion
    C. Heat stroke
    D. Hypothermia
    E. Raynaud's phenomenon

120. Which pulse should always be assessed with any injury to the lower extremity?
    A. Carotid pulse
    B. Brachial pulse
    C. Axillary pulse
    D. Radial pulse
    E. Dorsal pedal pulse

121. What type of shock is commonly referred to as fainting?
    A. Respiratory shock
    B. Cardiogenic shock
    C. Metabolic shock
    D. Anaphylactic shock
    E. Psychogenic shock

122. When a minor is injured and it is a life-threatening situation, the athletic trainer must try to contact the parents of the child. If the parents of the child cannot be contacted and they did not give consent in writing before the child began participation, the athletic trainer still has the right to give the child emergency care. Which type of consent is this?
    A. Informed
    B. Implied
    C. Complied
    D. Restrictive
    E. None of the above

123. Which of the following is a sign of heat stroke?
    A. Pale, cold, clammy skin
    B. Unequal pupils
    C. Hot and relatively dry skin
    D. Slow pulse
    E. Diaphoresis

124. Which of the following is not a sign of a diabetic coma?
    A. Fast and weak pulse
    B. Deep and sighing respirations
    C. Livid, later pale, skin
    D. Slow and weak pulse
    E. Fruity-smelling breath

125. What are the two most common sites to apply direct pressure to control severe bleeding of the upper and lower extremities?
    A. Brachial artery and femoral artery
    B. Popliteal artery and radial artery
    C. Brachial artery and suprascapular artery
    D. Brachial vein and femoral vein
    E. Carotid artery and femoral artery

126. _____ shock is a widely disseminated infection in many areas of the body, with the infection being borne through the blood from one tissue to another.
    A. Cardiogenic
    B. Septic
    C. Psychogenic
    D. Metabolic
    E. Hypovolemic

127. Which of the following is not a sign of hypovolemic shock?
    A. Low blood pressure
    B. Rapid and weak pulse
    C. Shallow and extremely rapid respiration
    D. Slow and weak pulse
    E. Agitation

128. How long can the brain be deprived of oxygen until brain cells begin to die?
    A. 10 to 15 minutes
    B. 1 to 3 minutes
    C. 4 to 6 minutes
    D. 17 to 20 minutes
    E. 12 to 16 minutes

129. Which of the following is a sign of inadequate breathing?
    A. Steady rise and fall of the chest
    B. The sound of air passing through the athlete's nose or mouth
    C. The sensation of the athlete breathing on the side of your face
    D. Noisy respiration, such as wheezing or gurgling
    E. None of the above

130. A football helmet should be removed only under which of the following circumstances?
    A. The injured athlete is not moving
    B. The injured athlete is no longer comfortable and says the helmet is hurting his neck
    C. You cannot gain adequate access to the airway
    D. If the EMTs think it is a great idea
    E. Never remove the helmet

131. What is a common bony process broken during adult CPR?
    A. Olecranon process
    B. The clavicle
    C. Styloid process
    D. Mastoid process
    E. The xyphoid process

132. Profuse sweating, dizziness, and nausea are signs and symptoms of which of the following?
    A. Heat stroke
    B. Heat exhaustion
    C. Hypothermia
    D. Frostbite
    E. Heat cramps

133. Which of the following things would you not want to do for someone who has gone into shock?
    A. Maintain the airway
    B. Keep the athlete calm
    C. Provide care for specific injury
    D. Give food or drink to the athlete
    E. Monitor their vital signs

134. An athlete with a skull fracture will have which of the following?
    A. Battle's sign
    B. Raccoon eyes
    C. Tenderness in the hard palate
    D. All of the above
    E. None of the above

135. Where would you place direct pressure on a wound that is bleeding?
    A. Directly on the wound
    B. On the right side of the wound
    C. Above the wound
    D. Below the wound
    E. On the closest artery

136. What is the first thing you should do if you suspect a spinal injury?
    A. Place the athlete on a spine board with assistance
    B. Hold in-line stabilization
    C. Help the athlete to sit up
    D. Have the athlete move his or her head
    E. Have the athlete move his or her legs

137. Which of the following is not included in a rehabilitation program after an injury?
    A. Plyometrics
    B. Proprioceptive neuromuscular facilitation
    C. Agility drills
    D. Immobilization
    E. Joint mobilizations

138. With ice application during the initial care of an acute injury, all of the following occur except:
    A. Increased metabolism in the area
    B. Inhibition of the hypoxic response
    C. Disruption of the pain/spasm cycle
    D. Reduction of edema
    E. Decreased nerve conduction

139. Which of the following carries impulses toward the central nervous system?
    A. Synaptic connections
    B. Afferent pathways
    C. Efferent pathways
    D. Dendrites
    E. Efferent axons

140. Deep stroking during massage is known as what?
    A. Tapotement
    B. Vibration
    C. Pétrissage
    D. Effluerage
    E. Friction massage

141. To determine if a victim is breathing you should do all of the following except:
    A. Place your ear over the victim's mouth to listen for breath sounds
    B. Observe the chest
    C. Feel for the rise and fall of the chest
    D. Ask the athlete to say his or her name
    E. A and C

142. _____ pupils indicate possible shock, hemorrhage, or cardiac arrest.
    A. Unequal
    B. Constricted
    C. Dilated
    D. Discolored
    E. Closed

143. Which of the following does not occur when an individual is in shock?
    A. Skin is pale and cool
    B. Blood pressure (BP) is high
    C. Pulse is rapid
    D. BP is low
    E. Respiration is shallow

144. Frostbite includes which of the following signs?
    A. Skin appears blotchy white to yellow-gray
    B. Skin is purple
    C. Skin is pale
    D. Skin is warm
    E. All of the above

145. The athletic trainer should do which of the following when dealing with an athlete with heat exhaustion?
     A. Administer cool fluids
     B. Remove unnecessary clothing
     C. Move to a cool place
     D. All of the above
     E. None of the above

Treatment, Rehabilitation, and Reconditioning

1. What does "extension lag" mean?
   A. Ability to only flex the knee
   B. Inability to fully backward bend (lumbar movement)
   C. One leg drags behind the other during gait
   D. Inability to fully extend the knee
   E. Inability to fully extend hip

2. What is the best method of determining the recovery status of the hand and forearm after a flexor injury?
   A. Use of a KT-1000 arthrometer
   B. Assessing the strength of a handshake
   C. Manual muscle testing of the wrist
   D. Use of a hand dynamometer
   E. EMG Testing

3. Which of the following is the correct sequence of tissue healing?
   A. Cellular response, regeneration, remodeling
   B. Remodeling, regeneration, cellular response
   C. Rejection, regeneration, resolution
   D. Regeneration, resolution, remodeling
   E. None of the above

4. What amount of time may it take for complete remodeling of tissues to occur after a soft tissue injury?
   A. 1 to 3 months
   B. 6 to 9 months
   C. 4 to 6 weeks
   D. 12 to 24 months
   E. Up to one year

5. Where is the primary location for adenosine triphosphate (ATP) production in skeletal muscle?
   A. Sarcomere
   B. Sarcoplasm
   C. Sarcolemma
   D. Sarcoplasmic reticulum
   E. Mitochondria

6. Sensory receptors located at the musculotendinous junction, which monitor active tension generated by the muscle during a contraction, are called:
   A. Pacinian corpuscles
   B. Ruffinian receptors
   C. Golgi tendon organs
   D. Muscle spindles
   E. Contractile sensory receptors

7. Which of the following describes a neurapraxia?
   A. Demyelination of the axon sheath that leads to a conduction block. Usually heals in approximately 1 to 2 weeks
   B. Loss or disruption of the axon and myelin sheath. The epineurium is still intact
   C. An injury to the endoneurium, perineurium, and epineurium with a permanent neurological deficit
   D. A crush injury to a nerve causing damage to the epineurium. The perineurium is intact
   E. None of the above

8. Bone grows via a process of apposition and resorption on its surface. Which of the following cells are responsible for the resorption of bone during its growth or repair?
   A. Osteoblasts
   B. Osteocytes
   C. Osteophils
   D. Osteoclasts
   E. None of the above

9. Why is the repair response so limited in the articular cartilage of a joint after an injury in the adult athlete?
   A. Articular cartilage cells do not undergo mitosis in the mature athlete
   B. Articular cartilage has a poor venous supply
   C. Articular cartilage has a low water content
   D. There are fewer mitochondria present in articular cartilage than in hyaline cartilage
   E. All of the above

10. What are the four sensations an athlete will experience with the application of cryotherapy?
    A. Cold, burning, cramping, numbness
    B. Pain, aching, stinging, cold
    C. Aching, burning, pain, numbness
    D. Cold, burning, aching, numbness
    E. Cold, burning, stinging, aching

11. The effects of treating a subacute musculoskeletal injury with a warm whirlpool include all of the following except:
    A. Analgesia
    B. Stimulation of local circulation
    C. Decreased muscle spasm
    D. Increased deep tissue temperature
    E. Decreased joint stiffness

12. Which cells are active after an injury to begin building collagen?
    A. Osteocytes
    B. Osteoblasts
    C. Granulocytes
    D. Osteoclasts
    E. Fibroblasts

13. Heat is dissipated in the body by all of the following except:
    A. Shivering
    B. Convection
    C. The lungs
    D. Sweat evaporation
    E. Vasodilation

14. External muscular force available for useful work is the result of all of the following factors except:
    A. The velocity of muscular shortening
    B. Whether the muscle is fast or slow twitch
    C. The angle of the pull of the muscle
    D. The length of the muscle
    E. C and D

15. Balance and coordination are critical for athletic performance. Feedback from the muscles as to what they are doing during a particular activity is known as _____. The area of the brain that assists in controlling movement is the _____.
    A. Proprioception, brainstem
    B. Muscle perception, medulla
    C. Kinesthesia, cortex
    D. Proprioception, cerebellum
    E. Kinesthesia, cerebrum

16. What is a stretching exercise that consists of a "stretch and hold" position called?
    A. Static stretch
    B. PNF pattern
    C. Ballistic stretch
    D. Warm-up
    E. B and C

17. If hyperventilation does not adequately increase the oxygen supply in the blood during aerobic exercise, what must occur to meet the gas exchange demands?
    A. Increased cardiac output
    B. Decreased cardiac output
    C. Supplemental iron pills must be provided
    D. The activity must be discontinued
    E. None of the above

18. An injured athlete is led through a therapeutic mental process in which he pictures himself being evaluated by the athletic trainer and assured the injury is not serious. He then pictures himself moving through rehabilitation, recovering nicely, and, finally, returning to his sport fully healed. What is this therapeutic approach to the recovery process called?
    A. Regression
    B. Thought stopping
    C. Biofeedback
    D. Meditation
    E. Visualization

19. What must the athletic trainer establish with the athlete prior to and during the rehabilitation in order for the rehabilitation of an injured athlete to be successful?
    A. A good rapport
    B. A position of dominance
    C. A deadline by which the athlete must return to full-time participation in his or her sport
    D. The understanding that the coach has the final decision in his or her rehabilitation sessions
    E. B and C

20. A basketball player who has sprained her ankle for the second time in 3 months reports to the athletic training room for her third treatment session. The athletic trainer notices she is demanding and wants to know why the athletic trainer "did not fix her ankle the right way the first time." She becomes somewhat threatening, stating that she will find someone else to help her if she is not successfully helped this time. What would be the best response to an attention-seeking athlete?
    A. Give up and let her seek help elsewhere
    B. Work with the athlete as long as necessary to satisfy her need for attention
    C. Set specific but reasonable time limits with the athlete per treatment session so the athletic trainer is not overtaxed
    D. Encourage the athlete to take a more positive position on her rehabilitation and use humor to divert her attention away from the injury
    E. None of the above

21. If an athlete needs to lose weight for health reasons, how many calories must his or her daily diet be reduced by in order to lose 1 to 2 pounds per week?
    A. 250 to 500 calories/day
    B. 1000 to 2000 calories/week
    C. 1000 to 2000 calories/day
    D. 500 to 1000 calories/day
    E. None of the above

22. Which modality would be best utilized if the desired therapeutic effect is decreased pain, edema, and inflammation?
    A. Moist heat packs
    B. Ultrasound
    C. Diathermy
    D. Fluidotherapy
    E. Ice packs

23. What are heat-producing currents in the body that are formed by a magnetic field that is externally applied in short-wave diathermy called?
    A. Induction currents
    B. Magnetic currents
    C. Eddy currents
    D. Alternating currents
    E. Interferential currents

24. High-voltage pulsed monophasic generators (HVPG) deliver current to deep tissues without damaging superficial tissues and are used for pain modulation. What type of waveform is used with this type of stimulator?
    A. Asymmetrical biphasic spiked pulse
    B. Monophasic squared pulse
    C. Symmetrical biphasic pulses
    D. Monophasic spike delivered in pairs
    E. None of the above

25. A moist heat pack causes all of the following effects except:
    A. Higher superficial tissue temperatures
    B. Increases in muscle tissue temperatures
    C. Sedation
    D. Reduction of muscle spasms
    E. Vasodilation

26. What physiological effects occur under the cathode of an electrical stimulator?
    I. Vasodilatation
    II. Vasoconstriction
    III. Tissue softening
    IV. Irritation

    A. I, III, IV
    B. II, III, IV
    C. I, II, III
    D. I, II, IV
    E. None of the above

27. All of the following are contraindications for using cryotherapy except:
    A. Raynaud's phenomenon
    B. Inflammation
    C. Vasculitis
    D. Cold urticaria
    E. A and D

28. What would be a functional skill for an athlete in an ankle rehabilitation program?
    A. Gastrocnemius flexibility
    B. Single-leg hopping
    C. Lifting tolerance
    D. Anterior tibialis strengthening
    E. All of the above

29. When rehabilitating a musculoskeletal injury, what is the proper progression of treatment?
    A. Range of motion, strength, endurance, proprioception
    B. Pain relief, agility, range of motion, strength
    C. Range of motion, pain relief, endurance, proprioception
    D. Proprioception, range of motion, strength, endurance
    E. Range of motion, endurance, strength, proprioception

30. Which of the following PNF techniques is not a strengthening technique?
    A. Slow reversal
    B. Rhythmic stabilization
    C. Slow-reversal-hold-relax
    D. Rhythmic initiation
    E. All of the above

31. During a lower extremity D1 flexion PNF pattern, what movements are taking place at the hip?
    A. Extension, abduction, internal rotation
    B. Flexion, abduction, internal rotation
    C. Extension, adduction, external rotation
    D. Flexion, adduction, external rotation
    E. Flexion, abduction, external rotation

32. During a D2 extension pattern of the upper extremity, what is the proper timing sequence?
    A. Shoulder extension, forearm pronation, finger flexion
    B. Shoulder flexion, scapular retraction, finger extension
    C. Shoulder abduction, forearm supination, finger extension
    D. Shoulder extension, forearm supination, finger flexion
    E. None of the above

33. According to Maitland's five grades of joint motion, which grade would be most appropriate when joint movement is limited by pain and spasm?
    A. I
    B. II
    C. III
    D. IV
    E. V

34. An athlete is seen by the athletic trainer 4 weeks postoperatively after shoulder arthroscopy. During the athletic trainer's assessment, it is found that the athlete has limited abduction secondary to capsular stiffness. Which of the following joint glides would be appropriate to improve this motion?
    A. Inferior humeral glide
    B. Anterior humeral glide
    C. Posterior humeral glide
    D. Superior humeral glide
    E. All of the above; combined glides

35. Which of the following statements accurately describes isokinetic training?
    A. Generation of a muscular force with no visible joint movement
    B. Generation of a muscular force with visible joint movement that occurs at a constant speed but with variable external resistance
    C. Generation of a muscular force with visible joint movement at a variable speed but with a fixed external resistance
    D. Generation of a muscle force during muscular lengthening
    E. None of the above

36. Which of the following massage techniques is a method of tapotement?
    A. Cupping
    B. Hacking
    C. Pinching
    D. All of the above
    E. None of the above

37. When massage is utilized to induce a sedative effect, which type of massage technique is indicated?
    A. Tapotement
    B. Vibration
    C. Pétrissage
    D. Danish
    E. Effleurage

38. What conditioning component is needed to perceive the position of the foot as it lands on the ground after the swing phase of gait?
    A. Agility
    B. Balance
    C. Proprioception
    D. Kinesthesia
    E. Eccentric stretching

39. Descending hills during running requires what type of muscular contraction by the quadriceps to decelerate the body?
    A. Positive
    B. Concentric
    C. Isokinetic
    D. Isometric
    E. Eccentric

40. What should a postseason conditioning program specifically focus on?
    A. Endurance activities
    B. Strengthening and flexibility exercises
    C. Sport-specific activities
    D. Identifying and improving the areas of conditioning in which the athlete is deficient
    E. All of the above

41. During the acute phase of an ankle injury, the water temperature of a whirlpool should be set at what temperature?
    A. 37°C to 37.7°C
    B. 55°F to 65°F
    C. 30°F to 35°F
    D. 70°F to 80°F
    E. 40°C to 50°C

42. Before returning an athlete to full activity, all of the following criteria should equal those taken from the uninvolved side at the end of the rehabilitation program except:
    A. Strength of each muscle group
    B. Girth measurements at 6 inches above and below the joint line
    C. Proprioception of both extremities
    D. Flexibility of the involved muscle groups
    E. C and D

43. Which of the following components of a rehabilitation program is most often overlooked by the athletic trainer during rehabilitation?
    A. Endurance
    B. Flexibility
    C. Proprioception
    D. Functional testing prior to returning to the sport
    E. Strength

44. What type of exercises may be safely initiated immediately after knee surgery?
    A. Closed-chain eccentric exercises
    B. Isotonic exercises
    C. Isometric exercises
    D. Functional exercises
    E. None of the above

45. When rehabilitating an athlete who has been diagnosed with "jumper's knee," which muscle group should eventually be strengthened?
    A. Hamstrings
    B. Quadriceps
    C. Hip adductors
    D. Hip extensors
    E. Triceps surae

46. When treating an athlete with trochanteric bursitis, flexibility should be increased in which of the following muscles?
    A. Gluteus maximus
    B. Tensor fascia latae
    C. Iliacus
    D. Piriformis
    E. Lumbar

47. A tight Achilles' tendon can cause _____ or _____ in order to allow the lower leg to move over the foot during running.
    A. Late heel-off, early heel strike
    B. Early heel-off, excessive supination
    C. Late heel-off, late toe-off
    D. Early heel-off, excessive pronation
    E. Early heel-off, early heel strike

48. Which of the following is not a factor in designing an appropriate treatment program?
    A. The stage of tissue healing
    B. Pain with joint motion
    C. The severity of the injury
    D. How soon the coach feels the athlete should return to play
    E. A and B

49. When rehabilitating a cervical strain, what must the athletic trainer maintain the integrity of?
    A. Shoulder girdle
    B. Lower back
    C. Upper arm
    D. Hand
    E. Kyphosis of the thoracic spine

50. Which of the following sequences is appropriate steps in rehabilitating a grade II ankle sprain?
    A. RICE, stretching the Achilles' tendon, isometric exercises, proprioceptive exercises, isotonic exercises
    B. RICE, isotonic exercises, hopping exercises, stretching the Achilles' tendon, active range-of-motion exercises
    C. RICE, isotonic exercises, isokinetic exercises, active range of motion exercises
    D. RICE, treadmill ambulation, active range of motion exercises, figure-eight exercises, stretching of the Achilles' tendon, foot intrinsic exercises
    E. None of the above

51. When is the best time to begin a rehabilitation program after an injury?
    A. Immediately
    B. After the injured part is "healed"
    C. After the inflammation is under control
    D. Once the pain subsides
    E. All of the above

52. When following the DAPRE technique of progressive resistive exercise, the first set of 10 repetitions is performed with a weight that is ____ of the weight that will be lifted in set three.
    A. 10%
    B. 25%
    C. 100%
    D. 75%
    E. 50%

53. When rehabilitating an athlete with patellofemoral pain syndrome, which muscle groups should be strengthened?
    A. Quadriceps, hamstrings
    B. Hip abductors, hamstrings
    C. Hip adductors, quadriceps
    D. Hip flexors, hip external rotators
    E. Iliotibial band, hip external rotators

54. Which of the following exercises are appropriate in attempting to decrease the symptoms of thoracic outlet syndrome?
    A. Cervical range of motion exercises, anterior shoulder strengthening
    B. Cervical range of motion exercises, cervical isometrics
    C. Anterior chest wall strengthening, cervical isometrics
    D. Stretching the anterior chest wall, strengthening the posterior midthoracic area
    E. None of the above

55. What are the most appropriate exercises for a diagnosis of lumbar spinal stenosis?
    A. Kegel exercises
    B. McKenzie extension exercises
    C. Lumbar stabilization exercises
    D. Postural awareness exercises
    E. Williams' flexion exercises

56. Which of the following exercises does not address proprioception?
    A. Recumbent stationary bicycling
    B. Mini-trampoline exercises
    C. Stork-standing exercises with the eyes open
    D. Treadmill exercises
    E. All of the above

57. When rehabilitating a shoulder, in what area should strengthening exercises be initiated first?
    A. Rotator cuff musculature
    B. Cervical musculature
    C. Scapular musculature
    D. Shoulder abductors, flexors, and internal rotators
    E. A and D

58. When rehabilitating an athlete who has undergone an anterior cruciate ligament reconstruction, which of the following muscle groups must be strengthened to support the graft?
    A. Triceps surae
    B. Hip adductors
    C. Quadriceps
    D. Gluteals
    E. Hamstrings

59. Which of the following pieces of equipment is not considered closed kinetic chain?
    A. Treadmill
    B. Leg-press machine
    C. Upper body ergometer
    D. Isokinetic knee extension machine
    E. BAPS Board

60. When rehabilitating the lateral epicondylitis, which muscle group needs to be strengthened?
    A. Wrist flexors
    B. Wrist extensors
    C. Elbow flexors
    D. Elbow extensors
    E. Shoulder abductors

61. When rehabilitating an athlete with a recent herniated lumbar disc, which of the following exercises are most appropriate?
    A. Williams' flexion exercises
    B. McKenzie extension exercises
    C. Lumbar stabilization exercises
    D. Posterior pelvic tilts and knee-to-chest exercises
    E. PNF stretching exercises

62. An athlete needs instruction on how to properly perform an abdominal sit-up. What should the athletic trainer recommend?
    A. Place his hands behind his head, take a deep breath and hold it, and pull his torso up toward his bent knees
    B. Cross his arms across his chest, tuck in his chin, bend his knees, inhale, and then exhale as he pulls his torso up toward his knees
    C. Place his hands behind his head, bend his knees, exhale completely first, and inhale deeply as he pulls his torso up toward his knees
    D. Keeping his arms down by his sides, bend his knees, inhale deeply, and hold it as he pulls his torso up toward his knees
    E. None of the above

63. Knee braces can be classified as either functional, prophylactic, or rehabilitative. Which type of brace might be worn for 1 to 2 weeks after a grade II medial collateral ligament tear?
    A. Functional
    B. Prophylactic
    C. Rehabilitative
    D. Custom fit
    E. No brace is necessary for this injury

64. In terms of specificity of training, which type of exercise would be appropriate during the late phases of rehabilitation of a soccer player?
    A. Stairmaster
    B. Swimming
    C. Stationary bicycle
    D. Leg press
    E. Treadmill exercise

65. Which of the following conditions is not indicated for mechanical traction?
    A. An acute interspinous sprain
    B. Degenerative joint disease
    C. Herniated discs or protrusions
    D. Degenerative disc disease
    E. Muscle spasm

66. Which of the muscle groups listed below are involved during a bench press?
    I.   Anterior deltoid
    II. Rhomboids
    III. Triceps
    IV. Pectoralis major
    V.   Latissimus dorsi
    VI. Upper trapezius

    A. I, II, III, IV
    B. III, IV, V, VI
    C. I, III, IV, V
    D. II, III, IV, VI
    E. I, II, III, V

67. Which of the following muscle groups are involved during a full squat with weights?
    I.   Quadriceps
    II. Hamstrings
    III. Erector spinae
    IV. Middle deltoid
    V.   Gluteus maximus
    VI. Serratus anterior

    A. I, II, IV, V
    B. II, III, IV, V
    C. I, II, III, V
    D. II, III, V, VI
    E. All of the above

68. Which of the following muscles are involved in a seated military press?
    I.   Trapezius
    II. Latissimus dorsi
    III. Pectoralis major
    IV. Serratus anterior
    V.   Posterior deltoid
    VI. Triceps

    A. II, III, VI
    B. I, III, IV, V
    C. I, IV, V, VI
    D. I, III, IV, VI
    E. All of the above

69. Which of the following describes a grade III joint mobilization technique?
    A. Small amplitude movement at the end range
    B. Large amplitude movement throughout the full available range of motion of the joint
    C. Small amplitude movement in the beginning of the range of motion
    D. Thrusting movement done at the anatomical limits of the joint
    E. None of the above

70. When rehabilitating an athlete, it is important that the area being rehabilitated is stressed with a variety of intensities and durations during conditioning. The body responds to these stresses by adapting to the specific demands imposed on it. What is this principle known as?
    A. The SAID principle
    B. The DAPRE principle
    C. The RICE principle
    D. The SITS principle
    E. None of the above

71. Which of the following is not an example of an isotonic device?
    A. Free weights
    B. A Total Gym
    C. A squat rack
    D. Wall pulleys
    E. A wall

72. When stretching during a warm-up routine, which type of stretching should not be encouraged because it may lead to an injury?
    A. Ballistic
    B. Active
    C. Static
    D. Plyometric
    E. Proprioceptive neuromuscular facilitation

73. In which of the following sports would plyometric training be beneficial?
    A. Rock climbing
    B. Cross-country
    C. Volleyball
    D. Archery
    E. Swimming

74. Which of the following exercises improves proprioceptive feedback when rehabilitating a lower extremity injury?
    A. Stationary bicycling
    B. Single-leg standing on a mini-trampoline
    C. Using a knee extension machine
    D. Bilateral calf raises
    E. All of the above

75. An athlete is recovering from a partial meniscectomy performed 5 days ago. All of the following actions would be appropriate at this time except:
    A. Achilles' stretching
    B. Four quadrant straight leg raises
    C. Stationary bicycling with minimal/no resistance
    D. Eccentric quadriceps strengthening
    E. Hip flexor strengthening

76. Which of the following exercises should be avoided in the early stages (phase I) of anterior cruciate reconstruction rehabilitation?
    A. Full knee extension exercises
    B. Resisted hip abduction
    C. Toe raises
    D. Hamstring curls
    E. Isometric contraction of the quadriceps

77. Two exercises that are designed to stabilize the lumbar spine during low back rehabilitation include _____ and _____.
    A. Single knee-to-chest exercise, double knee to chest
    B. Hamstring stretching, bridging exercises
    C. Partial sit-ups, active trunk extension in prone
    D. Resisted hip abduction exercise, iliotibial band stretching
    E. Hamstring stretching, piriformis strengthening

78. An athletic trainer working in a sports medicine clinic may have to read a SOAP note. In what section would a finding such as a positive Lachman's test be recorded?
    A. Subjective (S)
    B. Objective (O)
    C. Assessment (A)
    D. Plan (P)
    E. Special tests (S)

79. Bracing for scoliosis of the spine may be effective with all ages except:
    A. 5 year olds
    B. 10 year olds
    C. 18 year olds
    D. 14 year olds
    E. Bracing is not effective at any age

80. Ultrasound is based on the _____ effect.
    A. Resonance
    B. Sounding
    C. Cavitation
    D. Phoresor
    E. Reverse piezoelectric

81. What medium does not transmit ultrasound waves?
    A. Water
    B. Gel
    C. Body lotion
    D. Steroid creams
    E. Air

82. What kind of heating method does a warm whirlpool utilize?
    A. Conduction
    B. Convection
    C. Radiation
    D. Evaporation
    E. All of the above

83. What is the term used in ultrasound to describe the time that sound waves are being emitted during one pulse period?
    A. Ultrasound frequency
    B. Cavitation
    C. Attenuation
    D. Duty cycle
    E. Intensity

84. A moist heat pack offers what type of thermotherapy?
    A. Superficial
    B. Deep
    C. Cutaneous
    D. Surface
    E. None of the above

85. "Conventional TENS" uses a frequency in the _____ pulses per second range with a phase duration of _____ μseconds.
    A. 50 to 100, 250
    B. 50 to 100, 2 to 50
    C. 2 to 4, >150
    D. >100, 20 to 30
    E. <10, 50

86. What is one of the most serious adverse reactions during iontophoresis treatment?
    A. Galvanic burns
    B. Anaphylactic shock
    C. Dermatitis
    D. Histamine reaction
    E. None of the above

87. Paraffin bath therapy is commonly used on the hands and feet as a method of superficial heating. To keep the paraffin mixture in a molten state, the temperature should be maintained between:
    A. 100°F to 115°F
    B. 80°F to 105°F
    C. 126°F to 130°F
    D. 118°F to 125°F
    E. 140°F to 150°F

88. The therapeutic conversion of electrical energy into high-frequency sound energy above the audible range to create heat in the tissues is the definition of what modality?
    A. Diathermy
    B. Ultrasound
    C. Electric stimulation
    D. TENS
    E. Interferential current

89. Ultrasound waves are reflected by _____ and absorbed by _____.
    A. Bone, skin
    B. Skin, connective tissue
    C. Skin, blood
    D. Bone, muscle
    E. Nerve, muscle

90. Which of the following are contraindications to massage?
    I. Inflammation
    II. Pregnancy
    III. Hemorrhage
    IV. Infection
    V. Phlebitis

    A. I, II, III, IV
    B. I, III, IV, V
    C. II, III, IV
    D. II, III, IV, V
    E. All of the above

91. Which of the following is not an indication for diathermy?
    A. To increase local circulation
    B. Reduction of spasms
    C. Pain relief
    D. Cardiac abnormalities
    E. Osteoarthritis

92. Which of the following is not a contraindication or precaution for the use of ultrasound?
    A. Scarring
    B. Acute hemorrhage
    C. Anesthesia
    D. Treating over the endocrine gland
    E. Open wounds

93. Which physical law is applied with the use of an infrared lamp?
    A. Joule's law
    B. Inverse square law
    C. Wolff's law
    D. Ohm's law
    E. Newton's law

94. _____ and _____ are two means that deliver medication via sound waves and electricity.
    A. Ultrasound, iontophoresis
    B. Ultrasound, phonophoresis
    C. Micromassage, phonophoresis
    D. Phonophoresis, iontophoresis
    E. High volt electric stimulation, iontophoresis

95. What is a primary indication for cervical traction?
    A. Muscle spasm
    B. Hemorrhage
    C. Muscle weakness
    D. Vertigo
    E. None of the above

96. The athletic trainer of a collegiate women's swimming and diving team suspects one of his athletes might have a severe eating disorder. After lengthy discussions with both the coach and athlete, the athletic trainer decides it would be best for the athlete if she is referred for professional help. To which of the following professionals should the athlete be referred?
    A. An endocrinologist
    B. A chiropractor
    C. A registered dietitian
    D. A registered nurse
    E. A psychologist

97. One of your male athletes notices a tingling sensation in his urethra followed by a discharge of greenish yellow pus from his penis. He is also complaining of pain during urination. You suspect which sexually transmitted disease and recommend which of the following actions?
    A. Syphilis; have the athlete take Zovirax for 7 to 10 days
    B. Trichomoniasis; have the athlete drink acidic fluids, call his family physician, and have the athlete refrain from all sexual contact
    C. Genital candidiasis; have the athlete apply a fungicide to his penis
    D. Gonorrhea; refer the athlete to a physician and have him refrain from all sexual contact
    E. Genital herpes, have the athlete take Diflucan

98. During the rehabilitation of a knee injury, the athletic trainer decides the use of neuromuscular stimulation is indicated. As the athletic trainer is applying the electrodes to the athlete's thigh, the athlete says he has never had electric stimulation and is scared of electricity. Which of the following would be an appropriate response by the athletic trainer?
    A. Tell him he is being childish
    B. Demonstrate how it works
    C. Teach him about the general principles of electric stimulation
    D. Tell a joke about electricity to relax him
    E. Do not use an electrotherapeutic modality on the athlete

99. A cross-country runner comes to you because he would like to begin a strength-training program for general body development. He informs you that he "has never really lifted weights before." How would you instruct him regarding his breathing pattern during a lift?
    A. Have the athlete inhale deeply at the beginning of the lift and then forcefully exhale at the end of the lift
    B. Have the athlete hold his breath during the lift
    C. Have the athlete inhale during the lift and hold his breath at the end of the lift
    D. Have the athlete breathe in, blow out, and breathe in again at the end of the lift
    E. Breathe normally

100. What should the athletic trainer do when teaching an athlete how to properly use crutches?
    A. Make sure the athlete's weight is fully supported on his or her hands and armpits
    B. Caution the athlete not to lean on the crutches so that his or her weight is on the crutches' axillary pads
    C. Teach him or her how to use a cane first
    D. Teach the athlete a four-point gait
    E. Teach the athlete a five-point gait

101. You suspect one of your soccer players is experiencing "training staleness." Which of the following should you assess when developing a counseling approach with the athlete?
    A. The level of the athlete's ability to play the sport
    B. The relationship between the athlete and his family
    C. The athlete's training schedule and diet
    D. The athlete's competition schedule
    E. The relationship between the athlete and coach

102. When rehabilitating an athlete following a ligamentous wrist injury, once the ligament has healed enough where active motion can be initiated, it is important to educate the athlete to exercise only:
    A. Isometrically
    B. In water
    C. While using a prophylactic brace
    D. First thing in the morning
    E. In a pain-free range

103. One of your athletes has been diagnosed with Larsen-Johansson disease. Which of the following is not appropriate when advising the athlete in regard to minimizing his symptoms?
    A. To increase the strength of the vastus medialis obliqus muscle (VMO) with isotonic quadriceps strengthening exercises
    B. Use ice packs frequently to minimize pain and swelling
    C. Avoid stressful activities, such as running, for approximately 6 months
    D. Avoid deep squatting
    E. All of the above

104. When counseling an athlete about the proper way to self-administer a medication, it is important that the athletic trainer make the athlete aware of what two factors?
    A. Any side effects and, in detail, how the drug works on the body
    B. If the drug may be addictive and how long the effects will last
    C. If the drug may cause depression and, in detail, how the drug works on the body
    D. When to take the medication and what foods/drugs not to mix with it
    E. B and C

105. An athlete experiences a catastrophic injury in which she is permanently unable to return to playing the only sport with which she is familiar. What would be the athletic trainer's appropriate response when discussing the injury with the athlete?
    A. Tell her it is not appropriate to deny her condition and that it is best to accept her limitations
    B. Tell her it is OK for her to feel a variety of emotions and to openly express her needs and concerns
    C. Tell her to speak to her coach about her future in athletics
    D. Tell her to seek psychological counseling until she is no longer angry about her injury
    E. Tell her it happens all of the time and eventually she will get used to her situation

106. When advising an athlete about his year-long strength-training program, the athletic trainer should have the athlete limit his heavy lifting workouts to which periods?
    A. In-season and postseason
    B. Preseason and in-season
    C. Postseason and off-season
    D. Off-season and preseason
    E. None of the above

107. A swimmer reports to the athletic training room complaining of symptoms related to Scheuermann's disease. Which type of exercise(s) is beneficial in trying to diminish the symptoms during the early stages of the disease?
    A. Cervical range of motion exercises
    B. Extension and postural exercises
    C. Williams' flexion exercises
    D. Hughston exercises
    E. Deep breathing exercises

108. When rehabilitating an athlete following a lumbar strain, the athletic trainer should emphasize the significance of having the athlete improve the flexibility of all of the following structures except:
    A. The abdominals
    B. The iliopsoas
    C. The paraspinals
    D. The hamstrings
    E. The hip extensors

109. One of your basketball players often complains about localized lumbar "backaches." After performing your evaluation on this athlete, it appears his primary problem is postural. All of the following are actions that the athlete can take to prevent low back pain except:
    A. When standing for long periods of time, rest one foot on a stool if it is available
    B. Avoid sleeping in sidelying position with the knees slightly bent
    C. Carry objects at waist level when possible
    D. Sit on chairs with a firm seat and straight back
    E. Keep his abdominals strong

110. Which of the following individuals should the athletic trainer advise and consult with when developing a reconditioning program for an athlete following a musculoskeletal injury while playing football?
    A. The team physician
    B. The school nurse
    C. The head football coach
    D. The athlete's parents if he is a minor
    E. The team strength and conditioning coach

111. _____ and _____ are important qualities that an athletic trainer must possess when counseling an athlete during a time of distress.
    A. Empathy, humor
    B. Sympathy, pity
    C. Confidence, logic
    D. Objectivity, decisiveness
    E. Logic, detachment

112. If the athlete complains of a burning sensation during an ultrasound treatment, all of the following may be the source of the problem except:
    A. The intensity is too high
    B. Not enough ultrasound medium is being used
    C. Too much ultrasound gel is being used
    D. The movement of the transducer head is too slow
    E. B and D

113. Pain occurring at a site distant to damaged tissue that does not follow the course of a peripheral nerve describes what type of pain?
    A. Muscular
    B. Referred
    C. Radicular
    D. Visceral
    E. Parasympathetic

114. Which of the following is not a contraindication to the use of diathermy?
    A. Acute inflammation and joint effusion
    B. Muscle spasm
    C. Pregnancy
    D. Open wounds
    E. C and D

115. What occurs during a joint mobilization technique when a convex surface moves on a concave surface?
    A. Roll and glide occur in opposite directions
    B. Glide and spin occur in opposite directions
    C. A shearing force occurs at the joint surface
    D. Roll and glide occur in the same direction
    E. Straight glide in same direction

116. Contraindications to cervical traction include all of the following except:
    A. A positive vertebral artery test (VAT)
    B. A positive ALAR ligament test
    C. Disc herniation
    D. Increased radicular symptoms with treatment
    E. Nystagmus

117. Which of the following is a manual technique in which an injured athlete's muscles are actively contracted against a counterforce in a specific position?
    A. Myofascial release
    B. Muscle energy techniques
    C. Joint mobilization
    D. Strain-counterstrain
    E. Multi-angle isokinetics

118. Delayed-onset muscle soreness (DOMS) normally occurs how long after a strenuous exercise session?
    A. 1 hour after exercise
    B. 12 hours after exercise
    C. 24 to 72 hours after exercise
    D. 4 to 6 hours after exercise
    E. Immediately after exercise

119. Physiologic adaptations of the respiratory system during aerobic endurance training include all of the following except:
    A. Reduced submaximal heart rate
    B. Enhanced oxygen exchange within the lungs
    C. Decreased submaximal pulmonary ventilation
    D. Improved circulation throughout the lungs
    E. B and D

120. Which of the following muscles are involved in a seated row exercise?
    I. Latissimus dorsi
    II. Teres minor
    III. Teres major
    IV. Middle trapezius
    V. Rhomboids
    VI. Pectoralis major

    A. I, III, IV, VI
    B. II, III, IV, V
    C. I, IV, V, VI
    D. I, III, IV, V
    E. I, II, III, IV

121. Which of the following muscles are the primary muscles involved when performing a resisted wrist curl (palms up)?
    I. Flexor digitorum longus
    II. Flexor digiti minimi
    III. Adductor pollicis
    IV. Flexor carpi radialis
    V. Flexor carpi ulnaris
    VI. Brachialis

    A. I, II, IV
    B. I, IV, V, VI
    C. II, III, IV, VI
    D. IV, V
    E. III, IV, V

122. Which of the following structures is responsible for relaying information regarding muscle dynamics to the conscious and subconscious parts of the central nervous system?
    A. Muscle spindle
    B. Proprioceptors
    C. Golgi tendon organs
    D. Type III muscle fibers
    E. Brain stem

123. Which of the following is the most effective motivator for compliance to rehabilitation of an athletic injury?
    A. Coercion
    B. Bribery
    C. Fear
    D. Collaboration
    E. Goal setting

124. Which of the following types of exercise can produce a spike in systolic blood pressure that can result in a potentially life-threatening cardiovascular accident?
    A. Isometric
    B. Plyometric
    C. Isotonic
    D. Eccentric
    E. Isokinetic

125. Which of the following is an example of muscle spindle activity?
    A. Nystagmus
    B. Babinski's reflex
    C. Knee-jerk reflex
    D. Moro's reflex
    E. None of the above

126. When the length of a muscle prevents full range of motion at the joint or joints over which the muscle crosses, it is known as what?
    A. Adhesive capsulitis
    B. Passive insufficiency
    C. Hypomobility
    D. Muscle contracture
    E. None of the above

127. All of the following principles must be considered before the athletic trainer begins an activity designed to improve balance except:
    A. Multiple planes of motion must be stressed
    B. The activities must progress to sport-specific activities
    C. The activity should incorporate a unisensory approach
    D. The exercises must be safe but challenging
    E. A and B

128. Which of the following positions must be avoided when rehabilitating an athlete who has posterior instability of the glenohumeral joint?
    A. Abduction with external rotation
    B. Full forward flexion
    C. Internal rotation with horizontal adduction and flexion
    D. Internal rotation with shoulder extension
    E. A and B

129. When developing a functional progression for an athlete who is undergoing a rehabilitation program, all of the following factors need to be considered except:
    A. The physician's expectations for the athlete's return to activity
    B. The athlete's expectations for his or her return to activity
    C. The severity of the athlete's disability
    D. The length of the rehabilitation program
    E. The athlete's position in the sport

130. Upper extremity closed kinetic chain exercises are used primarily for strengthening and improving proprioception of which of the following structures?
    A. Muscles that stabilize the shoulder girdle
    B. Ligaments that stabilize the glenohumeral joint
    C. Tendons that support the joints of the cervical spine, shoulder, and elbow
    D. The articular surfaces of the glenohumeral and acromioclavicular joints
    E. The articular surfaces of the acetabulum and femoral head

131. Hans Selye's phenomenon of the general adaptation syndrome (GAS), which occurs when an individual responds to a stressful situation, includes which three stages of the stress response?
    A. Fright, flight, exhaustion
    B. The alarm stage, resistance stage, exhaustion
    C. The alarm stage, flight stage, acceptance stage
    D. Anger stage, bargaining stage, acceptance stage
    E. The alarm stage, flight, exhaustion

132. What is the temperature range of an ice bath?
    A. 35°F to 50°F
    B. 70°F to 75°F
    C. 65°F to 70°F
    D. 50°F to 60°F
    E. 60°F to 80°F

133. Which of the following actions may help to decrease skin-electrode resistance when performing an electrotherapy treatment?
    A. Moisten the electrodes with water
    B. Cool the skin first with an ice pack
    C. Place the electrodes on skin that has excessive hair
    D. Use a plastic-meshed cloth electrode
    E. Apply body lotion on the skin

134. Which of the following acoustical interfaces is most reflective of ultrasound energy?
    A. Water–soft tissue
    B. Soft tissue–fat
    C. Soft tissue–bone
    D. Soft tissue–air
    E. None of the above

135. Which of the following electrode placement techniques is most commonly used when treating an individual with "brief-intense" TENS?
    A. Direct placement
    B. Dermatome placement
    C. Stimulation point placement
    D. Continuous placement
    E. Bracket method

136. It is important to set specific short- and long-term goals when developing a treatment program. Goals serve all of the following purposes except:
    A. Insure full reimbursement from a third-party payer
    B. Identify outcomes
    C. Measure the effectiveness of the treatment protocol
    D. Establish timeliness of the treatment program
    E. Allows the athlete to be a part of the treatment

137. When using short wave diathermy, which of the following objects should not be located within the treatment area?
    A. Towels
    B. Wooden treatment tables (metal-free)
    C. A container of ultrasound gel
    D. Swiss balls and theraband
    E. Metal stools

138. _____ and _____ are two medications that can be combined when utilizing iontophoresis.
    A. Acetic acid, lidocaine
    B. Dexamethasone, lidocaine
    C. Dexamethasone, epinephrine
    D. Hydrocortisone, Medrol
    E. Antibiotic creams, lidocaine

139. How often should an ultrasound unit be calibrated to ensure the safe application of ultrasound?
    A. Every 3 months
    B. Every month
    C. Every other year
    D. Every 5 years
    E. At least once a year

140. An athlete presents to the athletic training room complaining of a "sore spot" on the back of his neck. It appears as a dark red, hard area, which later develops as a lesion discharging yellowish-red pus from numerous areas. The athletic trainer suspects the athlete has what type of infection?
    A. Viral
    B. Fungal
    C. Systemic
    D. Parasitic
    E. Bacterial

141. Herpes simplex labialis is caused by which of the following?
    A. Virus
    B. Fungus
    C. Bacteria
    D. Parasite
    E. None of the above

142. Pediculosis is most effectively treated with which of the following?
    A. Mouthwash
    B. An antibiotic
    C. Time
    D. An antifungal
    E. A parasiticide

143. Which of the following may occur as a result of a puncture wound that has not been properly treated?
    A. A tetanus infection
    B. A streptococcus infection
    C. A spirochete infection
    D. A staphylococcus infection
    E. Dissemination of the wound

144. How quickly may the adaptations in skeletal muscle reverse if strength training is discontinued or interrupted during rehabilitation?
    A. 24 hours
    B. 36 hours
    C. 48 hours
    D. 1 week
    E. 4 weeks

145. Circuit training is an effective training technique if the athletic trainer desires to improve _____ and _____.
    A. Agility, endurance
    B. Strength, flexibility
    C. Agility, proprioception
    D. Power, endurance
    E. Strength, power

146. The athletic trainer should look for all of the following features when purchasing a stationary bicycle except:
    A. A comfortable seat
    B. An easily modified workload
    C. Good construction
    D. An on-board computer for easy programming
    E. Adjustable to fit all athletes

147. All of the following are contraindications for the use of aquatic therapy except:
    A. An excessive fear of the water
    B. An open wound
    C. An athlete who is unable to tread water
    D. Urinary tract infection
    E. A skin infection

148. Which of the following medications is not a medication that could predispose an athlete to heat illness?
    A. Decongestants
    B. Antihistamines
    C. Diuretics
    D. NSAIDs
    E. Beta-adrenergic blockers

149. How long does it take for an athlete's heart rate to plateau at a given level during a cardiorespiratory training session?
    A. 10 minutes
    B. 30 seconds
    C. 45 seconds
    D. 5 minutes
    E. 2 to 3 minutes

150. What is the efferent response to sensory information called?
    A. Kinesthesia
    B. Neuromuscular control
    C. Proprioception
    D. Coordination
    E. Parathesia

151. What type of fracture fails to heal spontaneously within a normal time frame?
    A. Malunion
    B. Oblique
    C. Osteogenesis
    D. Nonunion
    E. Spiral

152. Which is not a thermal effect of ultrasound?
    A. Increased blood flow
    B. Secretion of chemotactics
    C. Reduction of muscle spasm
    D. Edema reduction
    E. Muscular heating

153. Which of the following modalities results in the movement of ions into the body through the use of an electrical current?
    A. Iontophoresis
    B. Pulsed diathermy
    C. Phonophoresis
    D. Direct coupling
    E. Ultrasound

154. _____ is a method of massage that involves the lifting and kneading of the skin, subcutaneous tissue, and muscle with the fingers or hand.
    A. Friction
    B. Tapotement
    C. Effleurage
    D. Rolfing
    E. Petrissage

155. Which of the following is a cardinal sign of inflammation?
    A. Cyanosis
    B. Loss of function
    C. Cold skin
    D. Numbness
    E. None of the above

156. What is a vascular reaction to cold that results in a white, red, or blue discoloration of the extremities?
    A. Neurapraxia
    B. Analgesia
    C. Raynaud's phenomenon
    D. Hypothermia
    E. Cyanosis

157. All of the following are indications for the use of a warm whirlpool except:
    A. Cleaning large, open wounds
    B. Relieving pain
    C. Initial edema reduction
    D. Increasing range of motion
    E. Reflexation

158. The most common form of hyperthyroidism identified by tremors, weakness, difficulty in swallowing/speaking, and facial/eye tics is known as:
    A. Graves' disease
    B. Legg-Calvé-Perthes disease
    C. Paget's disease
    D. Reye's syndrome
    E. Sarcoidosis

159. What is air hunger marked by labored or difficult breathing called?
    A. Dysuria
    B. Dystrophy
    C. Diaphoresis
    D. Dysphagia
    E. Dyspnea

160. A stretch injury to a nerve resulting in transient symptoms of paresthesia and weakness is known as what?
    A. Neurotmesis
    B. Neurapraxia
    C. Neurofibromatosis
    D. Nerve gliding
    E. Mypraxia

161. All of the following muscles form the pes anserinus muscle group except:
    A. Semimembranosus
    B. Semitendinosus
    C. Gracilis
    D. Sartorius
    E. B and D

162. What is the internal reaction or resistance of tissue to an external load called?
    A. Mechanical failure
    B. Strain
    C. Stress
    D. Yield point
    E. Threshold

163. An involuntary muscle contraction characterized by alternate contraction and relaxation in rapid succession is known as which of the following?
    A. Tonic contraction
    B. Alternating contraction
    C. Eccentric contraction
    D. Clonic contraction
    E. Phasic contraction

164. Which of the following is a term that refers to a group of techniques used for the purpose of relieving soft tissue from the abnormal grip of tight fascia?
    A. Glides
    B. Traction
    C. Myofascial release
    D. Therapeutic massage
    E. Joint mobilization

165. The rate at which a drug disappears from the body through metabolism, excretion, or both is known as which of the following?
    A. Biotransformation
    B. Half-life
    C. Efficacy
    D. Bioavailability
    E. Expiration rate

166. A type of training that employs a series of stations that consist of various combinations of weight training, flexibility, calisthenics, and brief aerobic exercise is known as which of the following?
    A. Isokinetic training
    B. Circuit training
    C. Plyometrics
    D. Progressive resistance exercises
    E. Specificity training

167. Diaphoresis is also known as which of the following?
    A. Rapid heart beat
    B. Body odor
    C. Bad breath
    D. Slow heart beat
    E. Sweating

168. Joint mechanoreceptors are found in all of the following structures except:
   A. Ligaments
   B. The brain
   C. Menisci
   D. Fat pads
   E. Musculotendinous junction

169. Cognitive function may be affected by all of the following conditions except:
   A. Dehydration
   B. Malnutrition
   C. Abnormal body temperature
   D. Depression
   E. Medication

170. Polydipsia is also known as which of the following?
   A. Excessive urination
   B. Excessive hunger
   C. Excessive blood glucose
   D. Low urine pH
   E. Excessive thirst

171. The progression for strengthening exercises is usually in what order?
   A. Isometric, isokinetic, isotonic, plyometric
   B. Isokinetic, isometric, plyometric, isotonic
   C. Isotonic, plyometric, isokinetic, isometric
   D. Isometric, isotonic, isokinetic, plyometric
   E. Plyometric, isometric, isotonic, isokinetic

172. Isotonic external rotation of the glenohumeral joint during shoulder rehabilitation focuses on what muscles?
   A. Infraspinatus
   B. Teres minor
   C. Posterior deltoid
   D. All of the above
   E. None of the above

173. Injury or disease of the pancreas creates pain in which quadrant of the abdomen?
   A. Lower right quadrant
   B. Upper right quadrant
   C. Upper left quadrant
   D. Lower left quadrant
   E. Central quadrant

174. Where is a Morton's neuroma most commonly located?
   A. Between the first and second metacarpals
   B. Between the third and fourth metatarsals
   C. Between the second and third metacarpals
   D. Between the second and third metatarsals
   E. Plantar surface of the heel

175. An excessive valgus force to the knee may result in an injury to which ligament?
   A. Lateral collateral ligament (LCL)
   B. Medial collateral ligament (MCL)
   C. Anterior cruciate ligament (ACL)
   D. Posterior cruciate ligament (PCL)
   E. Arcuate ligament

176. The female athletic triad describes the simultaneous presence of which of the following?
   A. An eating disorder, amenorrhea, and osteoporosis
   B. Depression, premenstrual syndrome (PMS), and osteoporosis
   C. An MCL, ACL sprain with meniscus tear
   D. Menstrual cramping, overeating, and PMS
   E. Dysmenorrhea, eating disorder, and osteoporosis

177. All of the following are tests for glenohumeral instability except:
   A. Clunk test
   B. Anterior apprehension
   C. Anterior glide
   D. Load and shift
   E. Neer's test

178. Which of the following involves the use of ice or a cold spray before performing a stretch?
   A. Cryokinetics
   B. Cryostretch
   C. Cold therapy stretching
   D. Dynamic stretching
   E. Cryogenics

179. Indications for ultrasound include all of the following except:
   A. Bursitis
   B. Fasciitis
   C. Acute hemorrhage
   D. Plantar warts
   E. Tendinitis

180. Which of the following are braces used after rehabilitation?
   A. Functional
   B. Prophylactic
   C. Patellofemoral
   D. Rehabilitative
   E. Postoperative

181. _____is a type of electrotherapy used to re-educate muscle.
    A. Interferential
    B. Russian
    C. Iontophoresis
    D. Premodulated
    E. Low intensity

182. What is a protective spasm of the muscular abdominal wall called?
    A. Gas pains
    B. Rigidity
    C. Myositis
    D. Splinting
    E. Very painful

183. What does the production of black, tar-like stools indicate?
    A. Upper gastrointestinal (GI) bleeding
    B. Infection
    C. Lower GI bleeding
    D. A diet that is too high in iron
    E. Colon cancer

184. Which of the following devices is more effective in decreasing skin temperature during a cryotherapy treatment?
    A. A microwaveable pack
    B. A chemical spray
    C. A cold towel
    D. An ice pack
    E. A fan

185. A dry, nonproductive cough is most often caused by which of the following?
    A. Lung infection
    B. Bronchitis
    C. Allergies
    D. Pneumothorax
    E. Cancer

186. A dynamic program of prescribed exercise for preventing or reversing the destructive effects of inactivity while returning an individual to his or her former level of competition is known as what?
    A. Pilates'
    B. Rehabilitation
    C. A DAPRE program
    D. Cardiovascular program
    E. Yoga

187. What is an upward force experienced by a body in a fluid that acts in the opposite direction of gravity and is responsible for the feeling of weightlessness in water?
    A. Specific gravity
    B. Viscosity
    C. Hydrostatic pressure
    D. Buoyancy
    E. None of the above

188. Electrical stimulating currents are classified into three categories. Which of the following is not one of these categories?
    A. Interferential current
    B. Direct current
    C. Pulsed current
    D. Alternating current
    E. Galvanic current

189. All of the following are contraindications for electrical stimulation electrode placement except:
    A. Stimulation across the heart
    B. Stimulation over an acute thrombophlebitis
    C. Control of labor pain by stimulation of the lower back
    D. Stimulation over the temples
    E. Directly over the spine

190. "Like charges repel while unlike charges attract each other." This is known as what law?
    A. Ohm's
    B. Coulomb's
    C. Murphy's
    D. Wolff's
    E. Horner's

191. All of the following are indications of ice massage application except:
    A. Subacute injuries
    B. Contusions
    C. Anesthetized skin
    D. Muscle spasm
    E. Overuse injuries

192. Which of the following types of electrical stimulators is considered "subsensory?"
    A. Interferential stimulator
    B. Low intensity stimulator
    C. TENS
    D. Diathermy
    E. High intensity stimulator

193. Which of the following is defined as an uninterrupted direct current?
    A. Interferential current
    B. Microcurrent
    C. Galvanic current
    D. Pulsed current
    E. None of the above

194. The amount of power generated by an ultrasound unit is defined as what?
    A. Frequency
    B. Duty cycle
    C. Duration
    D. Intensity
    E. An ohm

195. When using fluidotherapy, the treatment temperature range is normally set at which of the following temperatures?
    A. 60°F to 70°F
    B. 85°F to 100°F
    C. 100°F to 113°F
    D. 75°F to 96°F
    E. 40°F to 60°F

196. The D2 flexion pattern of the hip works which group of muscles?
    A. Abductors, flexors, internal rotators
    B. Abductors, flexors, external rotators
    C. Adductors, flexors, internal rotators
    D. Adductors, extensors, external rotators
    E. The abductors and flexors only

197. Strengthening of which muscle is vital in the throwing athlete?
    A. Lower trapezius
    B. Pectineus
    C. Serratus posterior
    D. Obliques
    E. Rhomboids

198. Treatment for facet dysfunction consists of all of the following except:
    A. Facet joint mobilization
    B. Passive rotation
    C. Pelvic rock exercises
    D. McKenzie extension exercises
    E. Abdominal strengthening

199. Which muscle does not need to be strengthened after a rotator cuff repair?
    A. Supraspinatus
    B. Biceps
    C. Teres minor
    D. Sternocleidomastoid
    E. Triceps

200. When a muscle is stretched to a point where a mild discomfort is felt and the limb is held in one position, it is known as what type of stretch?
    A. Ballistic
    B. PNF
    C. Static
    D. Dynamic
    E. None of the above

201. What is a form of exercise that helps develop eccentric control during dynamic movements?
    A. Isometric
    B. PNF
    C. Hydraulic training
    D. Isokinetics
    E. Plyometric

202. An athlete presents with an acute injury of the foot and has an antalgic gait pattern. Which of the following should you do first?
    A. Have the athlete run half speed on a treadmill for cardiorespiratory health
    B. Give the athlete crutches
    C. Instruct the athlete in a heel-to-toe gait pattern
    D. Observe/palpate the injured area for gross deformity and point tenderness
    E. Have the athlete wear an open toe shoe

203. The athletic trainer should perform which of the following tests for PCL laxity?
    A. Apley's distraction test
    B. Jerk test
    C. Apley's compression test
    D. Pivot shift test
    E. Posterior drawer test

204. When palpating the knee joint after an injury, the athletic trainer should be sure to palpate which of the following structures?
    A. Anterior superior iliac spine
    B. The navicular
    C. Medial condyle of the femur
    D. The tibial crest
    E. Dorsalis pedis

205. An athlete presents with insidious pain along the posterior aspect of the thigh. Which of the following steps should be performed first by the athletic trainer?
    A. Palpate the muscle bellies of the posterior thigh
    B. Ask how and when the pain started
    C. Manual muscle test the hamstring muscles
    D. Perform a functional test
    E. Assess sensation of the hip

206. Articular cartilage has limited ability to heal because of which of the following reasons?
    A. Constant movement of the joint does not allow for healing
    B. Cartilage has limited or no direct blood supply
    C. The high incidence of aseptic necrosis
    D. Poor results with NSAID treatment
    E. None of the above

207. Which of the following is the least occurring type of shoulder subluxation/dislocation?
    A. Superior
    B. Inferior
    C. Anterior
    D. Posterior
    E. C and D

Organization and Administration

1. All of the following forms are critical parts of the athlete's permanent medical record and should be completed before the athlete is permitted to participate in the first team practice except:
    A. Permission-to-treat form
    B. Preparticipation physical examination form
    C. Release form for athletes subjected to high risk
    D. Coach's injury report form
    E. Medical history form

2. How would you define a policy?
    A. A specific plan for members of an organization to follow
    B. A broad statement of an intended action
    C. An organizational plan that provides program direction for 1 or 2 years
    D. A mission statement of an organization
    E. A vision statement of an organization

3. The floor of an athletic training room can be comprised of all the following materials except:
    A. Vinyl
    B. Ceramic tile
    C. Concrete
    D. Rubber
    E. Wood

4. Maintaining up-to-date records is extremely important. How often should the athletic trainer document?
    A. Monthly
    B. Weekly
    C. Daily
    D. Every 6 months
    E. Every two weeks

5. An athletic trainer can release an athlete's medical records to which of the following?
    A. Professional athletic team organizations
    B. Insurance companies
    C. The media
    D. No organization or individual without the consent of the athlete or legal guardian
    E. B and C

6. A high school athlete is pitching during a baseball game and is hit in the head with a line drive. He is seriously injured. The assistant coach is also the athlete's father. In this situation, who is legally responsible for the athlete's immediate care?
    A. The head coach
    B. The assistant coach/parent
    C. The athletic trainer
    D. The high school at which the event is taking place
    E. All of the above

7. _____ is a form of record keeping that allows the athletic trainer to list the athlete's injury information, the actions taken by the athletic trainer, and the response of the athlete to the athletic trainer's treatment in column form.
    A. SOAP notes
    B. Focus charting
    C. Charting by exception
    D. Computerized documentation
    E. WOTS UP

8. You have been given the opportunity to assist in hiring a new team physician. What type of agreement should be drawn up between the school and the physician?
    A. School emergency systems agreement
    B. A noncompete agreement
    C. A medical consent agreement
    D. A physician's letter of agreement
    E. Liability contract agreement

9. Which of the following best describes an athletic trainer in a nontraditional athletic training setting?
    A. Controller
    B. Organizer
    C. Director
    D. Planner
    E. Manager

10. You are employed at a local high school as an athletic trainer and have been asked by your principal to refer any ill students to your school nurse. Who is responsible for the care of the student athletes in this situation?
    A. School nurse
    B. School physician
    C. Athletic trainer
    D. School principal
    E. B and D

11. What guidelines does the athletic trainer have to follow regarding maintaining proper hygiene and sanitation in the athletic training room?
    A. Joint Commission on Accreditation of Healthcare Organizations (JCAHO)
    B. American Medical Association (AMA)
    C. Rehabilitation Accreditation Commission (CARF)
    D. Occupational Safety and Health Administration (OSHA)
    E. Commission of the Accreditation of Athletic Training Education (CAATE)

12. Which of the following organizations establishes standards of quality for organizations that provide rehabilitative services?
    A. JCAHO
    B. AMA
    C. APTA
    D. OSHA
    E. CARF

13. All of the following are components of a well-written SOAP note except:
    A. It is legible, clear, and concise
    B. It contains many objective measurements
    C. Progress is expressed in functional terms
    D. It is written with the intent to mislead an insurance company
    E. It describes a clear plan of treatment

14. Which of the following documents would be most likely subpoenaed during a civil litigation suit against an athletic trainer?
    A. Equipment inventory
    B. Treatment log
    C. Budget reports
    D. Sporting event schedules
    E. Proof of ATC credentials and certifications

15. Fixed payments made on a monthly basis to a managed care provider are known as what type of reimbursement?
    A. Point-of-service plan
    B. Fee for service
    C. Third-party reimbursement
    D. Capitation
    E. Managed Care Option

16. Which of the following forms should the athletic trainer fill out to gain the quickest reimbursement from an insurance company?
    A. HCFA-1500 form
    B. CPT 1-A form
    C. UCR form
    D. An incident report form
    E. None of the above

17. The athletic trainer may use any of the following to treat an injured or ill athlete except:
    A. Prescription drug
    B. Hydrotherapy
    C. Cryotherapy
    D. Electrotherapy
    E. Massage

18. Maintaining accurate medical records is the responsibility of which of the following individuals in the high school setting?
    I. Athletic trainer
    II. Athletic director
    III. Principal
    IV. School nurse
    V. Team physician

    A. I, II, III
    B. II, IV, V
    C. III, IV, V
    D. I, IV, V
    E. All of the above

19. What type of analysis would be considered a useful tool in the strategic planning of an existing athletic training program?
    A. The HICFA analysis
    B. The strengths/weaknesses analysis
    C. The WOTS-UP analysis
    D. The Samson analysis
    E. Flow chart analysis

20. What is the primary care physician who is appointed by an insurance company to oversee the medical care given to an athlete and assigns any specialty and ancillary services called?
    A. The gatekeeper
    B. The participating provider
    C. The third-party administrator
    D. The policy holder
    E. None of the above

21. The _____ is a charge that represents the maximum amount that an insurance company will pay a provider.
    A. HCFA
    B. NCR
    C. ADA
    D. CPT
    E. UCR

22. The _____ is a nongovernmental, nonprofit organization that gathers injury data from a number of sources including educational institutions.
    A. National Safety Council
    B. NOCSAE
    C. ACSM
    D. OSHA
    E. ISS

23. Which organization must certify face masks that are used in ice hockey helmets?
    A. Canadian Standard Association (CSA)
    B. Hockey Equipment Certification Council (HECC)
    C. NOCSAE
    D. ASTM
    E. NCAA

24. _____ supplies include such items as adhesive tape, gauze pads, and bandages.
    A. Permanent
    B. Capital
    C. Nonexpendable
    D. Nonfixed
    E. Expendable

25. _____, _____, and _____ must be taken into consideration when developing a risk management plan.
    A. Security, liability, competence
    B. Security, fire safety, management of emergency injuries
    C. Insurance procedures, policies/procedures, materials
    D. Licensing, certifications, administrative policy
    E. Employees, liability, security

26. Large purchases for an educational institution are usually done through a process known as what?
    A. Direct purchase
    B. Indirect purchase
    C. Soliciting
    D. Bid process
    E. None of the above

27. Which of the following best describes a copayment?
    A. An occasional payment made by a policy holder to an insurance company
    B. The amount owed yearly by the policy holder before the insurance company will begin to pay for services
    C. The amount of money that both an employee and employer share when paying for medical benefits
    D. A percentage of the total amount the policy holder is required to pay for medical services rendered
    E. The amount of money that a provider offers as a discount for services

28. You are in the position to hire an assistant athletic trainer. You have a specific person in mind, but your athletic director implies he is not comfortable with this person's gender. Which level of the law mandates the hiring and firing of employees?
    A. State
    B. Local
    C. City
    D. District
    E. Federal

29. Which piece of information is not part of the athletic trainer's daily documentation?
    A. Treatment technique
    B. Playing status
    C. Daily injury log
    D. Athlete's insurance information
    E. Objective information

30. All of the following are important steps in avoiding legal problems when administering care to the athlete except:
    A. Keeping accurate records
    B. Staying familiar with the health history of the athlete
    C. Following orders of the team physician
    D. Allowing the coach to decide when the athlete should return to play after injury
    E. B and C

31. Which of the following is not a responsibility of the athletic trainer?
    A. Counsel and advise the athlete about health care
    B. Diagnose and treat illnesses
    C. Administer first aid as necessary
    D. Supervise proper equipment fitting
    E. Organize and set-up pre-participation physical exams

32. Which of the following is not characteristic of a managed care organization?
    A. They require provider accountability
    B. They promote the use of a physician as a "gatekeeper"
    C. They are based on a fee-for-service model
    D. They utilize various strategies
    E. They utilize specific providers

33. All of the following are reasons why an insurance claim might be denied except:
    A. Lack of patient progress
    B. The duration of care is considered excessive
    C. Improper coding
    D. The goals are based on functional outcomes
    E. Treating beyond the approved number of visits

34. What is the series of codes used by insurance agencies and providers alike to identify a patient's diagnosis for reimbursement purposes called?
    A. International classification of diseases or ICD-9 codes
    B. Interclinician codes of diagnoses or ICD-5 codes
    C. Third-party payer codes
    D. International procedure and diagnoses code or IPD-9 codes
    E. None of the above

35. All of the following are reasons why good documentation skills are an absolute necessity for the athletic trainer except:
    A. To protect the legal rights of the athlete and athletic trainer
    B. To improve the communication between the athletic trainer and other health care providers
    C. To enhance the care given by the athletic trainer and to determine when release from the athletic trainer's immediate care is appropriate
    D. To improve the athletic trainer's position for financial gain through reimbursement by the insurance company
    E. To keep an accurate log of treatment as a means of evaluating successful outcomes

36. You are part of a planning committee that has been given the responsibility of designing the new athletic training room at your school. You have been through the initial process of conducting a needs assessment and selecting an architect/contractor. You now are meeting with the architect to begin the development of the schematic drawings that will be submitted for approval. _____ and _____ are two major elements that must be addressed in these schematic drawings.
    A. Plumbing, electrical layouts
    B. Space needs, traffic patterns
    C. Field access, escape routes
    D. Aesthetics, large equipment positioning
    E. Color, furniture location

37. When acquiring capital equipment for your athletic training room, a decision must be made regarding leasing or purchasing the equipment. What might be a possible advantage in leasing the equipment?
    A. Less risk that the equipment will become obsolete
    B. Lower overall cost
    C. Outright ownership of the equipment
    D. Purchased equipment has little resale value
    E. All of the above

38. As the director of a free-standing sports medicine clinic, it is important to keep accurate records of an employee's personnel record. All of the following should be included in this file except:
    A. Performance evaluation records
    B. Salary and promotion records
    C. Time-off request sheets
    D. Employee contracts
    E. B and D

39. In athletic training, database software has been primarily used to perform what function?
    A. Write letters and produce forms
    B. Perform simple calculations and integrate text with graphics
    C. Store and retrieve information regarding athletic injury and treatment
    D. Merge lists and develop spread sheets
    E. All of the above

40. Which of the following describes an insurance "rider?"
    A. A supplementary clause to an insurance contract that covers the cost of conditions that extend beyond those associated with the standard policy
    B. The usual fee charged by a health care provider for a particular service
    C. A policy that pays for medical expenses only after all of the athlete's other medical insurance policies have reached their limit
    D. A universally accepted insurance claim form used by hospitals
    E. None of the above

41. All of the following are methods of enhancing a budget plan except:
    A. Keep an accurate inventory on all disposable and nondisposable supplies
    B. Figure out how much of your disposable supplies have been used and estimate how much more will be needed to finish out the fiscal year
    C. Consult with a certified public accountant (CPA) or professional financial advisor and follow his or her direction regarding the development of a budget plan
    D. Consult with several vendors to get an estimate of how much prices will rise in the upcoming year
    E. Determine how many athletes will be receiving care

42. When developing an emergency plan, all of the following should be established except:
    A. The athletic trainer and coaches should have the appropriate keys to important gates and locks
    B. There should be a phone accessible for immediate use
    C. The athletic trainer should be familiar with the community emergency medical system
    D. Who will accompany the injured athlete to the hospital, if necessary
    E. A and C

43. Which of the following is a prudent action that the athletic trainer should take prior to an emergency arising?
    A. The athletic trainer should arrange a meeting between him- or herself, the local rescue squad, team physician, and any other individual involved in handling an injured athlete at least once a year to establish and practice procedures that will be used in the event of an emergency
    B. Make sure all the golf carts are fully charged and ready to roll
    C. Make sure the athletic director and school nurse are on campus
    D. Know all of the emergency routes of the campus and have directions to the nearest hospital
    E. B and D

44. Which of the following is the biggest budgetary obstacle that many high school athletic trainers must face?
    A. Lack of a room and special facilities/equipment necessary to operate an adequate athletic training program
    B. Lack of athletic tape and wraps, athletic training kits, and a table
    C. Location of the athletic training room
    D. Lack of a student athletic trainers' program, which would provide the certified athletic trainer with free help
    E. Lack of a budget plan

45. There are different models of supervision that may be used by a head athletic trainer when managing an athletic training staff. Two of these models are known as _____ and _____ supervision.
    A. Monarchial, sovereign
    B. Clinical, directional
    C. Transitional, directional
    D. Inspection-production, administrative
    E. Clinical, developmental

46. Which of the following is not one of the three phases of the needs assessment as it is related to budget planning?
    A. Exploration
    B. Information gathering
    C. Negotiation
    D. Decision making
    E. A and B

47. What is the process in which health care practitioners are reimbursed by a policyholder's insurance?
    A. Primary-party reimbursement
    B. Secondary-party reimbursement
    C. Third-party reimbursement
    D. Tertiary-party reimbursement
    E. Direct reimbursement

48. Which of the following is a growing concept in the insurance industry stressing cost control through coordination of medical services?
    A. A primary care provider
    B. Health maintenance organization (HMO)
    C. Exclusive provider organization (EPO)
    D. Preferred provider organization (PPO)
    E. Managed care

49. Which of the following is not an error when planning the design of a sports medicine facility?
    A. Concentrating on function rather than style
    B. The use of wood for the main flooring material
    C. Having the adaptive access on the other side of the building
    D. Non-ground-fault interrupter (GFI) receptacles placed within the hydrotherapy area
    E. Having only one entrance and exit

50. Which of the following is not a type of insurance policy that is offered to organizations seeking to purchase insurance for athletic teams?
    A. Accident insurance
    B. Indemnity policy
    C. Basic medical coverage
    D. Group insurance
    E. Capitation

51. What is one of the most important steps an athletic trainer needs to take when starting a new high school athletic training program?
    A. Make an emergency plan
    B. Make sure there is enough tape and first-aid kits
    C. Have uniforms made for the athletic training staff so they may be identified by the coaches
    D. Meet with the school's booster clubs to begin fund-raising
    E. Network with local physical therapists

52. Which of the following is a priority when developing a sports medicine center for the local community?
    A. An area for massage therapy
    B. A mission statement
    C. An open house
    D. An educational seminar for coaches
    E. All of the above

53. The codes that were established by the AMA for healthcare providers to receive third-party reimbursement are CPT codes. What does CPT mean?
    A. Current procedural treatments
    B. Current provider terminology
    C. Consensus procedural treatments
    D. Current provider treatments
    E. Current procedural terminology

54. What is a type of organizational culture characterized by autonomy in decision making and problem solving?
    A. Organizational culture
    B. Collegial culture
    C. Personalistic culture
    D. Informal culture
    E. Independent culture

55. All of the following are basic steps in the purchasing process except:
    A. Request a quotation
    B. Negotiation
    C. Purchase order
    D. Bid requests
    E. Quality control

56. Which of the following is not a type of managed care organization?
    A. HMO
    B. Point-of-service
    C. Exclusive provider organization
    D. Third-party organization
    E. Preferred provider organization

57. When developing preparticipation physical examination forms, it is important to make sure all athletes have all of the following included in their medical folders except:
    A. Treatment consent form signed by their parents if the athlete is 18 years of age or older
    B. History of any previous conditions documented
    C. Documentation of medications being taken
    D. Assumption-of-risk forms
    E. C and D

58. In developing your emergency action plan, who should make all of the decisions about transporting an athlete?
    A. Athletic trainer
    B. Team physician
    C. Athletic director
    D. School nurse
    E. Paramedics

59. What is the state law that gives an individual the length of time (in years) to file a claim?
    A. Foreseeable harm
    B. Liability negligence
    C. Statute of limitations
    D. Tort
    E. Statute of suitability

60. If an athlete, who is covered by an HMO insurance policy, needs to see a specialist, who must make the referral in most cases?
    A. Athletic trainer
    B. The specialist
    C. Primary care physician
    D. Athlete
    E. None of the above

61. According to program management theory, which of the following is defined as a decision-making process in which a course of action is determined in order to bring about a future state of affairs?
    A. Vision statement
    B. Mission statement
    C. Planning
    D. Program evaluation
    E. Implementation evaluation

62. Which of the following describes a person or organization that supports a program but has a history of untrusting behavior (these people tend to be manipulative in their dealings)?
    A. Opponents
    B. Challengers
    C. Allies
    D. Adversaries
    E. Bedfellows

63. The process by which something is done in a sports medicine program is defined as a(n) _____.
    A. Procedure
    B. Policy
    C. Agreement
    D. Chain of command
    E. Protocol

64. What are cost-based providers contracted by the federal government and charged with reviewing Medicare claims made by hospitals called?
    A. An intermediary
    B. An insurance "carrier"
    C. A joint review board
    D. An insurance network
    E. Business manager

65. What is the potential to influence the behavior of a superior called?
    A. Superior power
    B. Position power
    C. Counter power
    D. Subordination power
    E. Personal power

66. Which of the following is not a type of budget?
    A. Fixed budgeting
    B. Variable budgeting
    C. Laissez-faire budgeting
    D. Lump-sum budgeting
    E. Line item budgeting

67. Primary coverage is defined as which of the following?
    A. "Self-pay" insurance
    B. A coverage that begins to pay for covered expenses after the deductible has been met
    C. Protection for an individual against future loss of earnings because of injury
    D. The invoiced cost of an insurance policy
    E. Third party payment

68. Medical records are defined as which of the following?
    A. Cumulative documentation of a person's medical history and health care interventions
    B. Widely accepted principles that are intended to guide the professional activities of the health care practitioner
    C. The act of recording health care assessments or treatment on cassette tapes or directly into a computer for later transcription
    D. A method of recording details of an athlete's assessment and treatment using a detailed prose-based format
    E. All of the above

69. Which of the following is not part of a SOAP note?
    A. Subjective information
    B. Objective information
    C. Assessment
    D. Participation level
    E. Plan

70. All of the following are ways athletic trainers can help keep insurance premiums to a minimum except:
    A. Insist that the athletes purchase their own personal insurance
    B. Adopt and communicate policies that increase the institution's financial obligations to those injuries that are covered by the school's insurance policy
    C. Spread the risk among all concerned parties
    D. Pass the cost or some fraction of the cost to the athlete
    E. Have the team physician see athletes in the athletic training room

71. Which of the following is a contract between a policyholder and an insurance company to reimburse a percentage of the cost of the policyholder's medical bills?
    A. An insurance "claim"
    B. Point-of-service insurance
    C. A promissory note
    D. Medical insurance
    E. Treatment agreement

72. All of the following are exceptions to the rule of confidentiality except:
    A. When the media desires information regarding the athlete's health status
    B. When there is clear and imminent danger to the athlete
    C. When there is clear and imminent danger to other persons
    D. When legal requirements demand that confidential information be released
    E. C and D

73. Athletic training equipment can be either leased or bought. Which of the following is an advantage to leasing equipment?
    A. Higher overall cost
    B. No ownership
    C. Lower initial cost
    D. Higher effective interest rate than traditional financing
    E. None of the above

74. Which of the following is a type of organizational culture characterized by consensus, teamwork, and participatory decision making?
    A. Transformational
    B. Personalistic
    C. Formulistic
    D. Organizational
    E. Collegial

75. Which of the following is the correct order for the steps in recruiting and hiring sports medicine personnel?
    A. Request for position, application collection, position request approval
    B. Application collection, position vacancy notice, offer of contract
    C. Request for position, telephone interviews, hiring
    D. Hiring, offer of contract, request for position
    E. Application collection, interview, request position

76. Which of the following is a method that allocates a fixed amount of money for an entire program without specifying how the money will be spent?
    A. Lump-sum budgeting
    B. Request for quotation
    C. Lump-sum bidding
    D. Line-item budgeting
    E. Need-based budgeting

77. Which type of budgeting model requires justification for every budget line item without reference to previous spending patterns?
    A. Fixed
    B. Variable
    C. Zero-based
    D. Performance
    E. Need-based budgeting

78. What is a type of tort in which an athletic trainer fails to act as a reasonably prudent athletic trainer would act under the same circumstances?
    A. Breach of contract
    B. Omission
    C. Abandonment
    D. Negligence
    E. Foreseeable harm

79. Which of the following standards are performance evaluation standards intended to help foster practicality in the employee appraisal process?
    A. Accuracy standards
    B. Feasibility standards
    C. Utility standards
    D. Propriety standards
    E. Quality standards

80. You were just given permission to hire a new staff athletic trainer. What order should these components follow when conducting staff selection activities?
    I. Retention
    II. Hiring
    III. Promotion
    IV. Performance evaluation
    V. Demotion

    A. III, V, IV, II, I
    B. II, III, I, IV, V
    C. I, II, III, IV, V
    D. IV, I, V, III, II
    E. I, II, IV, V, III

81. Which one of these is not a step for recruiting and hiring sports medicine personnel?
    A. Placing a position vacancy notice on the NATA Placement Vacancy Notices
    B. Interviewing
    C. Creating program goals
    D. Hiring a head athletic trainer
    E. All of the above are steps for recruiting and hiring staff

82. An "operational plan" is a plan that defines organizational activities in the short-term and should be no longer than which of the following?
    A. 10 years
    B. 15 years
    C. 25 years
    D. 7 years
    E. 2 years

83. The equal employment operating chief works with employees who have filed what type(s) of complaint?
    A. Discrimination
    B. Sexual harassment
    C. Racism
    D. All of the above
    E. None of the above

84. An athlete with a disability should not be discriminated against, but he or she must have documentation that supports his or her condition. How can he or she justify the disability?
    A. He or she tells you about the condition
    B. He or she has a record of such impairment with medical documentation
    C. He or she has trouble performing in class or in the sport
    D. All of the above
    E. None of the above

85. You are beginning to lay the foundation for your new athletic training room at North High School. In order to expedite the process and cut down on the amount of individuals you must deal with you have decided to use one of the following construction process models. Which of the following uses only one firm to both design and construct the new building?
    A. Lump-sum bidding model
    B. Construction development model
    C. Design/build model
    D. Contractor supply model
    E. None of the above

86. Which of the following would help an athletic trainer determine space needs when planning to build a sports medicine center?
    A. Enlisting the help of a doctor who is in private practice
    B. Developing a traffic pattern chart
    C. Buying the equipment first and then determining space needs
    D. Performing site visits at various gyms to get ideas
    E. All of the above

87. Which of the following methods for funding public sector sports medicine facilities utilizes an institution's assets in cash and investments not normally used for operational purposes?
    A. Capital campaign
    B. Tax exempt bonds
    C. An endowment
    D. Commercial loans
    E. Unrestricted loans

88. Which of the following is covered in a "rider" in an athletic accident insurance policy?
    A. Acute traumatic injuries
    B. Chronic overuse injuries
    C. Long-term permanent disabilities
    D. None of the above
    E. All of the above

89. Catastrophic insurance usually begins coverage after the first _____ of medical bills have been reached.
    A. $5000
    B. $15,000
    C. $100,000
    D. $50,000
    E. $25,000

90. What is a type of athletic insurance that pays for covered medical expenses only after all other insurance policies have reached their limits?
    A. Self
    B. Primary coverage
    C. Secondary coverage
    D. Catastrophic
    E. Liability coverage

91. What organization publishes CPT codes on an annual basis?
    A. AMA
    B. NATA
    C. Commission on Accreditation of Allied Health Education Programs (CAAHEP)
    D. BOC
    E. None of the above

92. What would be included in the capital expenses of an athletic training program?
    A. Staff salaries
    B. Equipment under $500
    C. Athletic training supplies
    D. Buildings and room construction
    E. All of the above

93. A properly organized athletic training room should have separate, designated areas for all the following except:
    A. Modality area
    B. Hydrotherapy area
    C. Storage facilities
    D. Changing room for the athletes
    E. Physician treatment

94. What is a practical, effective size for most school athletic training rooms?
    A. 900 sq ft
    B. 1000 to 1200 sq ft
    C. 2000 to 3000 sq ft
    D. 800 to 1000 sq ft
    E. 500 to 800 sq ft

95. How high should the electrical outlets be placed above the floor in the athletic training room?
    A. 2 to 3 ft
    B. 4 to 5 ft
    C. 6 ft
    D. 1 to 2 ft
    E. None of the above

96. Which of the following could present a problem for the athletic trainer when using a computer to store medical records?
    A. Maintaining security
    B. Retrieving specific information
    C. Loading files
    D. Using email
    E. All of the above

97. How far from the nose should the face mask of a football helmet be located?
    A. 1 inch
    B. Two finger widths
    C. Three finger widths
    D. 0.75 inch
    E. 3 inches

98. Thermomoldable plastics, such as Orthoplast or Aquaplast, may be indicated for many different situations. Which of the following conditions might benefit from the use of this type of material?
    A. Genu recurvatum
    B. Thoracic outlet syndrome
    C. Quadriceps contusion
    D. Anterior cruciate sprain
    E. Genu varum

99. Which organization has identified the domains of athletic training as defined by the Role Delineation Study?
    A. AMA
    B. American Physical Therapy Association (APTA)
    C. BOC
    D. NATA Ethics Committee
    E. CAATE

100. Which of the following pieces of information are important for the athletic trainer to keep on record in the athletic training room?
    A. Injury reports
    B. Injury evaluations and progress notes
    C. Daily treatment logs
    D. All of the above
    E. None of the above

101. Which type of budget allocates a fixed amount of money for specific program functions and activities?
    A. Lump-sum budgeting
    B. Fixed budgeting
    C. Need-based budgeting
    D. Variable budgeting
    E. Line-item budget

102. Which of the following is the most restrictive form of regulation for the profession of athletic training?
    A. Exemption
    B. Certification
    C. Registration
    D. Licensure
    E. Reciprocity

103. To be a successful athletic trainer, an individual must possess all of the following personal qualities except:
    A. The ability to adapt to a changing environment
    B. A good sense of humor
    C. An interest in making money
    D. Empathy
    E. B and D

104. Which of the following best describes the function of the school nurse in the sports medicine program of a high school?
    A. As a liaison between the athletic director and the athletic trainer
    B. The direct supervisor of the "health" services
    C. As the "first assistant" to the team physician
    D. As a liaison between the athletic trainer and the school health services
    E. All of the above

105. Which of the following organizations was established in 1950 and created a code of ethics and standards for the profession of athletic training?
    A. American Orthopaedic Society for Sports Medicine
    B. American College of Sports Medicine
    C. American Physical Therapy Association
    D. National Athletic Trainers' Association
    E. National Academy of Sports Medicine

Professional Development and Responsibility

1. You find out that a certified athletic trainer in your conference is selling an herbal substance to his athletes on a regular basis for personal profit. Which of the following codes is this individual violating?
    A. APTA *Code of Honor*
    B. NASM *Code of Ethics*
    C. NCAA *Code of Honor*
    D. ACSM *Code of Medicine*
    E. NATA *Code of Ethics*

2. When explaining to a parent the difference between an athletic trainer and a physical therapist, the expertise of a physical therapist might best be described by which of the following?
    A. Expertise in the rehabilitation of the handicapped individual
    B. Those health care professionals trained in the rehabilitation of orthopedic injuries
    C. Those individuals trained in the rehabilitation of a diverse population
    D. Expertise in the rehabilitation of athletic, geriatric, and neurologically impaired populations
    E. None of the above

3. Over the past 6 months, you notice one of the athletic trainers on your staff exhibiting some behaviors that are out of character for that individual. You recognize these behaviors as signs of "burnout." Which of the following are signs of job burnout?
    I.   Insomnia
    II. Angry behavior
    III. Manic behavior
    IV. Self-preoccupation
    V.   Attentiveness
    VI. Daily feelings of exhaustion

    A. I, II, IV, VI
    B. I, III, IV, V
    C. II, III, V, VI
    D. II, III, IV, VI
    E. All of the above

4. Which of the following is not among the best means by which an athletic trainer may educate the general public and other health care workers regarding the profession of athletic training?
    A. Organizing professional seminars and conferences
    B. Providing high quality care to the physically active individual
    C. Publishing articles in professional journals and participating in research
    D. Developing television advertisements
    E. A and C

5. What is the most important thing an athletic trainer should do when taking a history from an athlete after an injury has occurred or when a problem arises?
    A. Be an active listener
    B. Make sure the athlete "gets to the point"
    C. Find out when the injury occurred
    D. Be sure to ask plenty of leading questions
    E. Ask what type of insurance policy they have

6. When assisting the general public in understanding the term sports medicine, the definition should include which of the following descriptors?
    A. Strength training
    B. Physician
    C. Rehabilitation
    D. Fitness
    E. Multidisciplinary

7. Which of the following qualities is needed in order to be an effective educator in an athletic training program?
    A. Competence in classroom teaching methods
    B. Competence in speech writing and communication skills
    C. A background in sociology
    D. Competence in computer language and audiovisual technology
    E. All of the above

8. "Torts" are legal wrongs committed against a person or his or her property. Such wrongs may be a direct result of _____ or _____.
    A. Negligence, commission
    B. Negligence, liability
    C. Omission, commission
    D. Omission, negligence
    E. Commission, liability

9. Athletic trainers should carry what type of insurance?
    A. Catastrophic event insurance
    B. Professional liability insurance
    C. Accident insurance
    D. Life insurance
    E. Primary insurance

10. Which of the following models of supervision for a head athletic trainer could be described as a "mentoring" approach?
    A. Developmental supervision
    B. Inspection supervision
    C. On-field supervision
    D. Clinical supervision
    E. None of the above

11. You have been asked to initiate an athletic training education program in the high school in which you work. One of the areas you are covering is sexually transmitted diseases. The following topics relating to AIDS should include all of the following except:
    A. Blood-borne pathogens
    B. HIV testing
    C. Universal precautions
    D. Bacterial infections
    E. OSHA guidelines

12. An athletic trainer discovers that he is infected with HIV. All of the following would be prudent steps for the athletic trainer to take except:
    A. Avoid seeking medical care
    B. Inform, if or when it becomes appropriate to do so, his patients, coworkers, or supervisors of his status
    C. Take the necessary steps to avoid the possibility of infecting others
    D. Make sure he has ongoing medical evaluations
    E. B and D

13. The statute of limitations involving a negligence suit has a limit of how many years?
    A. Up to 2 years
    B. 4 to 5 years
    C. 7 to 10 years
    D. 10 to 15 years
    E. 1 to 3 years

14. Which type of insurance should the athletic trainer carry in case of a criminal complaint involving negligence?
    A. General secondary insurance
    B. Catastrophic insurance
    C. Accident insurance
    D. Professional liability insurance
    E. Primary insurance

15. An athlete and his coach from your wrestling program have been trying to convince you that the athlete, who has been diagnosed with impetigo, can return early to wrestle. Your response should be based upon which NATA *Code of Ethics* principle?
    A. I: "Members shall respect the rights, welfare and dignity of all individuals."
    B. II: "Members shall comply with the laws and regulations governing the practice of athletic training."
    C. III: "Members shall accept responsibility for the exercise of sound judgment."
    D. V: "Members shall not engage in any form of conduct that constitutes a conflict of interest or that adversely reflects on the profession."
    E. None of the above

16. Which of the following are types of state regulation statuses for athletic trainers?
    I. Certification
    II. Licensing
    III. Active
    IV. Registration
    V. Inactive

    A. I, II, V
    B. II, III, IV
    C. I, II, IV
    D. II, IV, V
    E. I, II, III

17. All of the following are steps an athletic trainer can take to avoid litigation except:
    A. Develop a comprehensive emergency plan
    B. Establish a detailed, written job description
    C. Establish a yearly plan for modality maintenance
    D. Keep accurate records of all prescription medications dispensed
    E. A and B

18. An athletic trainer is working in a clinical setting. Which of the following populations is the athletic trainer best suited to treat?
    A. Neurologically impaired
    B. Mentally impaired
    C. Burn patients
    D. Geriatric patients
    E. Physically active

19. All of the following are violations of the BOC standards of practice except:
    A. Practicing as an athletic trainer without a license in a state that has an athletic trainer regulation
    B. Representing oneself as a BOC-certified athletic trainer using another individual's certification number
    C. Divulging the contents of a section of the certification exam to another certified athletic trainer or to a prospective student
    D. Functioning as a clinical athletic trainer in a sports medicine clinic within the confines of the individual state's practice act
    E. Prescribing medication

20. According to the 2006 to 2011 continuing education guidelines, how many CEUs may be obtained by a certified athletic trainer who participates in the certification examination as a board of certification (BOC) examiner/model?
    A. 2 CEUs per year
    B. 5 CEUs per year
    C. 10 CEUs per year
    D. 15 CEUs per year
    E. 20 CEUs per year

21. What is the state of being legally responsible for the harm one causes another person?
    A. Criminal intention
    B. Foreseeable harm
    C. Tort
    D. Negligence
    E. Liability

22. An athlete steps out of a whirlpool onto a slippery, wet floor and slips and falls, fracturing his wrist. The athletic trainer may be considered _____ in this case.
    A. Negligent
    B. Immune
    C. A plaintiff
    D. A witness
    E. Not guilty

23. The athletic trainer can avoid the risk of litigation by doing all the following except:
    A. Keep medical records confidential
    B. Establish positive personal relationships with athletes
    C. Create a safe playing environment with documentation of such
    D. Keep an updated resumé on file with the athletic director
    E. B and C

24. To attain certification as an athletic trainer, one must fulfill all of the following core requirements except:
    A. The applicant must have a high school diploma
    B. Maintain a 3.25 grade point average (GPA) as an undergraduate
    C. Proof of graduation at the baccalaureate level from an accredited college or university
    D. Have the certification application endorsed by a BOC-certified athletic trainer
    E. A and D

25. What is the main reason for the historically "uncomfortable" relationship between the physical therapist and the certified athletic trainer?
    A. The "aggressive" nature of physical therapists
    B. The identification of the athletic trainer as a "water boy"
    C. No such discomfort exists between the two professions
    D. The role confusion of both groups regarding the rehabilitation of injuries
    E. A and B

26. A certified athletic trainer is observed to be intoxicated while at work at a major university. This is in violation of which principle of the NATA *Code of Ethics?*
    A. I: "Members shall respect the rights, welfare, and dignity of all individuals."
    B. II: "Members shall comply with the laws and regulations governing the practice of athletic training."
    C. III: "Members shall accept responsibility for the exercise of sound judgment."
    D. IV: "Members shall maintain and promote high standards in the provision of services."
    E. None of the above

27. A certified athletic trainer refuses to treat an athlete based on the athlete's ethnic race. This is in violation of which principle of the NATA *Code of Ethics?*
    A. I: "Members shall respect the rights, welfare, and dignity of all individuals."
    B. III: "Members shall accept responsibility for the exercise of sound judgment."
    C. IV: "Members shall maintain and promote high standards in the provision of services."
    D. V: "Members shall not engage in any form of conduct that constitutes a conflict of interest or that adversely reflects on the profession."
    E. None of the above

28. Sports medicine is a term that includes all of the following specializations related to study of sport except:
    A. Exercise physiology
    B. Biomechanics
    C. Sports psychology
    D. Sports nutrition
    E. Recreational therapy

29. In what year were certified athletic trainers recognized by the AMA as "Allied Health Care Professionals?"
    A. 1988
    B. 1997
    C. 1994
    D. 2000
    E. 1991

30. Athletic training scope of practice parameters set by legislation fall into all of the following areas except:
    A. Restrictions regarding site of practice
    B. Modality use restrictions
    C. Restrictions regarding classroom teaching
    D. The definition of athletic training or athletic trainer
    E. Supervision of athletic trainers

31. Which of the following health care providers would be known as a primary care provider?
    A. A physical therapist
    B. An orthopedic technician
    C. A nurse
    D. An athletic trainer
    E. A physician

32. _____ and _____ are two states that license athletic training.
    A. Delaware, New Mexico
    B. Idaho, Kansas
    C. Arizona, Connecticut
    D. Minnesota, Colorado
    E. Colorado, Hawaii

33. Which of the following states restrict the practice of athletic training to the "traditional setting" (ie, scholastic, collegiate, or professional sport athletic training rooms)?
    A. Arkansas and Indiana
    B. Hawaii and Nebraska
    C. Alabama and Ohio
    D. Kentucky and New York
    E. None of the above

34. When taking a history from an athlete during the initial evaluation after an injury, at which of the following "levels of listening" should the athletic trainer be functioning?
    A. Passive
    B. Active
    C. Courteous
    D. Appreciative
    E. Analytical

35. _____ and _____ are two major components of "professionalism."
    A. Commitment, open-mindedness
    B. Status, narcissism
    C. Procrastination, decisiveness
    D. Job titles, upward mobility
    E. Dedication, upward mobility

36. CEUs may be obtained through all of the following methods except:
    A. Attending a BOC-approved seminar
    B. Completing a NATA journal quiz
    C. Completing postgraduate course work
    D. Writing a medical column in a local newspaper or popular magazine
    E. Home study courses

37. The only individuals who should have access to databases containing an athlete's medical records should be the _____ and _____.
    A. The athletic trainer, team physician
    B. The athletic trainer, school nurse
    C. The team physician, athletic director
    D. The parents, school nurse
    E. The athletic trainer, coach

38. _____ and _____ are two signs of occupational "burnout."
    A. Exhaustion, anger
    B. Excitement, creativeness
    C. Confusion, anxiety
    D. Paranoia, skepticism
    E. Anger, forgetfulness

39. Which of the following professionals possesses an expertise in the analysis of human motion?
    A. A physiatrist
    B. An exercise physiologist
    C. A strength and conditioning specialist
    D. A biomechanist
    E. An athletic trainer

40. One of your athletes is having significant pain as a result of a hallux valgus deformity. Which of the following individuals should the athletic trainer consult with in the care of this athlete?
    A. A hand surgeon
    B. A physical therapist
    C. A podiatrist
    D. A dentist
    E. A neurologist

41. Although an athletic trainer has successfully passed the BOC certification examination, he or she must be educated on the rules and regulations of the states in which he or she intends to practice. The individual must be knowledgeable of the state's:
    A. Certification guidelines
    B. Code of ethics
    C. Medical practice act
    D. Board of directors directives
    E. OSHA guidelines

42. Which of the following should a certified athletic trainer be concerned with when treating athletes?
    A. Foreseeable harm
    B. Tort
    C. Malfeasance
    D. The good samaritan act
    E. Malpractice

43. One of your high school baseball players is having elbow surgery at the end of the season. He is a major league prospect, and a scout has asked you to detail the surgery and outline the anticipated rehabilitation. When answering the scout's questions, the athletic trainer should do which of the following?
    A. Refer the scout to the athletic director
    B. Refer the scout to the team physician
    C. Refer the scout to the athlete
    D. None of the above
    E. All of the above

44. As a head athletic trainer at a division I university, you are charged with designing a drug testing procedure. It is up to you how to design, implement, and select the individuals being tested. The best way to select subjects is to use which of the following methods?
    A. Random timing
    B. Announced testing
    C. Preseason testing
    D. Random selection
    E. Scheduled weekly testing

45. All athletes should be required to participate in a preparticipation physical examination prior to any athletic related activity. During this exam, an athlete should also be required to fill out pertinent paperwork. What is one of the most important forms the athlete must complete?
    A. Previous athletic experience form
    B. Assumption of risk form
    C. Statutes of limitations form
    D. Personal information form
    E. Health insurance form

46. All of the following are ways of reducing risk of injury except:
    A. Assess activity areas for safety
    B. Frequent handwashing
    C. Proper equipment maintenance
    D. Documentation of treatments
    E. All of the above

47. The NATA *Code of Ethics* is defined as which of the following?
    A. Moral legal privileges inherent in being a member of a community
    B. Violation of commitment to privacy and protection of information or communications
    C. A set of rules by which an athletic trainer should conduct him- or herself
    D. The basis or explanation for an action taken by an athletic trainer
    E. None of the above

48. Which of the following is a way for an athletic trainer to protect him- or herself from negligence?
    A. Good documentation
    B. Testimony in court
    C. Sovereign immunity
    D. Having good malpractice insurance
    E. All of the above

49. Which of the following is a form of state credential, established by statute and intended to protect the public, that regulates the practice by specifying who may practice and what duties they may perform?
    A. Licensure
    B. Exemption
    C. Certification
    D. Registration
    E. None of the above

50. Which of the following is not one of the five principles of the NATA *Code of Ethics*?
    A. Members shall comply with the laws and regulations governing the practice of athletic training
    B. Members shall maintain and promote high standards in the provision of services
    C. Members may engage in conduct that constitutes a conflict of interest if the BOC board of supervisors grants prior written approval
    D. Members shall respect the rights, welfare, and dignity of all individuals
    E. A and C

51. Which of the following is a legal defense that attempts to claim that an injured plaintiff understood the risk of an activity and freely chose to undertake the activity regardless of the hazards associated with it?
    A. Sovereign immunity
    B. Comparative negligence
    C. Assumption of risk
    D. Statutes of limitations
    E. None of the above

52. Which of the following is not necessary when obtaining insurance information for an athlete's medical records?
    A. The insured's name
    B. The insured's mother's maiden name
    C. The insurance company's phone number
    D. Policy numbers
    E. The insurance company's address

53. Which of the following is not an approach to ethical decision making?
    A. Egoism
    B. Utilitarianism
    C. Formalism
    D. Socialism
    E. A and C

54. Sports medicine encompasses all of the following fields of study related to sport except:
    A. Biomechanics
    B. Massage therapy
    C. Sports nutrition
    D. Sport psychology
    E. Coaching

55. All of the following are considered support personnel that work along with the athletic trainer to ensure the health and safety of the athlete except:
    A. Nurse
    B. Sport psychologist
    C. Social worker
    D. All of the above
    E. B and C

56. All of the following are guidelines and position statements released by the NATA except:
    A. Helmet removal
    B. Fluid replacement for athletes
    C. Eye safety in sports
    D. Blood-borne pathogens
    E. Asthma in athletics

57. All of the following are considered members of the primary sports medicine team except:
    A. Coach
    B. Athletic trainer
    C. Physical therapist
    D. Team physician
    E. A and D

58. When was the NATA officially formed?
    A. 1948
    B. 1953
    C. 1955
    D. 1962
    E. 1950

59. Who is responsible for compiling medical histories and conducting physical examinations for each athlete on a team?
    A. The athletic trainer
    B. The team physician
    C. The athletic director
    D. All of the above
    E. None of the above

60. Which of the following is a possible employment setting for an athletic trainer?
    A. Industrial setting
    B. High school setting
    C. Hospital setting
    D. College or university
    E. All of the above

61. Which of the following is not a classification of regulation utilized when allowing an athletic trainer the right to practice within a specific state?
    A. Certification
    B. Licensing
    C. Delegation
    D. Exemption
    E. Registration

62. Who is the accrediting body for athletic training education programs?
    A. CAATE
    B. Joint Review Committee on Athletic Training (JRC-AT)
    C. NATA-EC
    D. BOC
    E. CAAHEP

63. Which of the following is not a domain of athletic training?
    A. Immediate care
    B. Diagnosis of athletic injuries
    C. Prevention
    D. Treatment, rehabilitation, and reconditioning
    E. Organization and administration

64. Athletic trainers are which type of decision maker?
    A. Primary
    B. Secondary
    C. Tertiary
    D. Supplemental
    E. Definers

65. What is negligence?
    A. A situation in which an athletic trainer fails to act as a reasonably prudent athletic trainer would act under the same circumstances
    B. A legal wrong, other than breech of contract, for which a remedy will be provided, usually in the form of monetary damage
    C. An unexcused failure to perform the duties specified in a contract
    D. Liability generating conduct associated with the adverse outcome of a patient treatment
    E. None of the above

66. Part of professional development is networking within your profession. This is accomplished by which of the following?
    A. Going to professional meetings
    B. Having a professional appearance at all times
    C. Arriving late to a conference
    D. Not keeping in contact with colleagues in your profession
    E. All of the above

67. The NATA requires medical documentation of all physician referrals, initial evaluation, assessment, treatments, and dates of follow-up care for all athletes. This is a good idea for all of the following reasons except:
    A. Professional standards of practice
    B. Legal protection if sued
    C. Improved communication between the team or family physician
    D. Protection against a possible malpractice suit
    E. B and C

68. All of the following are true about certification and licensure with respect to athletic trainers except:
    A. Certification is a less restrictive form of professional regulation than licensure
    B. Licensure does not prohibit anyone from performing the tasks of an athletic trainer under state law
    C. The BOC is recognized as the certifying board
    D. Licensure is the most restrictive form of state credentialing
    E. A and C

69. The rules, standards, and principles that dictate proper conduct among members of a society or profession are known as which of the following?
    A. Rights of conduct
    B. Code of conduct
    C. Morality
    D. Professional demeanor
    E. Ethics

70. Which of the following is not one of the five principles of the NATA *Code of Ethics*?
    A. Members shall respect the rights, welfare, and dignity of all individuals
    B. Members shall not engage in any form of conduct that constitutes a conflict of interest or that adversely reflects on the profession
    C. Members shall not release confidential information under any circumstance
    D. Members shall accept responsibility for the exercise of sound judgment
    E. A and B

71. All of the following are components of outcome assessment methods from the Agreement-Trust Matrix except:
    A. Patient chart documentation
    B. Internal chart audits
    C. Randomized clinical trials
    D. Patient review
    E. A and D

72. All of the following are advantages of inspection-production supervision except:
    A. Helps ensure goal achievements
    B. Sets well-defined limits on job behavior
    C. Documents input and output of a sports medicine clinic
    D. Enhances common understanding of athletic roles
    E. A and D

73. What does it mean when one fails to act when there is a legal duty to do so?
    A. Negligence
    B. Malpractice
    C. Commission
    D. Misdemeanor
    E. Omission

74. Which word defines a person that is highly cooperative in a support plan?
    A. Bedfellow
    B. Opponent
    C. Plaintiff
    D. Adversary
    E. Ally

75. Athletic directors, owners, staff, and _____ are all part of a major inside interest group.
    A. Parents
    B. Clients
    C. Coaches
    D. Professional groups
    E. None of the above

76. A sports medicine program should include which of the following in order to be successful?
    A. Provide the best possible health care
    B. Good communication among members of the sports medicine team
    C. Good communication between the athletic trainer and parents
    D. All of the above
    E. None of the above

77. One of your soccer players is requesting to play in the conference championship in 2 days. This athlete is 2 days post a grade one concussion. Who makes the final decision of an athlete's eligibility for participation in organized athletic activity in this situation?
    A. Coach
    B. Athlete
    C. Athletic trainer
    D. School nurse
    E. Physician

78. The athletic administrator's role includes which of the following?
    A. Establishes the chain of command for the sports medicine team
    B. Makes certain that each member has appropriate credentials
    C. Is responsible for having appropriate personnel for the appropriate positions
    D. All of the above
    E. None of the above

RELATED ATHLETIC TRAINING SUBJECT MATTER

Human Anatomy

1. What is inflammation of the common flexor origin of the forearm musculature called?
    A. Lateral epicondylitis
    B. Cycler's wrist
    C. Tennis elbow
    D. Pronation overuse syndrome
    E. Medial epicondylitis

2. Where is the olecranon process located?
    A. Ulna
    B. Tibia
    C. Vertebrae
    D. Sternum
    E. Clavicle

3. Which muscle does not assist in plantar flexion of the ankle?
    A. Peroneus tertius
    B. Posterior tibialis
    C. Plantaris
    D. Soleus
    E. Gastrocnemius

4. Which muscle does the axillary nerve innervate?
    A. Deltoid
    B. Latissimus dorsi
    C. Pectoralis minor
    D. Trapezius
    E. Scalenes

5. The collateral ligaments of the knee are taut in which of the following?
    A. Flexion
    B. Extension
    C. Extension and flexion
    D. Genu varus
    E. Genu valgum

6. Which cranial nerve is injured if the athlete complains of a decrease in the sense of smell after a high velocity head injury?
    A. II
    B. IV
    C. III
    D. V
    E. I

7. The rotator cuff consists of all the following muscles except:
    A. Supraspinatus
    B. Infraspinatus
    C. Teres major
    D. Subscapularis
    E. Teres minor

8. The rectus femoris muscle performs what two actions?
    A. Hip flexion and knee extension
    B. Hip extension and knee flexion
    C. Hip flexion and hip internal rotation
    D. Knee extension and hip internal rotation
    E. None of the above

9. The pes anserinus is made up of the tendons of what three muscles?
    A. Biceps femoris, gracilis, semitendinosus
    B. Iliotibial band, sartorius, semimembranosus
    C. Sartorius, gracilis, semimembranosus
    D. Sartorius, gracilis, semitendinosus
    E. Tensor fasciae latae, gracilis, semitendinosus

10. The subscapularis muscle originates on the _____ and inserts into _____.
    A. Subscapular fossa, the lesser tubercle of the humerus
    B. Supraspinous fossa, the greater tubercle of the humerus
    C. Distal two-thirds of the humerus, the coronoid process of the ulna
    D. Scapula, the middle third of the humerus
    E. None of the above

11. The gluteus maximus is responsible for what following motion(s)?
    A. Flexion and internal rotation of the thigh
    B. Extension of the hip
    C External rotation of the hip
    D. Extension and external rotation of the hip
    E. Abduction of the hip

12. What is the nerve root that affects elbow extension?
    A. C4
    B. C8
    C. C5
    D. C6
    E. C7

13. Holding a vibrating tuning fork next to the athlete's ear to determine air conduction of sound is a test for the _____ cranial nerve.
    A. VIII
    B. VI
    C. V
    D. X
    E. III

14. To test the hypoglossal nerve, the athletic trainer should request the athlete to perform what action?
    A. Shrug his or her shoulders
    B. Stick his or her tongue out
    C. Open his or her mouth wide
    D. Smile
    E. None of the above

15. "Handlebar palsy," which occurs in cyclists, presents with motor weakness of what nerve(s)?
    A. Ulnar
    B. Median
    C. Musculocutaneous
    D. Ulnar and median
    E. Radial

16. Where is the scaphoid bone of the wrist palpated?
    A. Proximal to the radial head
    B. Lateral to the cuboid bone
    C. Just distal to the styloid process of the radius
    D. Just distal to the styloid process of the ulna
    E. Just proximal to the styloid process of the ulna

17. All of the following muscles are innervated by the ulnar nerve except:
    A. Flexor carpi ulnaris
    B. Adductor pollicis
    C. All the hypothenar muscles
    D. Extensor carpi ulnaris
    E. None of the above

18. What type of joint is the hip joint?
    A. Fibrous
    B. Amphiarthrotic
    C. Synarthrotic
    D. Diarthrotic
    E. Semiarthrotic

19. Flexion and extension of the knee joint occurs in the _____ plane around a _____ axis.
    A. Sagittal, transverse
    B. Sagittal, coronal
    C. Frontal, anterior-posterior
    D. Transverse, longitudinal
    E. Sagittal, longitudinal

20. Which of the following describes an impacted fracture?
    A. A fracture that telescopes one part of the bone on the other
    B. The bone splits along its length
    C. The fracture is at a right angle to the shaft
    D. A fracture consisting of three or more fragments at the fracture site
    E. None of the above

21. Which of the following joints is classified as a uni-axial diarthrodial joint?
    A. The interphalangeal joints of the fingers
    B. Hip joint
    C. Carpometacarpal joint of the thumb
    D. Scapulothoracic joint
    E. None of the above

22. Which of the following muscles does not flex the hip?
    A. Tensor fascia latae
    B. Pectineus
    C. Iliopsoas
    D. Rectus femoris
    E. Biceps femoris

23. Which of the following movements is greatest in the thoracic region?
    A. Lateral flexion of the spine
    B. Flexion and extension of the spine
    C. Rotation and extension of the spine
    D. Flexion of the spine
    E. None of the above

24. Which structures are located in the lateral compartment of the lower leg?
    A. Extensor digitorum longus, peroneus longus, and peroneus brevis muscles
    B. Peroneus longus and brevis muscles, the superficial branch of the peroneal nerve, and the peroneal artery
    C. Posterior tibialis muscle, posterior tibial artery, and the deep peroneal nerve
    D. Extensor digitorum longus, peroneal brevis, and peroneal tertius muscles
    E. Anterior tibialis, peroneal brevis, and Achilles tendon

25. Where would a Baker's cyst be located?
    A. In the popliteal fossa
    B. In the groin area
    C. On the breast
    D. On the lip
    E. The wrist

26. Which of the joints below comprise the shoulder girdle?
    I. Sternoclavicular
    II. Acromioclavicular
    III. Glenohumeral
    IV. Scapulothoracic
    V. Costoclavicular
    VI. Scapulohumeral

    A. I, II, VI
    B. I, II, III, IV
    C. III, IV, V, VI
    D. III, V, VI
    E. I, II, V

27. The coracoclavicular ligaments consist of the _____ and _____ ligaments.
    A. Trapezoid, conoid
    B. Coracoacromial, conoid
    C. Acromioclavicular, trapezoid
    D. Costoclavicular, conoid
    E. Trapezoid, glenoid

28. Which of the following joints is a "mortise" joint?
    A. First metatarsophalangeal
    B. Elbow
    C. Sacroiliac
    D. Knee
    E. Ankle

29. What two structures pass through the tunnel of Guyon?
    A. The ulnar nerve and ulnar artery
    B. The radial and ulnar nerves
    C. The radial nerve and radial artery
    D. The ulnar nerve and radial artery
    E. None of the above

30. Which muscle is usually affected with tennis elbow?
    A. Extensor carpi radialis brevis
    B. Flexor carpi radialis
    C. Extensor carpi ulnaris
    D. Extensor pollicis brevis
    E. Coracobrachialis

31. All of the following muscles are intrinsic muscles of the hand except:
    A. The lumbricals
    B. The muscles of the thenar eminence
    C. The interossei
    D. The multifidi muscles
    E. All of the above are intrinsic muscles of the hand

32. What are the primary actions of the psoas major?
    A. Abduction of the hip
    B. Extension and internal rotation of the hip
    C. Hip flexion and internal rotation
    D. Trunk flexion
    E. Lateral flexion of the trunk

33. Where is the origin of the vastus lateralis located?
    A. Gerdy's tubercle
    B. The anterior inferior iliac spine
    C. The greater trochanter of the femur
    D. The lateral aspect of the femur
    E. Lister's tubercle

34. Which of the following muscle tendons form the borders of the anatomical snuff-box?
    I. Extensor hallucis longus
    II. Extensor pollicis brevis
    III. Flexor pollicis longus
    IV. Abductor pollicis longus
    V. Extensor pollicis longus

    A. I, III, V
    B. I, II, IV
    C. III, IV, V
    D. II, IV, V
    E. I, II, III

35. What is the structure that carries deoxygenated blood from the head and upper body to the heart?
    A. Descending aorta
    B. Superior vena cava
    C. Ascending aorta
    D. Jugular vein
    E. None of the above

36. At which of the following structures does gas exchange occur in the lungs?
    A. Terminal bronchiole
    B. The parietal pleura
    C. The pulmonary arteries
    D. The pulmonary veins
    E. The alveoli

37. All of the following structures pass through the popliteal fossa except:
    A. Tibial nerve
    B. Popliteal artery
    C. Popliteal vein
    D. Common peroneal nerve
    E. Peroneal artery

38. Where is the odontoid process located?
    A. Base of the sacrum
    B. Proximal end of the ulna
    C. Off the second cervical vertebrae
    D. Base of the skull
    E. Distal to the olecrenon process

39. Which of the following bones is not a carpal bone of the wrist?
    A. Lunate
    B. Cuneiform
    C. Hamate
    D. Pisiform
    E. Scaphoid

40. The plantar fascia or plantar aponeurosis is located where in the body?
    A. Base of the neck
    B. Lumbar region
    C. Lateral side of the thigh
    D. Sole of the foot
    E. Cervical spine

41. The sternocleidomastoid muscle originates on the _____ and inserts into the _____.
    A. Clavicle, mastoid process
    B. Clavicle and sternum, mastoid process
    C. Manubrium, occipital protuberance
    D. Manubrium, clavicle
    E. Third cervical vertebrae, clavicle

42. Which of the following muscles is a strong extensor of the trunk?
    A. Gluteus maximus
    B. Erector spinae
    C. Quadratus lumborum
    D. Iliacus
    E. None of the above

43. Which structures pass through the femoral triangle?
    A. Femoral artery, femoral vein, femoral nerve
    B. Femoral artery, femoral nerve, iliac vein
    C. Deep circumflex vein, femoral nerve
    D. Great saphenous vein, femoral vein, iliac vein
    E. Superficial circumflex vein, femoral artery, femoral nerve

44. Which artery is closely involved with the brachial plexus and becomes the brachial artery at the lower border of the tendon of the teres major muscle?
    A. Subclavian
    B. Radial
    C. Axillary
    D. Subscapular
    E. None of the above

45. Which of the following muscles does not dorsiflex the ankle?
    A. Extensor digitorum longus
    B. Peroneus tertius
    C. Tibialis anterior
    D. Peroneus brevis
    E. A and C

46. Which of the following is not a bone of the middle ear?
    A. Malleus
    B. Cochlea
    C. Stapes
    D. Incus
    E. All of the above

47. Where is the C3,4 dermatome located?
    A. The top of the head
    B. Over the posterior upper arm area
    C. Over the lateral upper arm area
    D. The superior aspect of the shoulders and posterior neck area
    E. Anterior chest area

48. In what abdominal quadrant is the spleen located?
    A. Central
    B. Lower right
    C. Lower left
    D. Upper right
    E. Upper left

49. Your athlete comes to the athletic training room after injuring his neck and left arm. You suspect involvement of the C5,6 nerve root. Which of the following actions would not be involved with an injury to a muscle with this innervation?
    A. Little finger abduction
    B. Elbow flexion
    C. Shoulder abduction
    D. Forearm supination
    E. Shoulder flexion

50. A soccer player has been kicked in the upper right quadrant of his abdomen. Which of the following internal organ(s) could have sustained a significant injury?
    A. Kidney
    B. Ureters
    C. Spleen
    D. Appendix and sigmoid colon
    E Liver and gallbladder

Human Physiology

1. The bottom number of a blood pressure reading is the _____ pressure.
    A. Intrinsic
    B. Systolic
    C. Ejection fraction
    D. Venous
    E. Diastolic

2. The optimum time an ice pack should be applied to a body part is 10 minutes. This is to avoid the _____ response.
    A. Vasomotor
    B. Blocking
    C. Moro
    D. Belle
    E. Hunting

3. Redness and swelling during the inflammation process are caused by all of the following except:
    A. Histamine
    B. Prostaglandins
    C. Serotonin
    D. Acetylcholine
    E. Bradykinin

4. What is the level of desirable total cholesterol?
    A. Less than or equal to 200 mg/100 mL
    B. Greater than 250 mg/100 mL
    C. 55 mg/100 mL
    D. Less than 100 mg/100 mL
    E. None of the above

5. Which of the following is known as the separation of electrically charged particles causing a transmembrane electrical potential difference?
    A. Resting membrane potential
    B. Membrane permeability threshold
    C. Electrogenic pump
    D. Depolarization threshold
    E. Ion interference

6. When sodium ions move into a cell and the transmembrane potential is reduced (approaches zero), and when potassium ions rush out of the cell and the transmembrane potential is gradually re-established, an action potential is created. The two phases described above are known as what?
    A. Depolarization and repolarization
    B. Repolarization and depolarization
    C. Stimulation and propagation
    D. Propagation and repolarization
    E. Permability and repolarization

7. What is the primary component of striated skeletal muscle?
    A. Sarcomere
    B. Muscle fiber
    C. Myofibril
    D. Fascicle
    E. None of the above

8. What does a motor unit consist of?
    A. A cell body, axon, and dendrites
    B. The axon and single muscle fiber it innervates
    C. A motor neuron and the group of muscle fibers it innervates
    D. The motor neuron, muscle fiber, and muscle group
    E. The dendrite, and the group of muscle fibers it innervates

9. What type of muscle fiber is more prevalent in a sprinter's lower extremity?
    A. Pink
    B. Type I
    C. Slow twitch
    D. Smooth
    E. Fast twitch

10. What mineral must be present in adequate amounts in the muscle fiber for a contraction to occur?
    A. Na+
    B. Ca++
    C. Cl-
    D. PO_4
    E. All of the above

11. In addition to the release of energy, the breakdown of ATP during a muscle contraction produces which of the following byproducts?
    A. $H_2O + CO_2$
    B. $Cr + PO_4$
    C. Adenosine diphosphate (ADP) + PO_4
    D. ADP + adenosinetriphosphatase (ATPase)
    E. Bilirubin

12. During aerobic metabolism, enzymes reduce large molecules of carbohydrates, fat, and protein into smaller particles so they can be oxidized in a chain of chemical reactions. What is this series of chemical reactions collectively called?
    A. The Krebs cycle
    B. Oxidative carboxylic acid cycle
    C. Thermocaloric cycle
    D. Phosphocreatine reaction
    E. Electron transport cycle

13. Deep pain may originate from three specific areas when a nerve is injured. These areas are known as sclerotomes, myotomes, and dermatomes. Sclerotomic pain is transported by what type of nerve fiber?
    A. Unmyelinated C fibers
    B. Unmyelinated D fibers
    C. Myelinated A-Delta fibers
    D. Myelinated C fibers
    E. Myelinated B-Delta fibers

14. Muscular fiber arrangements may be known as _____ or _____.
    A. Fusiform, pennate
    B. Oblique, striated
    C. Striated, smooth
    D. Multinuclear, uninuclear
    E. Transverse, longitudinal

15. What is amenorrhea?
    A. Diminished flow during menses
    B. Absence of flow during menses
    C. Painful menses
    D. Late onset of menses
    E. None of the above

16. What should be avoided by an athlete who has frequent episodes of constipation?
    A. Laxatives or enemas
    B. High fiber diet
    C. Bland diet
    D. Calcium supplements
    E. B and D

17. Hemophilia occurs when which of the following blood factors is missing?
    A. Granulocytes
    B. Hemoglobin
    C. Factor IV
    D. Rh factor
    E. Factor VIII

18. In addition to the partial pressure of oxygen in the alveolar gas of the lungs, what other factors influence the rate of diffusion of oxygen into the bloodstream?
    A. The respiratory rate and pleural surface area
    B. The amount of CO_2 present in the alveoli and the pulmonary veins
    C. The respiratory rate and CO_2 partial pressure
    D. The thickness of the alveolar capillary membrane and the amount of surface area available for diffusion
    E. All of the above

19. An athlete's pulmonary function is tested via spirometry. Several measurements are taken during this test. What is the maximum amount of air that can be expired after a maximum inspiration?
    A. Maximum expiratory flow rate
    B. Forced expiratory volume
    C. Residual volume
    D. Tidal volume
    E. Vital capacity

20. During what phase of the menstrual cycle does a graafian follicle mature?
    A. Second phase
    B. Ovulatory
    C. Luteal
    D. Menstrual
    E. Follicular

21. What are the two phases of menstruation?
    A. Anovulation, luteal
    B. Prolactin, menarche
    C. Follicular, luteal
    D. Menarche, follicular
    E. First phase, second phase

22. Which of the following structures is not innervated?
    A. Periosteum of bone
    B. Peritoneum of the abdomen
    C. Epithelium of the skin
    D. Enamel of a tooth
    E. All of the above are innervated

23. A football player sustained a large laceration to his lower leg 4 weeks ago. Which type of repair has taken place by this time?
    A. Callus formation
    B. Primary healing
    C. Margination
    D. Secondary healing
    E. Erythrocyte migration

24. Noxious stimuli that are created by musculoskeletal injury result in the release of endorphins and enkephalins during the mediation of pain. These opioids are produced by the stimulation of the _____ of the midbrain and _____ in the pons and medulla.
    A. Periaqueductal gray area, substantia gelatinosa
    B. Periaqueductal gray area, raphe nucleus
    C. Central cortex, substantia gelatinosa
    D. Raphe nucleus, red nucleus
    E. Periaqueductal white area, substantia gelatinosa

25. A female field hockey player reports to the athletic trainer complaining that her knee still hurts from a grade II medial collateral ligament sprain she suffered almost 3 months ago. How long may it take for a ligament to completely heal after a significant injury?
    A. Between 4 and 6 months
    B. Up to 1 year
    C. Up to 4 months
    D. Between 1.5 and 2 years
    E. Between 4 and 6 weeks

26. You are aware of a diabetic athlete who has just self-administered his morning dose of insulin and has basketball practice within the following hour. Which of the following would be a prudent action to suggest to this athlete before he begins exercising?
    A. Hyperhydrate prior to practice
    B. Eat a candy bar before practice
    C. Suggest the athlete eat a slice of bread with peanut butter or cheese prior to practice
    D. Drink a soft drink before exercising
    E. None of the above

27. All of the following are physiological responses to cryotherapy except:
    A. Increased metabolism
    B. Decreased muscle spasm
    C. Analgesia
    D. Increased joint stiffness
    E. B and D

28. An athlete falls on an outstretched hand and injures his wrist. After evaluating the injury, the athletic trainer suspects a scaphoid fracture. Because this area has a poor blood supply, which of the following conditions may occur if the injury is mistreated?
    A. DeQuervain's syndrome
    B. Aseptic necrosis
    C. Carpal tunnel syndrome
    D. Swan neck deformity
    E. Brunet's deformity

29. A soccer player gets kicked in the low back and is brought to the athletic training room. During his examination, he goes to the bathroom and reports that there is blood in his urine. Which of the following terms describes this sign of an internal injury?
    A. Hyperpnea
    B. Hematoma
    C. Hypernatremia
    D. Hemarthrosis
    E. Hematuria

30. Smooth muscle tissue is found in all of the following structures except:
    A. Lungs
    B. Arterial walls
    C. Colon
    D. Intestines
    E. Scalenes

31. While performing an isometric contraction, an athlete should be instructed to breathe normally to prevent the valsalva's effect. Which of the following occurs when the athlete produces the valsalva's effect?
    A. The athlete experiences dyspnea
    B. The athlete will hyperventilate
    C. The athlete becomes hypotensive
    D. There is a significant, rapid rise in blood pressure
    E. The athlete will pass out

32. During ballistic stretching, the Golgi tendon organs are unable to produce a relaxing effect of the muscle because of the constant stimulation of which of the following structures?
    A. Muscle spindles
    B. Posterior horn of the spinal cord
    C. The antagonist muscle
    D. Cerebral cortex
    E. None of the above

33. The adrenal glands secrete which of the following substances?
    I. Cortisol
    II. Epinephrine
    III. Serotonin
    IV. Aldosterone
    V. Estrogen
    VI. Human growth hormone

    A. I, II, III, VI
    B. I, II, IV, V
    C. II, III, V, VI
    D. III, IV, V, VI
    E. I, II, III, IV

34. A male athlete gets kicked in the groin area and sustains an injury to the testicles. The major function of the testes is to produce _____ and _____.
    A. Semen, urine
    B. Spermatozoa, testosterone
    C. Testosterone, estrogen
    D. Semen, spermatozoa
    E. Testosterone, progesterone

Exercise Physiology

1. What can be defined as the training effect on the cardiac system?
   A. Cardiac output (CO) = increased stroke volume (SV) + decreased heart rate (HR)
   B. CO = SV / HR
   C. CO = decreased SV – increased HR
   D. SV = CO x HR
   E. None of the above

2. When reading an exercise prescription, which of the following statements represents the frequency of exercise?
   A. Three sessions a week
   B. 45 minutes of continuous exercises
   C. Running or cycling
   D. 80% of VO_2 max
   E. None of the above

3. What three different lipoproteins make up total cholesterol?
   A. Triglycerides, high-density lipoproteins (HDL), and low-density lipoproteins (LDL)
   B. LDL, HDL, and very-low-density lipoproteins (VLDL)
   C. LDL, VLDL, and triglycerides
   D. Alpha lipoprotein, LDL, and triglycerides
   E. Triglycerides, omega-3 fatty acids, HDL

4. During vigorous activity, accessory muscles come into play to aid respiration. During inspiration, these muscles include the _____ and _____.
   A. Upper trapezius, levator scapulae
   B. Sternocleidomastoid, scalenes
   C. Intercostals, abdominals
   D. Intercostals, levator scapulae
   E. Abdominals, sternocledomastoid

5. In very cold environments, the athlete's body will attempt to produce heat through many different mechanisms. One of these methods is by hypothalamic stimulation of what?
   A. Posterior hypothalamus
   B. Sweat glands
   C. Pituitary glands
   D. Adrenal glands
   E. Thyroid gland

6. A basketball player comes limping off the court complaining of a hamstring spasm. Which of the following procedures would be the most effective in reducing the spasm?
   A. Massage the hamstring
   B. Moist heat pack followed by ultrasound
   C. Static stretch of the involved muscle
   D. Static stretch of the antagonistic muscle
   E. Ice massage followed by ballistic stretch

7. An athlete who is hyperflexible (mobile beyond the joint's normal range) is subject to what types of injuries?
   A. Tendinitis and bursitis
   B. Fractures and ligament tears
   C. Sprains and strains
   D. Fractures and dislocations
   E. Tendinitis and adhesive capsulitis

8. Interval training would be appropriate for all the following sports except:
   A. Football
   B. Soccer
   C. Volleyball
   D. Basketball
   E. Archery

9. During what season would it be beneficial for an athlete to participate in a sport (other than his or her primary sport) to maintain an adequate level of fitness?
   A. Off-season
   B. Postseason
   C. In-season
   D. Preseason
   E. Transition phase of in-season

10. Which of the following principles must be adhered to when designing a training program for an athlete in order to obtain optimal training effects?
    I. Overload
    II. Specificity
    III. Progression
    IV. Consistency
    V. Environmental factors
    VI. Psychological well-being

    A. I, III, IV, V
    B. II, IV, V, VI
    C. I, II, III, IV
    D. II, III, V, VI
    E. I, II, IV, VI

11. All of the following effects are true regarding changes that take place as a result of resistive exercise except:
    A. Increased ligament and tendon strength
    B. Improved elasticity of skeletal muscle
    C. Increased mineral content of bone
    D. Improved maximal oxygen uptake
    E. Increased tendon strength

12. Under which of the following conditions is the tension created in a muscle the greatest during exercise?
    A. When the interaction between the cross-bridges of the actin and myosin myofilaments are at a maximum
    B. When the muscle position is at its shortest
    C. When a muscle is at its most lengthened point
    D. When the muscle insertion is at a 90-degree angle to the shaft of a bone
    E. None of the above

13. _____ and _____ determine the amount of blood that is pumped through the heart in a given period of time.
    A. Cardiac output, heart rate
    B. Respiratory rate, ventricular filling rate
    C. Stroke volume, cardiac output
    D. Heart rate, stroke volume
    E. Respiratory rate, cardiac output

14. If a 20-year-old athlete is exercising at 80% of his maximal heart rate, his target heart rate could be calculated to equal what?
    A. 150 BPM
    B. 140 BPM
    C. 170 BPM
    D. 200 BPM
    E. 160 BPM

15. In order to improve an athlete's flexibility, PNF techniques may be incorporated into a training program. Which of the following techniques involves an isotonic contraction during the "push" phase?
    A. Hold-relax
    B. Contract-relax
    C. Slow-reversal-hold-relax
    D. Fast-reversal-hold-relax
    E. Slow-hold-relax

16. When bench-pressing a barbell, the triceps and pectoralis major musculature contract in what manner during the "lift" phase?
    A. Isokinetically
    B. Isometrically
    C. Eccentrically
    D. Concentrically
    E. None of the above

17. Which type of training program is most beneficial if the coach or athletic trainer is trying to improve muscular strength and flexibility?
    A. Plyometric training
    B. Anaerobic training
    C. Circuit training
    D. Power lifting
    E. All of the above

18. If an athlete is not well-hydrated, is in poor physical condition in the beginning of a sport season, and is exercising in a very hot, humid environment, he may be susceptible to heat injuries. What is the area of the body that is responsible for thermoregulation?
    A. Barioceptors
    B. Thymus
    C. Hypothalamus
    D. Pituitary gland
    E. Adrenal gland

19. Year-round sports conditioning is developed through the concept of periodization. Periodization is an approach that allows the athlete to train in stages so peak performance may be attained at the appropriate time and injuries are avoided. Which of the following describe the different phases in periodization?
    A. Fall season, winter season, spring season, off-season
    B. Postseason, off-season, preseason, in-season
    C. First, second, third, and forth quarters
    D. Preparation phase, active phase, maintenance phase
    E. Active phase, prepatory phase, competition phase

20. The purpose of a proper cool-down period after exercising is to _____ and _____.
    A. Decrease the heart rate, decrease cardiac output
    B. Increase ventilation, prevent dizziness
    C. Help the blood return to the heart to be reoxygenated, decrease muscular lactic acid build-up
    D. Improve flexibility, decrease body temperature
    E. Decrease heart rate, restore thermoregulation

21. Which type of exercise utilizes a rapid stretch of the muscle eccentrically followed by a rapid concentric contraction and is used to develop explosive movements?
    A. Ballistic
    B. Isokinetic
    C. Isotonic
    D. Internal
    E. Plyometric

22. Developing significant muscle bulk is dependent on the levels present in the body of which of the following hormones?
    A. Epinephrine
    B. Cortisol
    C. Norepinephrine
    D. Estrogen
    E. Testosterone

23. To help prevent an athlete from developing hypothermia while playing in very cold weather, what should the athletic trainer advise the athlete to do?
    A. Wear a hooded sweatshirt
    B. Only stay out in the cold for brief periods of time
    C. Wear layers of clothing
    D. Wear lined pants
    E. B and D

24. One of your lacrosse players has blonde hair, light green eyes, and a very fair complexion. You suggest she wear a sunscreen with which of the following levels of SPF?
    A. 4
    B. 6
    C. 10
    D. 30
    E. 8

25. An asthmatic athlete who lives and trains in an urban area is susceptible to the effects of air pollution. To avoid an asthma attack while training, the athletic trainer should recommend that the athlete train at which of the following times of day?
    A. Predawn hours
    B. Mid-day
    C. Late afternoon
    D. On weekends and the evening
    E. None of the above

26. You have an African-American athlete with known sickle-cell disease who is training in high altitudes for a long distance road race. This athlete might be at risk for which condition?
    A. Ruptured spleen
    B. Enlarged gallbladder
    C. Cystic fibrosis
    D. Tinea corporis
    E. Hypertension

27. Unlimited access to fluids is critical during hot weather because the athlete will sweat more. Sweat is hypotonic, which means what imbalance is the athlete likely to experience?
    A. Water loss in excess of salt loss
    B. Salt loss in excess of water loss
    C. Water loss is equal to salt loss
    D. Sugar loss in excess of water loss
    E. Sugar loss equal to water loss

28. Delayed-onset muscle soreness (DOMS) can occur with high-intensity exercise. Which of the following types of exercise is most likely to cause DOMS?
    A. Endurance
    B. Isometric
    C. Plyometric
    D. PNF
    E. Isotonic

29. If a joint capsule is stretched beyond its physiological limitations causing a reflexive muscle contraction, which of the following laws is being demonstrated?
    A. Ohm's
    B. Harrod's
    C. Wolff's
    D. Newton's
    E. Hilton's

30. When performing a urinalysis with a dipstick (such as Clinix Stix or a similar product) for abnormal glucose and protein levels, which of the following are considered abnormal findings in the adolescent?
    A. +2
    B. +3
    C. +4
    D. All of the above
    E. None of the above

31. Why are men generally much stronger than women?
    A. Women have a lower strength:body weight ratio
    B. Men have a lower strength:body weight ratio
    C. Men have a greater strength:muscle mass ratio
    D. Women have a greater strength:fat percentage ratio
    E. Women have a lower strength:body mass ratio

32. Which of the following physiological adaptations does not occur in skeletal muscle during endurance training?
    A. Increased aerobic enzyme activity
    B. Increased myoglobin levels
    C. Increased mitochondrial density
    D. Decreased mitochondrial density
    E. A and B

33. During a 400-meter sprint, which of the following energy systems is predominant?
    A. Lactic acid system
    B. ATP-CP system
    C. Anaerobic glycolysis system
    D. Aerobic metabolic system
    E. Anaerobic metabolic system

34. What affect does aerobic exercise have on an athlete's diastolic blood pressure?
    A. Diastolic blood pressure will increase at the same pace as systolic
    B. Diastolic blood pressure will significantly decrease at higher workloads
    C. It will remain closely the same level as at rest
    D. Diastolic blood pressure will significantly increase with increasing workloads
    E. None of the above

35. Footstrike anemia can be controlled by having the athlete wear well-cushioned shoes, limiting running to very soft surfaces, and teaching the athlete to land lightly on his or her feet while exercising. What is this condition called?
    A. Hemolysis
    B. Hyperkalemia
    C. Rubefacients
    D. Hemarthrosis
    E. Hemoptysis

Biomechanics

1. What is a contraction that occurs as the muscle shortens?
    A. Isotonic
    B. Eccentric
    C. Isometric
    D. Concentric
    E. Static

2. The foot becomes a "rigid lever" for push-off when it is in what position?
    A. Supination
    B. Pronation
    C. Dorsiflexion
    D. Adduction
    E. Plantarflexion

3. How many degrees of freedom does the knee have?
    A. 0
    B. 1
    C. 3
    D. 4
    E. 2

4. How many degrees of movement does the scapula contribute to shoulder abduction?
    A. 30
    B. 80
    C. 100
    D. 180
    E. 60

5. What role does the quadriceps musculature assume during active knee extension against gravity?
    A. Antagonist
    B. Agonist
    C. Synergist
    D. Stabilizer
    E. None of the above

6. In the human body, the point of attachment of the muscle causing the motion is almost always closer to the joint axis than the resisting motion. What type of lever system most commonly exists in the body?
    A. Fourth
    B. Second
    C. Fifth
    D. First
    E. Third

7. In what position will the movement arm of a force be the greatest?
    A. When the movement arm is at a 45-degree angle to the applied force
    B. When the force of gravity is 90 degrees to the applied force
    C. When the lever being moved is parallel to the applied force
    D. When the angle of application of the force is at 90 degrees to the lever being moved
    E. None of the above

8. Of the following statements, which is true about anatomic pulleys?
    A. Anatomic pulleys change the direction of the muscle force but not the magnitude of the force
    B. Anatomic pulleys always deflect the line of pull of a muscle away from the joint axis
    C. Anatomic pulleys change the direction and magnitude of the force
    D. Anatomic pulleys improve leverage and, therefore, increase the magnitude of the force
    E. None of the above

9. Muscular tension may be increased by increasing the _____ or _____.
    A. Frequency of motor units firing, the number of motor units that are stimulated
    B. External force, inert muscle force
    C. Contractile tension, viscoelastic tension
    D. Number of repetitions while weight lifting, the poundage of weight
    E. Angle of applied force, frequency of motor units firing

10. What three motions comprise pronation of the foot?
    A. Inversion, abduction, dorsiflexion
    B. Inversion, adduction, plantar flexion
    C. Eversion, abduction, dorsiflexion
    D. Eversion, adduction, plantar flexion
    E. Eversion, abduction, plantar flexion

11. What class lever does the gastrocnemius use during plantar flexion?
    A. First
    B. Second
    C. Third
    D. Fourth
    E. Fifth

12. Each lever has a _____, which is the perpendicular distance from the line of force to the axis, and a _____, which is the perpendicular distance from the resistance to the axis.
    A. Force arm, rotary arm
    B. Short arm, long arm
    C. Force arm, resistance arm
    D. Rotary arm, translatory arm
    E. Force arm, translatory arm

13. Running utilizes _____ motion of the entire body and _____ motion of the arms and legs.
    A. Decelerant, accelerant
    B. Vertical, horizontal
    C. Rotary, translatory
    D. Linear, angular
    E. Vertical rotary

14. Momentum is created by the combination of _____ and _____.
    A. Speed, weight
    B. Mass, velocity
    C. Acceleration, weight
    D. Torque, friction
    E. Acceleration, inertia

15. A sprinter who is in the "ready" position at the start of a race has a lot of potential energy. What is his potential energy converted into as he takes off when the gun is heard?
    A. Lactic acid
    B. Thermal energy
    C. Work energy
    D. Kinetic energy
    E. Aerobic energy

16. Which of the following describes the plane and axis for cervical rotation?
    A. Horizontal, vertical
    B. Horizontal, sagittal
    C. Sagittal, anterior-posterior
    D. Frontal, vertical
    E. Frontal, horizontal

17. When manually resisting the tibia during knee extension, all of the following statements regarding the torque produced are true except:
    A. The torque of an external force (ie, the hand against the anterior tibia) can be increased by increasing the magnitude of the applied force
    B. The torque of an external force can be increased by applying the force perpendicular to the tibial crest
    C. The torque of an external force can be increased by moving the force distally near the ankle
    D. The torque of an external force can be increased by applying the force parallel to the tibial shaft
    E. A and B

18. An avulsion fracture of a bone is caused by which type of tissue stress?
    A. Compression
    B. Bending
    C. Shearing
    D. All of the above
    E. None of the above

19. A lever is considered in rotational equilibrium when any muscle acting on that lever is neither shortening nor lengthening. This results in what kind of contraction?
    A. Isometric
    B. Isotonic
    C. Passive
    D. Concentric
    E. Eccentric

20. What type of joint is the carpometacarpal joint of the thumb?
    A. Pivot
    B. Ball and socket
    C. Hinge
    D. Plane
    E. Saddle

21. What is the maximum nmber of degrees of freedom a joint can possess?
    A. 2
    B. 5
    C. 4
    D. 6
    E. 3

22. Which of the following joints is an example of a hinge joint?
    A. Acromioclavicular
    B. Atlantoaxial
    C. Talocrural
    D. Shoulder
    E. Elbow

23. The frontal plane divides the body into _____ and _____ parts.
    A. Top, anterior
    B. Right, left
    C. Top, bottom
    D. Anterior, posterior
    E. Superior, lateral

24. What is an example of an activity taking place with the upper extremity in a closed-chain position?
    A. Swinging a bat
    B. Performing a push-up
    C. Throwing a ball
    D. Running with closed fists
    E. All of the above

25. What occurs at the knee joint during the screw-home mechanism?
    A. The tibia externally rotates on the femur during knee extension
    B. The femur externally rotates on the tibia during knee flexion
    C. The femur internally rotates on the tibia during knee extension
    D. The tibia internally rotates on the femur during knee extension
    E. The tibia externally rotates on the femur during knee flexion

26. What occurs at the articulating surfaces of a joint that is subjected to a compressive load?
    A. The joint surfaces are brought closer together
    B. The joint surfaces are forcefully separated
    C. There is a "twisting" movement at the joint surfaces
    D. There is a "bending" motion that occurs at the joint surfaces
    E. There is a "gliding" motion that occurs at the joint surfaces

27. Loading of a joint that is unstable due to a ligament rupture produces which of the following stresses on the joint cartilage?
    A. No change at all
    B. Rolling/pivoting stress
    C. Tension forces
    D. Abnormally low stress
    E. Abnormally high stress

28. Shoulder abduction occurs in the _____ plane and moves around a _____ axis.
    A. Frontal, sagittal
    B. Horizontal, vertical
    C. Frontal, anterior-posterior
    D. Sagittal, medial-lateral
    E. Frontal, superior-inferior

29. Hip internal/external rotation occurs in the _____ plane around a _____ axis.
    A. Sagittal, medial-lateral
    B. Horizontal, anterior-posterior
    C. Frontal, anterior-posterior
    D. Horizontal, vertical
    E. Sagittal, anterior-posterior

30. While covering a football game, a player gets tackled and sustains a spiral fracture of the tibial shaft. Which of the following force(s) comes into play when a bone is fractured in this manner?
    A. Compression, tension
    B. Torsion
    C. Compression, shearing
    D. Impaction
    E. Shearing, distraction

31. Repeated rubbing over the epidermis may cause which of the following conditions?
    A. Avulsion
    B. Blisters
    C. Contusions
    D. Bursitis
    E. Impetigo

Psychology

1. An athlete comes to the athletic trainer just prior to his first soccer game complaining of nausea and informs the athletic trainer he is really nervous. Which of the following is an appropriate method to relax a nervous athlete?
    A. Yoga
    B. Progressive muscle relaxation
    C. Have the coach calm the athlete
    D. Resting in a warm sauna for 10 minutes
    E. Pilates

2. The coach confers with the athletic trainer concerning a difficult athlete on his team. During his description of the athlete's behavior, he complains of the athlete's lack of assertiveness, procrastination, constant criticism of others, and evasiveness. What type of behavior does this profile?
    A. Obsessive-compulsive
    B. Passive-aggressive
    C. Anxiety disorder
    D. Depression
    E. Post-traumatic stress disorder

3. Which of the behaviors below are seen with abuse of anabolic steroids?
    I. Mania
    II. Depression
    III. Anxiety
    IV. Psychosis
    V. Hyperactivity
    VI. Insomnia

    A. III, V, VI
    B. I, II
    C. V, VI
    D. I, II, III, VI
    E. II, III, IV, V

4. Which of the following is not a stage of the general adaptation syndrome (response phases of stress)?
    A. Exhaustion
    B. Anger
    C. Resistance
    D. Alarm
    E. All of the above

5. An athlete who is "burned out" may display which of the following symptoms?
    A. Negative self-concept
    B. Chronic fatigue
    C. Negative attitude toward his teammates
    D. Headaches
    E. All of the above

6. At the time of injury the athlete experiences a great deal of stress. The athlete responds to this stressor by passing through three psychophysiological phases. During which of the following phases is the adrenal gland most active?
    A. Exhaustive
    B. Resistance
    C. Anger
    D. Alarm
    E. Frustration

7. You notice one of your basketball players is showing signs of overtraining. Which of the following would not be an appropriate response to an overtrained athlete by the athletic trainer?
    A. Listening to the athlete's fears
    B. A tapered decrease in training over a period of 1 week
    C. An abrupt cessation of training
    D. Counseling the athlete in relaxation techniques
    E. All of the above

8. Which of the following must the athlete feel if he or she is to have a good rapport with the athletic trainer?
    A. Neglect
    B. Empathy
    C. Pity
    D. Love
    E. Trust

9. How might an athletic trainer assist the athlete in helping him- or herself heal after an injury?
    A. Provide the athlete access to painkillers
    B. Help the athlete "visualize" the healing process through imagery
    C. Give the athlete articles to read about his or her injury
    D. Make sure therapeutic modalities are applied in the correct sequence
    E. Move the athlete through rehabilitation as rapidly as possible

10. After a wrestler is injured, you notice he has developed a very negative attitude and is generally depressed. Two methods of redirecting this athlete's negative and angry ideas are _____ and _____.
    A. Thought stopping, refuting irrational thoughts
    B. Meditation, progressive relaxation
    C. Therapeutic imagery, attention diversion
    D. Thought stopping, mediation
    E. None of the above

11. While rehabilitating an athlete, you find he is excessively willing to do "whatever it takes" to recover fully and as quickly as possible. In doing so, you often have to remind the athlete not to push himself too hard and do too much. Which of the following is not a possible cause of overcompliance?
    A. Obsessive-compulsive behavior
    B. Slight feelings of denial
    C. Masking an underlying fear
    D. Manic-depressive behavior
    E. B and C

12. During a football player's rehabilitation of a fractured lower leg, he will experience moments of intense pain. What may the athletic trainer suggest to the athlete as a means of controlling his own pain?
    A. Rehearse various plays in his mind
    B. Scream at the top of his lungs
    C. Tell the athletic trainer to stop when he feels a little discomfort
    D. Only come to therapy when no other athlete or coach is in the room
    E. Tell him it is going to hurt and not to complain

13. You notice after a severe wrist injury a gymnast you have been treating becomes sarcastic, loses her appetite, and appears unusually fatigued all the time. These are all symptoms of what?
    A. Denial
    B. Anxiety
    C. Bulimia
    D. Anorexia
    E. Depression

14. An athlete must be _____ and take _____ if he or she is to completely rehabilitate an injury.
    A. Emotionless, time off
    B. Passive, all prescribed medications
    C. Cooperative, responsibility
    D. Dependent, time off
    E. Aggressive, responsibility

15. Purging is a major symptom of what?
    A. Bulimia
    B. Anorexia nervosa
    C. Obsessive-compulsive disorder
    D. Manic depression
    E. None of the above

16. Just before a big game, one of your athletes is demonstrating symptoms of moderate anxiety. Which of the following responses would be appropriate when caring for the athlete?
    A. Tell the athlete to "get a grip on himself"
    B. Tell the athlete you feel sorry for him
    C. Tell the athlete to talk to the coach
    D. Tell the athlete it is okay to be nervous but to focus on his goal
    E. Tell the athlete you will ask the team physician to prescribe an anti-depressant

17. While treating an athlete for chronic patellar tendinitis, his coach tells you it is tough to get the athlete motivated to practice and his performance has significantly declined since the beginning of the season. What might the athletic trainer suspect the problem might be?
    A. Undertraining
    B. Staleness
    C. A personality disorder
    D. The athlete is accident-prone
    E. Bipolar disorder

18. An athlete who will be experiencing a long rehabilitation process and may have his position filled by another player may be at risk for which problem?
    A. Schizophrenia
    B. Mania
    C. Severe depression
    D. Bipolar disorder
    E. Personality disorder

19. What would be an appropriate action for the athletic trainer to take to relax an athlete who is very anxious about his injury?
    A. Teach the athlete about his injury
    B. Teach the athlete about controlled breathing
    C. Have the athlete speak with the school nurse
    D. Downplay the injury
    E. All of the above

20. An athlete is injured during an ice hockey game, and after being examined by the team physician is diagnosed with a complete anterior cruciate ligament tear. You have been told by the doctor this athlete cannot compete the rest of the season. When you see the athlete the next day he states, "The doctor doesn't know what he is talking about. I'll be fine." This athlete is demonstrating what behavior?
    A. Hysteria
    B. Depression
    C. Anger
    D. Bargaining
    E. Denial

21. Which of the following actions taken by the athletic trainer can help make the athlete more compliant with rehabilitation of an injury?
    A. Have the coach threaten to kick him off the team if he does not cooperate
    B. Have the athlete bring a friend to the rehabilitation session
    C. Plan the rehabilitation sessions around the athlete's daily routine
    D. Make the rehabilitation sessions "fun"
    E. All of the above

22. Which of the following factors has a significant impact on the amount of stress an athlete will experience during his or her recovery from an injury?
    A. Whether or not soothing music is played in the athletic training room
    B. Whether or not the coach is present during treatment
    C. Whether or not the same athletic trainer renders care
    D. The degree to which the athlete perceives he or she has control over his or her care
    E. The amount of pressure the athletes family places on him/her to play

23. An athlete who wipes off his golf clubs after every shot and constantly makes sure it is returned to exactly the same spot in his bag every time it is used is demonstrating which of the following behaviors?
    A. Obsessive-compulsive
    B. Anxiety disorder
    C. Staleness
    D. Overachievement
    E. Obsessive defiant disorder

24. Which of the following techniques allows the athlete to assess his or her own efforts at controlling a specific physiological response, such as muscular tension?
    A. Moist heat pack
    B. Biofeedback
    C. Massage
    D. PNF
    E. Imagery

25. The anorexic female is usually a _____ and an _____.
    A. Hypochondriac, underachiever
    B. Perfectionist, overachiever
    C. Type B individual, underachiever
    D. Neurotic individual, antisocial personality
    E. Type A individual, amusing personality

26. An athlete becomes hysterical after learning she has suffered a severe shoulder injury and cannot compete in her sport anymore. She is crying, screaming, and generally appears out of control. The appropriate response from the athletic trainer would be which of the following?
    A. Find her coach and have him deal with her
    B. Call her parents and have one of them calm her down
    C. Give the athlete "space"
    D. Allow the athlete to express her fears but remain calm and demonstrate understanding. Assist the athlete in seeing the problem in proportion to the situation
    E. Tell the athlete she is acting like a three year old

27. You have an athlete who comes to your office and is very depressed. He is not doing well academically, his parents are in the process of a divorce, and the coach just cut him from the baseball team after tryouts. He tells you he wants to kill himself. What is your appropriate response?
    A. Tell the athlete he should see a psychiatrist
    B. Listen to the athlete, take him seriously, and consult the team doctor immediately
    C. Tell the athlete he is not normal
    D. Ignore the athlete and hope he will not do anything
    E. Tell the athlete he is just looking for attention

Nutrition

1. In which of the following foods is a high concentration of vitamin A found?
    A. Liver, yogurt, milk
    B. Red meat, oranges, tea
    C. Nuts, cereals, fish
    D. Liver, carrots, greens
    E. None of the above

2. What is also known as vitamin C?
    A. Retinol
    B. Thiamin
    C. Ascorbic acid
    D. Niacin
    E. Folic acid

3. Besides sources such as fortified milk and fatty fish oils (such as in tuna fish), what is another major mode of obtaining vitamin D?
    A. Topical creams
    B. Sunlight
    C. Artichokes
    D. Fried beef liver
    E. None of the above

4. What is the conversion of glucose to lactic acid called?
    A. Photosynthesis
    B. Glycolysis
    C. Lactolysis
    D. The Krebs cycle
    E. Glycogenosis

5. When is the best time for an athlete to eat carbohydrate-rich foods?
    A. Within 2 hours after training
    B. 1 hour prior to training
    C. In small amounts while training
    D. A half-hour prior to training and throughout the training session
    E. Four to six hours after training

6. At low workloads, muscle cells use _____ for fuel, while _____ is used for periods of intense exercise of short duration.
    A. Fat, protein
    B. Carbohydrate, fat
    C. Fat, phosphocreatine
    D. Protein, carbohydrate
    E. Glycogen, protein

7. In which of the following foods would be a high concentration of the mineral phosphorus be found?
    A. Potatoes
    B. Dark green vegetables
    C. Oranges
    D. Table salt
    E. Milk and cheese

8. Which of the following are the "building blocks" of protein?
    A. Sugars
    B. Amino acids
    C. Triglycerides
    D. Sterols
    E. All of the above

9. The loss of _____ and _____ account for the greatest percentage of electrolytes lost through sweat.
    A. Potassium, chloride
    B. Magnesium, potassium
    C. Sodium, potassium
    D. Potassium, zinc
    E. Sodium, chloride

10. All of the following statements regarding fluid replacement during performance are appropriate except:
    A. The athlete should drink cold fluids to decrease body core temperature
    B. It is best for the athlete to consume small amounts of fluids frequently rather than large amounts of fluid infrequently
    C. Water is the ideal fluid replacement
    D. Do not force fluids on the athlete; he or she will seek out fluid replacement when thirsty
    E. A and B

11. Which of the categories below are not considered one of the six classes of nutrients?
    I.   Carbohydrates
    II. Proteins
    III. Antioxidants
    IV. Water
    V.   Fats
    VI. Vitamins

    A. I, IV
    B. II, V
    C. V, VI
    D. III
    E. I, II

12. Which of the following nutrients is absolutely necessary for every body chemical reaction to take place normally?
    A. Vitamins
    B. Amino acids
    C. Water
    D. Fats
    E. All of the above

13. Nutrition labels that are found on food packages allow the purchaser to compare nutritional values of food and are expressed in "percent daily values" (based on a 2000-calorie diet) that follow a new nutrient label, which used to be known as the US recommended daily allowance (US RDA). What new standards does the new label now follow?
    A. Recommended percent nutrients (RPN)
    B. US RDA
    C. Reference daily intakes (RDI)
    D. US advised allowances (US AA)
    E. None of the above

14. All of the following are methods of measuring body composition except:
    A. Measuring muscle and fat girths
    B. Hydrostatic weighing
    C. Electrical impedance
    D. Measuring skin-fold thickness
    E. C and D

15. Weight loss occurs when which of the following conditions exists?
    A. Less than 1000 calories are expended per day
    B. There is a negative caloric balance
    C. There is a positive caloric balance
    D. There is perfect caloric balance
    E. None of the above

16. Fat is a nutrient that is utilized as an energy source in the form of triglycerides. Triglycerides are stored in what type of cell?
    A. Striated
    B. Lypoma
    C. Beta
    D. White blood cells
    E. Adipose

17. A football player desires to increase his body weight and wants to know how he should go about it in a safe manner. To increase his muscle mass without causing negative results, both his _____ and _____ should increase appropriately.
    A. Fat intake, carbohydrate intake
    B. Muscular exercise, dietary intake
    C. Dietary intake, caloric expenditure
    D. Caloric expenditure, water intake
    E. None of the above

18. One of your female cheerleaders has been diagnosed by your team physician with a combination of anorexia, osteoporosis, and amenorrhea. You recognize this combination as signs of what?
    A. Marfan syndrome
    B. The unhappy triad
    C. Female triad syndrome
    D. Paget's disease
    E. Bone cancer

19. One of your gymnasts has had a bone density test that has come back positive for mild osteoporosis. Which of the following minerals should be supplemented to prevent osteoporosis in a high-risk athlete?
    A. Folate
    B. Niacin
    C. Folic acid
    D. Fluoride
    E. Calcium

20. One of your male cross-county runners is a committed lactovegetarian. Which of the following minerals may be deficient with this type of diet?
    A. Calcium, fluoride
    B. Iron, zinc
    C. Folic acid
    D. Copper, iron
    E. None of the above

21. One of your athletes goes out of his way to avoid eating carbohydrates, such as bread and potatoes, because of his fear of becoming fat. Which of the following substances will the body begin to utilize for energy if there is a significant lack of carbohydrates in the diet?
    A. Protein
    B. Fat
    C. Glucose
    D. Antioxidants
    E. None of the above

22. An athlete routinely complains of bloating, flatulence, and diarrhea after ingesting milk or ice cream. What might be the cause of this athlete's symptoms?
    A. Proteinuria
    B. Rickets
    C. Scurvy
    D. Lactase deficiency
    E. None of the above

23. Significant losses of electrolytes, such as sodium, chloride, potassium, or magnesium, during heavy exercise may lead to symptoms such as _____ or _____.
    A. Drop in pressure, diuresis
    B. Muscle strains, ligament strains
    C. Dyspnea, indigestion
    D. Muscular cramps, heat illness
    E. None of the above

24. Which two structures regulate water excretion?
    A. Kidneys, brain
    B. Kidneys, bladder
    C. Stomach, small intestines
    D. Kidneys, ureters
    E. Adrenal glands, thyroid

25. One of your baseball players reports he is having difficulty playing in the outfield under lights and has similar difficulty seeing at night while driving. While evaluating him you find out he hates vegetables and drinks milk infrequently. He "enjoys hamburgers and french fries." What substance might this athlete be lacking in his diet?
    A. Carbohydrates
    B. Protein
    C. Vitamin A
    D. Phosphorus
    E. None of the above

Pharmacology

1. Lomotil is what type of medication?
    A. Antibiotic
    B. Antidiarrheal
    C. Antifungal agent
    D. Antiemetic
    E. Antipyretic

2. Which of the following medications is often used for depression?
    A. Relafen
    B. Lithium
    C. Midol
    D. Ritalin
    E. Prozac

3. All of the following substances have stimulant properties except:
    A. Nicotine
    B. Theophylline
    C. Pseudoephedrine
    D. Caffeine
    E. Pepcid

4. Ibuprofen is available in which of the below dosages?
   I. 400 mg
   II. 200 mg
   III. 600 mg
   IV. 50 mg
   V. 100 mg
   VI. 800 mg

   A. II, IV, V
   B. II, III, V
   C. III, V, VI
   D. I, II, III, VI
   E. III, IV, V

5. What is the brand name for the NSAID diclofenac?
   A. Indocin
   B. Voltaren
   C. Orudis
   D. Feldene
   E. Relafan

6. What is the recommended dosage for the NSAID Naprosyn?
   A. 250 to 500 mg twice a day
   B. 500 to 750 mg twice a day
   C. 50 to 100 mg twice a day
   D. 200 mg once a day
   E. None of the above

7. Frequently abused drugs include stimulants such as amphetamines (speed), cocaine (coke or crack), and depressants (alcohol or downers). An athlete who has overdosed on a stimulant would manifest all of the following signs except:
   A. Agitation
   B. Decreased reaction time
   C. Rapid pulse and respirations
   D. Convulsions
   E. Arrythmias

8. Beta-blockers inhibit the action of catecholamines and decrease cardiac output. In which of the following sports would the effects of beta-blockers potentially enhance performance?
   A. Swimming
   B. Long-distance running
   C. Archery
   D. Baseball
   E. All of the above

9. In moderation, caffeine stimulates the _____ and _____ centers of the brain, causing increased alertness.
   A. Cerebral cortex, medulla
   B. Reticular formation, medulla
   C. Hypothalamus, midbrain
   D. Cerebellum, midbrain
   E. Brain stem, midbrain

10. Which of the following is not an adverse effect associated with the abuse of human growth hormone?
   A. Laryngeal thickening
   B. Hypercalciuria
   C. Hypertrophic neuropathy
   D. Mandibular growth
   E. Diarrhea

Physics

1. The area of the applicator that emits ultrasound and is expressed in square centimeters (cm^2) is known as what?
   A. The transducer head surface area
   B. Effective emitting area
   C. Effective radiating area
   D. Direct-contact area
   E. The sound head

2. What is the frequency range of therapeutic ultrasound?
   A. 1.0 to 3.0 MHz
   B. 0.1 to 1 MHz
   C. 10,000 to 20,000 Hz
   D. 10,000 to 30,000 Hz
   E. None of the above

3. An object immersed in water experiences an upward force that is equal to the weight of the water displaced by the object. What law of physics is this?
   A. Archimedes' principle
   B. Wolff's law
   C. Pascal's law
   D. Bernoulli's law
   E. Newton's third law

4. A TENS unit is based on the _____ of pain control.
   A. Counter irritant theory
   B. Gate control theory
   C. Beta-endorphin theory
   D. Opiate theory
   E. Distraction theory

5. A pulsed current may be _____ or _____.
    A. Monophasic, biphasic
    B. Alternating, direct
    C. Direct, monophasic
    D. Alternating, biphasic
    E. None of the above

6. What is the most commonly used frequency in short-wave diathermy?
    A. 10 MHz
    B. 27.33 MHz
    C. 4068 Hz
    D. 2450 MHz
    E. None of the above

7. Which modality produces electromagnetic radiation with a frequency above 300 MHz and a wavelength shorter than 1 m?
    A. Infrared diathermy
    B. Short-wave diathermy
    C. Microwave diathermy
    D. Induction field diathermy
    E. None of the above

8. All of the following may be settings on a TENS unit except:
    A. Modulating
    B. Burst
    C. Continuous
    D. Ramp
    E. Surge

9. What kind of current is needed for iontophoresis?
    A. Interferential
    B. Alternating
    C. Alternating or direct
    D. Ionized
    E. Direct

10. Which of the following is the correct definition of work?
    A. W = distance x velocity
    B. W = force x power
    C. W = force x distance
    D. W = pressure x distance
    E. None of the above

11. To perform iontophoresis, the medication used must be _____.
    A. Diluted
    B. Neutralized
    C. In powder form
    D. Mixed with a gel
    E. Ionized

12. According to Joule's law, heat produced by high-frequency electrical currents is directly proportional to all of the following except:
    A. Power output
    B. Square of the current strength
    C. Resistance of the conductor
    D. Time during which the current flows
    E. C and D

13. In the application of electrotherapy, the strength of an electrical current in a circuit is directly proportional to the applied electromotive force and inversely proportional to the resistance of the current. What law does this describe?
    A. Cosine's
    B. Cowling's
    C. Joule's
    D. Wolff's
    E. Ohm's

14. By what means does heat transfer to the skin with the use of a hot pack?
    A. Conduction
    B. Convection
    C. Radiation
    D. Evaporation
    E. All of the above

15. What type of waveform is produced when the current flow direction reverses on regular intervals?
    A. Galvanic current
    B. Pulsed current
    C. Alternating current
    D. Faradic current
    E. None of the above

16. The temperature of a thermometer reading is given in degrees Celsius. What formula must be used to convert the temperature from Celsius to Fahrenheit?
    A. (Temperature in Fahrenheit – 32) x 5/9
    B. (Temperature in Celsius – 32) x 5/9
    C. (Temperature in Celsius x 9/5) + 32
    D. (Temperature in Celsius + 32) x 5/9
    E. None of the above

17. What is the impedance of an electrical circuit?
    A. The pathway in which a current will flow
    B. The magnitude of the current flow
    C. The resistance within the circuit
    D. The direction of current flow
    E. The frequency of current flow

18. An athlete is evaluated by the athletic trainer and it is determined he has acute supraspinatus tendinitis. Which of the following modalities is not appropriate to decrease pain and inflammation of the tendon?
    A. Phonophoresis
    B. Iontophoresis
    C. Ice packs
    D. Ice massage
    E. Moist heat packs

19. The strength of a current flow is known as what?
    A. Rheobase
    B. Resistance
    C. Amperage
    D. Voltage
    E. None of the above

20. According to Poiseuille's law, the _____ and _____ of a blood vessel are very critical in terms of resistance to blood flow.
    A. Length, radius
    B. Muscle type, contractility
    C. Length, thickness
    D. Direction, temperature
    E. Direction, radius

21. Which of the following intensities is considered medium intensity when treating an area with ultrasound?
    A. 0.8 to 1.5 watts per square cm
    B. 1.5 to 2.0 watts per square cm
    C. 1.0 to 3.0 total watts
    D. 5.0 to 8.0 total watts
    E. < 0.8 watts per square cm

22. How far from the skin surface should the ultrasound transducer head be kept when utilizing the underwater technique?
    A. Between 1 and 3 in
    B. 3 in
    C. 5 in
    D. 0.5 to 1 in from the skin surface
    E. 3 to 5 inches

23. What is the polarity of an anode in an electrical stimulator?
    A. Disperse
    B. Negative
    C. Positive
    D. Neutral
    E. The anode has no polarity

WRITTEN SIMULATION SAMPLE QUESTIONS

Chapter 4

This section is used to evaluate your critical thinking and decision-making skills in a manner similar to what you have to do when taking the BOC certification exam. Six questions from this section can be accessed online. The intent of the computer-based Written Simulation questions is to provide you with feedback. In addition to feedback, this section will offer practice with computer-based testing. Please see the enclosed slip of paper for further information, URL, and password for the online test.

A passing mark for each section of the following questions must be 80%. The passing mark is arrived by the number of correct responses encompassing 80% of the total number of questions per section. The authors recommend that if you do not pass a section at an 80% level, that you review the material that is relevant to that particular section. Please note that the actual calculation used to score the simulation section of the BOC certification exam differs from the scoring presented in this text.

Assign the appropriate value from the list identified below:

KEY

++ = Most appropriate answer

+ = Appropriate, but not first priority

0 = No relevance to the problem

- = Not a priority/harmful

-- = Detrimental

For example: Opening scene: One of your wrestlers comes to the athletic training room complaining of severe itching and burning sensation of the top of his scalp. He has noticed a lot of skin flaking with some hair loss.

Section A

How will you begin your evaluation of this athlete's condition? (Please select and prioritize your choices).

___ 1. Ask the athlete if he has had this problem before.

___ 2. Put gloves on and examine the athlete's scalp.

___ 3. Ask the athlete if he has had a recent cold.

___ 4. Administer an oral antibiotic medication from your athletic training kit.

___ 5. Use the athlete's teammate's towel to clean the area.

Section A (answers)

The current situation: You know that your athlete has a dermatological problem.

Your immediate responsibility: To perform your initial evaluation to determine the type and extent of the problem.

1. +) It is appropriate to ask the athlete if he has had this problem before because he may be able to provide you with important information regarding this condition.

2. ++) It is necessary and proper to don gloves and examine the athlete's scalp to determine the type and extent of this lesion.

3. 0) Asking the athlete if he has had a recent cold has no relevance to this problem.

4. --) It is not within the athletic trainer's scope of practice to administer a prescription drug without the direction of a supervising medical doctor.

5. -) This is an inappropriate action because this condition could be contagious, and using another individual's towel is not sanitary.

PROBLEM I

Opening Scene

A gymnast injures his right lower leg after a dismount off the rings. He appears to be in a lot of pain and has not stood up. He is lying on his left side. You did not witness this event.

Section A

How will you begin your initial evaluation of the athlete's condition? (Please select and prioritize your choices.)

___1. Ask the athlete what happened.
___2. Ask the athlete if he heard a snap.
___3. Check the right knee range of motion.
___4. Observe the leg for edema or bleeding.
___5. Palpate the leg for deformity.
___6. Check the athlete's vital signs.
___7. Palpate the athlete's popliteal pulse.
___8. Place a moist heat pack directly on the injury.
___9. Elevate the right leg.
___10. Have a coach call for an ambulance.
___11. Check the rest of his body for any other injuries.
___12. Cut away the gymnast's pant leg (uniform).
___13. Immediately immobilize the lower right leg.

Section B

You have ruled out a compound fracture but suspect a fracture of both the tibia and fibula. With this information, how would you proceed at this time? (Please select and prioritize your choices.)

___14. If there is an obvious deformity of the bony shaft, try to reduce it to get good alignment.
___15. Remove the athlete from the mat to apply an immobilizer.
___16. Direct others to clear the area of people and equipment.
___17. Pack the right leg in ice.
___18. Check pulses in the ankle and foot.
___19. Check for Volkmann's contracture.

___20. Allow the competition to continue.
___21. Position the athlete in a supine position.
___22. Palpate the right hip joint.
___23. Elevate the entire leg.
___24. Check for crepitus.
___25. Immobilize the right lower leg.
___26. Massage the injured area.

Section C

The EMS team has arrived, and the athlete is about to be transported to the emergency room. What are your final steps before he leaves with the EMS team? (Please select and prioritize your choices.)

___27. Check the lower extremity for numbness.
___28. Have the athlete walk to the ambulance with crutches.
___29. Issue NSAIDs for swelling.
___30. Have the coach follow the athlete to the hospital.
___31. Allow the athlete to eat and drink whatever he wants.
___32. Notify the coach that the athlete will no longer be permitted to participate for the rest of the season.
___33. Call ahead to the emergency room to make arrangements for his arrival.
___34. Check the athlete for symptoms of shock.
___35. Assure the athlete he will be taken care of before he departs.
___36. Fit the athlete for crutches.
___37. Call the athlete's parents.
___38. Fill out an injury report.

PROBLEM II

Opening Scene

A field hockey player who is playing defense gets hit in the eye with a ball during a direct shot at the goal. She is lying on her side with her hands on her face.

Section A

How will you begin to evaluate the severity of the injury? (Please select and prioritize your choices.)

___1. Remove the face mask.
___2. Check that athlete's fine motor skills.
___3. Test the athlete's balance.
___4. Use an ammonia capsule to revive the athlete.
___5. Have the athlete walk off the field.
___6. Remove the mouthguard.
___7. Ask who made the shot.
___8. Ask the athlete where the pain is located.

Written Simulation Sample Questions   117

__9. Palpate the athlete's shoulders.

__10. Perform a primary survey.

__11. Gently palpate the area around the orbit and nose for crepitus.

__12. Don latex gloves.

__13. Observe for a "battle sign."

__14. Ask the athlete if she is a scholarship athlete.

__15. Check the area for bleeding and lacerations.

__16. Ask the athlete if her vision is blurred.

Section B

The athlete has a deep laceration above the left eyebrow. Based on this information, what are your next steps? (Please select and prioritize your choices.)

__17. Check the pupil for reflex movements with a penlight.

__18. Apply moist heat to the eye.

__19. Rinse the wound with saline solution.

__20. Apply antiseptic ointment to the laceration.

__21. Cover both eyes with gauze pads.

__22. Have the athlete tell you what happened.

__23. Apply ice to the injury.

__24. Use Steri-Strips to close the laceration.

__25. Ignore the athlete if she asks if there will be a scar.

__26. Use sutures to close the wound.

__27. Call for an ambulance.

__28. Have the athlete wait outside for the ambulance.

__29. Apply compression directly to the eye once you have "closed" the laceration.

__30. Perform a secondary survey.

Section C

You now have the laceration "closed" and are awaiting the ambulance. What are your final steps going to include? (Please select and prioritize your choices.)

__31. Keep the athlete calm.

__32. Announce the athlete's status over the public address system.

__33. Check the athlete's insurance plan.

__34. Call the school nurse to accompany the athlete to the hospital.

__35. Constantly change the bandage.

__36. Allow the athlete to speak to her coach.

__37. Allow the press access to the athlete.

__38. Wash your hands.

__39. Document the incident on an accident report form.

__40. Give the athlete a vitamin E pill.

__41. Report your findings and treatment plan to the athlete's coach.

PROBLEM III

Opening Scene

While covering a state track meet, you observe a high jumper land incorrectly on the crash mat. When you get to the high jump pit, you see him lying on his right side and he is not moving.

Section A

Given the above information, what would your initial steps be in evaluating the condition of this athlete? (Please select and prioritize your choices.)

__1. Call for an ambulance.

__2. Ask the athlete where he has pain.

__3. Do a primary survey.

__4. Make a mental note as to how the athlete is positioned.

__5. With assistance from an athletic training student, turn the athlete onto his back.

__6. Ask the athlete to wiggle his fingers and toes.

__7. Ask the athlete what occurred.

__8. Place an ice pack on the athlete's neck.

__9. Palpate the athlete's knees for deformity.

__10. Check the athlete for any areas of bleeding on his face.

__11. Send for the athlete's parents.

__12. Check the athlete's level of consciousness.

Section B

After speaking to the athlete and completing your initial evaluation, you suspect a potentially serious neck injury. What would your next steps be in caring for this athlete? (Please select and prioritize your choices.)

__13. With assistance, carry the athlete to the sidelines.

__14. To determine the severity of the injury, see if the athlete can rotate his head.

__15. Ask the athlete if he has any numbness or tingling down either upper extremity.

__16. Tell the athlete to not move his head.

__17. Check the athlete's pupillary response with a penlight.

__18. Do a check of cranial nerves IV through XII.

__19. With the assistance of at least two to four other people and while maintaining the head in neutral, log-roll the athlete into a supine position.

__20. Ask the officials to stop the meet.

__21. Secure the athlete on a spine board.

__22. Ask someone to call an ambulance.

__23. Place the athlete in a cervical collar.

__24. Monitor the athlete's vital signs.

Section C

The athlete is brought by ambulance to the hospital. What would your next actions be? (Please select and prioritize your choices.)

__25. Contact your team physician.

__26. Fill out an accident report form.

__27. Return to the meet and follow-up with the athlete at a later time.

__28. Check your records to see if the athlete is allergic to any medications.

__29. Check with the coach to see if the athlete is on a scholarship.

__30. Contact the athlete's parents to inform them of the accident.

__31. Follow the ambulance to the hospital and leave your senior athletic training student to cover the meet.

__32. Suggest to the athletic director that the school should eliminate the high jump event next time because it is too dangerous.

PROBLEM IV

Opening Scene

One of your female cross-country runners comes into the athletic training room complaining of chronic left anterior knee pain, which comes and goes with activity.

Section A

Your initial evaluation of this problem would include which of the following actions? (Please select and prioritize your choices.)

__1. Put an ice pack on the athlete's knee.

__2. Observe the athlete's posture.

__3. Palpate the anteromedial joint line for tenderness and swelling.

__4. Perform a bilateral Ober's test.

__5. Ask the athlete if she feels a popping sensation while walking or running.

__6. Ask the athlete if she has ever injured her foot before.

__7. Perform a Patrick's test.

__8. Ask the athlete if the knee hurts going up and down stairs.

__9. Tell the athlete to stop running when it hurts.

__10. See how the athlete responds to temporary orthotics.

__11. Observe the left knee for swelling.

__12. Palpate the patellar area for tenderness.

__13. Perform a KT-1000 test.

Section B

After your initial evaluation, you conclude this athlete has a chronically subluxing patella. What steps would you take at this time to treat this athlete? (Please select and prioritize your choices.)

__14. Recommend the athlete wear a soft brace to stabilize the patella during running.

__15. Teach the athlete exercises to strengthen her hamstrings.

__16. Teach the athlete exercises to strengthen her left VMO.

__17. Tell the athlete to perform deep squatting exercises two to three times per day.

__18. Evaluate the effect of patellar taping with activity.

__19. Teach the athlete iliotibial band stretching exercises.

__20. Tell the athlete to consistently stretch her hamstrings.

__21. Give the athlete Voltaren.

__22. Tell the athlete to avoid soft, flat surfaces while running.

Section C

To speed up this athlete's rehabilitation, you decide she should come to see you on a daily basis for treatment in the athletic training room. Which activities/treatments would you perform for this condition? (Please select and prioritize your choices.)

__23. Apply a TENS unit to the left knee for pain.

__24. Perform PNF exercises, which emphasize hip flexion, abduction, and internal rotation.

__25. Apply ultrasound treatments to promote healing.

__26. Instruct the athlete in plyometric activities.

__27. Have the athlete perform both open- and closed-chain quadriceps exercises.

__28. Evaluate the athlete's running gait on a treadmill.

__29. Have the athlete perform exercises that strengthen the hip adductors.

__30. Routinely apply ice packs to the affected knee after activity.

PROBLEM V

Opening Scene

The pitcher from your baseball team comes to the training room with complaints of a deep ache in his right shoulder, which occurs after pitching and lingers for a number of hours after he stops the activity. He also states his right arm feels unusually fatigued after throwing a short period of time. He reports his shoulder feels the best when he has his right hand in his pants pocket. You have seen him voluntarily sublux his shoulders in the past as he was telling his friends he is double-jointed.

Section A

What questions would be appropriate to ask during the history portion of your initial exam? (Please select and prioritize your choices.)

___ 1. How long he has had this problem.
___ 2. When the last time his right shoulder was injured.
___ 3. What specific actions/positions make the pain worse.
___ 4. If he is eating enough protein.
___ 5. If his shoulder feels like it slips with activity.
___ 6. If he is double-jointed.
___ 7. If he is taking his vitamins.
___ 8. What the intensity of the pain is on a scale of 0 to 10 (0 representing no pain, 10 representing excruciating pain).
___ 9. If his father had the same problem when he played baseball.
___ 10. If he is taking any medications for the pain.

Section B

With the information obtained from the history, which of the following special tests would be appropriate when examining his shoulder? (Please select and prioritize your choices.)

___ 11. Phalen's test.
___ 12. Clunk test.
___ 13. Pivot shift test.
___ 14. Patrick's test.
___ 15. Thompson's test.
___ 16. Apprehension test (anterior and posterior).
___ 17. Hawkins-Kennedy test.
___ 18. Neer's sign.
___ 19. Posterior drawer test (of the shoulder).
___ 20. Ober's test.
___ 21. Trendelenburg's test.
___ 22. Sulcus sign.

Section C

After completing your evaluation, you suspect the athlete has multidirectional instability of the right shoulder. Knowing what you do about this condition, which of the following exercises would be appropriate to specifically strengthen the scapular stabilizers and rotator cuff musculature? (Please select and prioritize your choices.)

___ 23. Shoulder shrugs.
___ 24. Biceps curls.
___ 25. Shoulder abduction exercises with free weights.
___ 26. Cervical isometric exercises.
___ 27. Internal/external rotation of the shoulder using a Theraband.
___ 28. Manual PNF exercises (D2 extension pattern).
___ 29. Triceps curls.
___ 30. Rowing exercises.
___ 31. Serratus anterior strengthening exercises.
___ 32. Partial sit-ups.
___ 33. Prone trunk extensions.
___ 34. Calf raises.

PROBLEM VI

Opening Scene

You are covering a tennis match when one player runs to the net for a volley, stops and sets for the shot, and suddenly falls to the court while grabbing his left lower leg. He is in severe pain.

Section A

With the information you have available, how will you begin your initial evaluation of this injury? (Please select and prioritize your choices.)

___ 1. Establish if the athlete is breathing.
___ 2. Ask the athlete to walk off the court.
___ 3. Ask the athlete what happened.
___ 4. Determine the athlete's level of consciousness according to the Glasgow Coma Scale.
___ 5. Check the athlete's leg for bleeding.
___ 6. Ask the athlete where the pain is located.
___ 7. Observe the left lower extremity for any deformity.
___ 8. Ask the athlete if he felt a snap or pop.
___ 9. Have an athletic training student apply an ice bag to the leg.
___ 10. Ask the athlete if he has ever injured his right leg before.
___ 11. Ask the athlete if he can hop on the left leg.

Section B

You assist the athlete off the court and have him sit on a bench. What actions would you perform at this time? (Please select and prioritize your choices.)

___12. Palpate the calf for pain, swelling, or deformity.

___13. Perform a Lachman's test bilaterally.

___14. Perform a Thomas test bilaterally.

___15. Check active range of motion of both ankles.

___16. Measure the Q-angle of the right leg.

___17. Check to see if the athlete has bunions.

___18. Perform a Thompson's test bilaterally.

___19. Perform a Hawkin's test bilaterally.

___20. Perform an anterior drawer test bilaterally on both ankles.

___21. Palpate the left femoral pulse.

___22. Test the patellar tendon reflex bilaterally.

___23. Manually muscle test the ankle plantar flexors bilaterally.

Section C

Based on your initial assessment, you determine the athlete has a torn gastrocnemius muscle. The athlete is transported to the athletic training room in a golf cart. What would your initial treatment consist of during week 1? (Please select and prioritize your choices.)

___24. Warm whirlpool treatments.

___25. Applying ice packs to the lower leg.

___26. Applying a compression wrap.

___27. High volt galvanic stimulation.

___28. Posterior lower leg splint.

___29. Range of motion exercises on the biomechanical ankle platform system (BAPS) board.

___30. Calf raises.

___31. Fitting the athlete with crutches.

___32. Applying an antibiotic ointment to the defect.

___33. Begin hamstring curls with weight.

___34. Start ultrasound treatments.

___35. Begin gentle active range of motion exercises for the right ankle.

Section D

Four weeks have passed since the initial injury. The athlete has minimal/no discomfort with active plantar flexion, but the movement is still weak against resistance (4/5). All other ankle and knee motions are within normal ranges. Which of the following exercises would be appropriate? (Please select and prioritize your choices.)

___36. Stationary bike.

___37. Uphill jogging.

___38. Push-ups.

___39. Progressive-resistance ankle exercises.

___40. Plyometric exercises.

___41. Upper body ergometer.

___42. Proprioception exercises.

___43. Calf raises.

___44. Partial squats.

___45. Progressive-resistance hamstring exercises.

___46. Progressive-resistance quadriceps exercises.

___47. General lower extremity flexibility exercises.

___48. Biceps curls.

___49. Shoulder press.

___50. Agility exercises.

Section E

Six weeks have passed since the initial injury. The athlete has done very well during his rehabilitation. What specific criteria would you use to determine that this athlete is fully recovered and ready to participate in tennis? (Please select and prioritize your choices.)

___51. The athlete can walk 50 feet without a limp.

___52. The athlete has no complaints of lower extremity pain at rest or during activity.

___53. There is no visible swelling or ecchymosis.

___54. There is no pain with palpation of the injured area.

___55. The athlete has no pain while performing a hamstring curl.

___56. The athlete has full ankle and knee range of motion.

___57. The coach demands the athlete's return to competition.

___58. The athlete can hop on the injured leg without pain.

___59. The athlete can jog on the treadmill for 20 minutes without pain.

___60. The athlete is getting bored with his rehabilitation program.

___61. The strength of the athlete's left ankle and leg is equal to the right side.

___62. The team physician clears the athlete to return to full activity.

___63. The athlete can bench press 50 pounds or more.

PROBLEM VII

Opening Scene

You are covering a men's varsity basketball game when one of your players is observed injuring his right knee while rebounding a ball. He is able to limp off the court unassisted. He reports his knee bent sideways when he landed. He states he felt a sharp pain but cannot recall feeling a pop or snap.

Section A

What actions would you take during your initial assessment of this injury? (Please select and prioritize your choices.)

___ 1. Ask the athlete to point to where he feels pain.

___ 2. Observe the right knee for swelling or deformity.

___ 3. Apply an ice pack to the knee.

___ 4. Apply a knee immobilizer to the injured extremity.

___ 5. Issue a cane to the athlete.

___ 6. Palpate the right knee anterolateral/anteromedial joint line.

___ 7. Palpate the right gluteus medius muscle.

___ 8. Have the athlete perform 10 calf raises.

___ 9. Check the range of motion of both knee joints.

___10. Ask the athlete if he has ever injured his right knee before.

___11. Manually muscle test the strength of the hip flexors bilaterally.

___12. Manually muscle test the strength of the quadriceps bilaterally.

___13. Manually muscle test the strength of the hamstrings bilaterally.

___14. Check the athlete's pupillary reaction.

Section B

What special tests would you perform during your evaluation of this injury? (Please select and prioritize your choices.)

___15. Lachman's test bilaterally.

___16. Vertebral artery test bilaterally.

___17. Tinel's test bilaterally.

___18. Valgus stress test bilaterally.

___19. Varus stress test bilaterally.

___20. Posterior drawer test bilaterally.

___21. Empty can test bilaterally.

___22. Finkelstein test bilaterally.

___23. Yergason's test bilaterally.

___24. McMurray's test bilaterally.

___25. Anterior drawer test bilaterally.

___26. Pivot shift test bilaterally.

___27. Patellar apprehension test bilaterally.

Section C

After being examined by the team physician, the athlete is diagnosed with a second-degree medial collat-

eral sprain. What actions would you take to control the pain and swelling and address the limitations in range of motion? (Please select and prioritize your choices.)

___28. Apply moist heat packs to the right knee.

___29. Massage the knee joint.

___30. Have the athlete use a rowing machine.

___31. Fit the athlete with crutches.

___32. Manually muscle test the quadriceps.

___33. Begin isotonic hamstring strength exercises.

___34. Apply ice packs to the knee.

___35. Have the athlete perform active knee extension and flexion range of motion exercises as tolerated.

___36. Have the athlete elevate his left leg during the course of the day.

___37. Give the athlete Tylenol with codeine for pain.

___38. Use high-volt galvanic stimulation.

Section D

The team physician recommends the athlete begin rehabilitation in 1 week. Knowing the athlete will be unable to return to basketball for approximately 4 to 5 weeks, how would you go about beginning a functional exercise program and maintaining his aerobic condition during weeks 1 to 2 postinjury? (Please select and prioritize your choices.)

___39. Swimming (regular crawl).

___40. Calf raises.

___41. Running on the treadmill.

___42. Stairmaster (low resistance).

___43. Upper body ergometer.

___44. Wall pulley exercises (upper extremity).

___45. Stationary bicycling.

___46. Fartlek training.

___47. Plyometric exercises.

___48. Rowing machine.

Problem VIII

Opening Scene

A soccer player jumps up to head a ball. While he is in the air, he is kicked in the abdominal area by an opponent. He curls up in pain on the ground.

Section A

What steps would you take during your initial evaluation of this athlete? (Please select and prioritize your choices.)

___ 1. Perform a primary survey.

___ 2. Give the athlete oxygen.

___3. Ausculate the athlete's heart.

___4. Palpate the abdominal area.

___5. Ask the athlete where the pain is located.

___6. Have the athlete stand and jog a little.

___7. Have the athlete count backward from 100.

___8. Have an athletic training student bring out a stretcher.

___9. Put on a glove before touching the athlete.

___10. Observe the abdominal area for edema or ecchymosis.

___11. Ask if the pain radiates anywhere.

Section B

Following your initial evaluation, you have determined this athlete has sustained a contusion to the lower right quadrant. What actions would you take at this time? (Please select and prioritize your choices.)

___12. Apply an ice pack to the injured area.

___13. Apply a compression wrap to the injured area.

___14. Massage the athlete's lumbar area.

___15. Massage the athlete's abdominal area.

___16. Assist the athlete to walk off the field if he is able to do so.

___17. Apply a neoprene rib belt.

___18. Position the athlete in supine with his knees bent.

___19. Monitor the athlete for any changes in pain intensity.

___20. Take the athlete's pulse and blood pressure.

Section C

You follow up with the athlete the next day in the training room. He states he is sore but has less pain today. How would you treat this athlete at this time? (Please select and prioritize your choices.)

___21. Continue to apply ice to the injured area.

___22. Begin to apply moist heat packs.

___23. Manually muscle test the abdominal muscles.

___24. Re-evaluate the injury.

___25. Have the athlete drink a glass of Gatorade.

___26. Pad the area for activity.

___27. Have the athlete begin exercises on an upper body ergometer.

Problem IX

Opening Scene

Two soccer players collide head-on during a game. You are called onto the field by the referee after your player does not get up off his back. You did not witness the collision.

Section A

How will you begin your initial evaluation of the athlete's condition? (Please select and prioritize your choices.)

___1. Ask the athlete where his pain is located.

___2. Immediately roll the athlete onto his side.

___3. Check to see if the athlete can move his fingers and toes.

___4. As you approach the field, ask any witnesses what occurred.

___5. Check the athlete for any areas that may be bleeding.

___6. Instruct an athletic training student to call for an ambulance.

___7. Evaluate the athlete's level of consciousness.

___8. Perform a primary survey.

___9. Ask the athlete if he has ever had a prior head injury.

___10. Note the position of the athlete.

___11. Ask if the athlete can stand and walk.

___12. Check the athlete's pupillary reactions with a penlight.

___13. Place an ice pack on the athlete's left shoulder.

___14. Remove the athlete from the playing field.

___15. Ask the athlete if he can remember what happened and ask him to explain.

___16. Assess the athlete's pulse rate and blood pressure.

___17. Ask the athletic training student to get a spine board.

___18. Sit the athlete up to make breathing easier.

Section B

The athlete is able to get up and walk off the field to the sidelines without assistance. Based on the information you now have, what would you do next? (Please select and prioritize your choices.)

___19. Perform a secondary survey.

___20. Ask the athlete if he knows where he is, the date, and the name of his coach.

___21. Escort the athlete to the athletic training room and let him sleep.

___22. Give the athlete aspirin for a headache.

___23. Palpate the athlete's cervical area.

___24. Palpate the athlete's left upper trapezius muscle.

___25. Check the athlete's bilateral grip strength.

___26. Tell the coach the athlete is not to return to the game.

__27. Observe the athlete's posturing as he walks off the field.

__28. Note the athlete's skin color.

__29. Ask the athlete's parents what type of medical insurance they have.

__30. Call the team physician to gain guidance.

__31. Call the athlete's parents to make sure they arrange a doctor's visit the next day.

__32. Elevate the athlete's feet.

__33. Give the athlete a pair of crutches.

Section C

Your athletic training staff has escorted the athlete to the athletic training room. You meet the athlete there and reassess his injury. (Please select and prioritize your choices.)

__34. Record the athlete's vital signs every 10 minutes.

__35. Manually muscle test the upper trapezius muscle.

__36. Perform an Adson's test.

__37. Manually muscle test the deltoids.

__38. Manually muscle test the rotator cuff musculature.

__39. Have the athlete sit with his head between his knees.

__40. Have the athlete do a couple of deep squats.

__41. Ask the athlete to count backward from 50.

__42. Check the deep tendon reflex of the triceps bilaterally.

__43. Give the athlete oxygen via a mask.

__44. Have the team physician come to the athletic training room to reassess the injury.

__45. Have the athlete drive himself home.

__46. Check the athlete's sensation of the left upper arm.

__47. Check the active range of motion of the athlete's neck.

__48. Test for a Tinel's sign.

__49. Palpate the lateral epicondyle of the elbow for any tenderness.

__50. Manually muscle test the biceps.

__51. Manually muscle test the triceps.

Section D

The team physician has arrived and re-evaluated the athlete. He determines the athlete has a first-degree concussion and a left-sided "burner." What would you do at this time? (Please select and prioritize your choices.)

__52. Put an ice pack on the athlete's left shoulder.

__53. Assess if the athlete still has sensory changes in his left upper arm or hand.

__54. Let the coach know the athlete has a minor injury and will play tomorrow.

__55. Have the physician write a note to keep the athlete home the next 2 days for observation by his parents.

__56. Give the athlete shoulder strengthening exercises.

__57. See if the athlete can do a few push-ups.

__58. Monitor the athlete the next few days for any changes in his condition.

__59. Make sure the team physician clears the athlete first before he returns to playing soccer.

__60. Give the athlete a soft neck collar to wear.

Problem X

Opening Scene

A wrestler from an opposing high school was elbowed in the nose prior to his arrival to your school for a county tournament. Throughout the tournament, he has been experiencing recurrent nosebleeds. He approaches you during an active nosebleed.

Section A

How will you begin your initial evaluation and treatment of the athlete's condition? (Please select and prioritize your choices.)

__1. Ask the athlete how hard he was hit.

__2. Ask the athlete if he has had a similar problem in the past.

__3. Ask the athlete if his parents are aware of his current problem.

__4. Ask the athlete if he has any allergies.

__5. Have the athlete put his head between his knees.

__6. Ask the athlete if he is dizzy.

__7. Take the athlete's pulse and blood pressure.

__8. Ask the athlete if his trainer has given him a noseguard.

__9. Place a warm compress on his nose.

__10. Ask the athlete if he has high blood pressure.

__11. Apply pressure to the athlete's right cheek.

__12. Palpate the athlete's nose and surrounding areas for pain and swelling.

__13. Observe the nose for swelling or deformity.

__14. Put an ice pack behind the athlete's neck.

__15. Allow the athlete to blow his nose to clear the nostril.

__16. Place a cotton nose plug under the athlete's top lip.

Section B

The nosebleed is beginning to stop. With this information, what would be your next steps? (Please select and prioritize your choices.)

__17. Perform a primary survey.

__18. Keep the athlete lying down with his legs elevated.

__19. Allow the athlete to apply finger pressure to the bridge of his nose.

__20. Allow your athletic training student to find the athlete's coach or a responsible adult so your assessment can be shared.

__21. Do not let the athlete return to the competition for the rest of the day.

__22. Apply a nose splint.

__23. Have the athlete sit with his head tilted back.

__24. Call the athlete's home athletic trainer.

__25. Use a cotton nose plug to stop the bleeding.

__26. Give the athlete aspirin for the swelling.

__27. Make sure there is no blood present on the athlete, his clothing, the mat, and the floor.

Section C

The nosebleed has stopped. What would be your final actions, and what instructions would you provide the athlete with at this time? (Please select and prioritize your choices.)

__28. Call your team doctor to report what happened.

__29. Call the athlete's team doctor to report what happened.

__30. Have the athlete's parents come to your training room.

__31. Limit the athlete's fluid intake.

__32. Allow the athlete to return to the competition.

__33. Send the athlete for x-rays.

__34. Call the athlete's athletic trainer to report what happened.

__35. Have the athlete do 10 sit-ups.

__36. Use a biohazard bag for any contaminated materials.

__37. Maintain close contact with the athlete during the remainder of the competition.

__38. Tell the athlete to keep an ice pack on his nose while he is not competing.

PROBLEM XI

Opening Scene

You are covering a basketball game when one of your players steps on another player's foot. You see the athlete twist his left ankle. He is jogging with an obvious limp. The coach calls a "time-out."

Section A

What will your initial evaluation include? (Please select and prioritize your choices.)

__ 1. Check the athlete's low back for an injury.

__ 2. Get a wheelchair.

__ 3. Check the athlete's hamstring flexibility.

__ 4. Observe both ankles for swelling/deformity.

__ 5. Have the athlete jog off the court.

__ 6. Gently bang on the heel of the injured ankle.

__ 7. Perform a Lachman's test.

__ 8. Perform an anterior draw test on both ankles.

__ 9. Palpate the ankle and foot for areas of tenderness.

__10. Check the range of motion of the left ankle.

Section B

You have completed your initial evaluation and suspect that he has a second-degree lateral sprain of his left ankle. With assistance, the athlete is brought into the training room. What is your initial treatment going to include? (Please select and prioritize your choices.)

__11. Keep the athlete in nonweightbearing.

__12. Dispense aspirin to the athlete.

__13. Begin RICE.

__14. Call the team doctor with your assessment.

__15. Begin ultrasound treatments.

__16. Place the left ankle in a hot whirlpool.

__17. Fit the athlete with crutches.

__18. Set up an appointment for an x-ray.

__19. Begin an upper body exercise program.

__20. After the game, present your findings to the coach.

__21. Begin a Theraband strengthening program for the left ankle.

Section C

The team doctor is scheduled to be in the athletic training room tomorrow morning. What instructions will you give the athlete for home? (Please select and prioritize your choices.)

__22. If he still has mild/moderate pain tonight, have the athlete go to the nearest emergency room.

___23. Call the athlete's parents with information on what happened.

___24. Begin lower extremity closed-chain exercises as tolerated.

___25. Keep ice packs on the ankle frequently and elevate it when the athlete is not ambulating.

___26. Keep a compression wrap on the ankle except when the athlete is sleeping.

___27. Have the athlete wear high-top sneakers.

___28. Have the athlete try to hop on the affected leg the next day to see if it still hurts.

PROBLEM XII

Opening Scene

The women's gymnastics coach reports to your office to discuss the behavior of one of her athletes. After reviewing what the coach has observed over the past month, you both suspect the athlete may be showing signs of anorexia nervosa.

Section A

With the information you now have available, how would you advise the coach to proceed? (Please select and prioritize your choices.)

___1. Confront the athlete with her problem and do not allow her to compete until the team physician evaluates her.

___2. Do not overemphasize the impact of lower body weight on the athlete's performance.

___3. Tell the coach to keep a diary of when the athlete eats.

___4. Have the coach encourage the athlete to maintain good nutritional habits to optimize her performance.

___5. Keep the athletic training staff informed if the athlete dramatically changes her behavior.

Section B

The athlete has talked with the coach and comes to your office to express her fear of being cut from the team. With the information available, how would you proceed? (Please select and prioritize your choices.)

___6. Assist the athlete in setting practical goals pertaining to safe means of dieting and determining a sensible target weight.

___7. Use "scare" tactics to discourage the use of laxatives and diuretics.

___8. Encourage the athlete to express her fears and concerns regarding her weight and athletic abilities.

___9. Address the issue with your athletic director.

___10. Discuss the athlete's options in case she is cut from the gymnastics team.

___11. Tell the athlete she has nothing to worry about and you will talk to the coach for her.

___12. Tell the athlete she should think about getting professional counseling to overcome her problem.

___13. Set up a meeting between the coach, athlete, and yourself to discuss what has been observed and how it will be managed.

Section C

The athlete concedes to the coach and the athletic trainer that she may have an eating disorder. With this information available, what are your next steps? (Please select and prioritize your choices.)

___14. Call the team physician.

___15. Set up an appointment with a psychologist.

___16. Put the athlete on a strict diet emphasizing weight gain.

___17. Weigh the athlete on a daily basis.

___18. Arrange for the athlete to be hospitalized for a week to force feed her.

___19. Arrange counseling meetings for the athlete with a sports nutritionist.

___20. Put the athlete on a diet consisting of Ensure, bananas, and red meat at least twice a day.

PROBLEM XIII

Opening Scene

You are traveling with your school's men's basketball team when one of your athletes comes to you complaining he has been having abdominal cramping and intermittent diarrhea for the past 2 days.

Section A

Based on the above information, how would you proceed with your initial assessment of this athlete? (Please select and prioritize your choices.)

___1. Ask the athlete what his diet has consisted of (food and drink) during the past 2 to 3 days.

___2. Ask the athlete if he is nervous about playing.

___3. Ask the athlete if he has had this problem before.

___4. Check the athlete's blood pressure.

___5. Take the athlete's oral temperature.

___6. Check the athlete's body fat levels.

___7. Palpate the athlete's abdomen.

___8. Have the athlete run on a treadmill for 20 minutes.

Section B

Assuming from your evaluation that this athlete has a gastrointestinal upset because of precompetition anxiety, what might your next steps be in assisting in this athlete's recovery? (Please select and prioritize your choices.)

__9. Speak with the coach and have the athlete refrain from practice until the symptoms disappear.

__10. Weigh the athlete before and after practices and games.

__11. Give the athlete antimotility drugs, such as Imodium.

__12. Make sure the athlete eats a lot of green vegetables, like broccoli and cabbage.

__13. Give the athlete milk, soda, or tea to rehydrate.

__14. Buy a water-testing kit and evaluate the hotel's drinking water.

__15. Have the athlete drink only bottled water.

PROBLEM XIV

Opening Scene

A soccer player injures his knee during practice. He is assisted into the training room by two teammates. Upon your initial observation, you notice he is limping and his right knee is visibly swollen.

Section A

Given the above information, how would you proceed with your initial evaluation of this athlete? (Please select and prioritize your choices.)

__1. Palpate the knee joint and surrounding areas for point tenderness.

__2. Ask the athlete if he can do a deep squat without pain.

__3. Ask the athlete what happened.

__4. Check the dorsalis pedis pulse of the affected limb.

__5. Ask the athlete if he heard or felt a snap or pop.

__6. Perform a Speed's test.

__7. Perform a Lachman's test.

__8. Check the knee for crepitus.

__9. Ask the athlete if he has had a prior injury to the affected knee.

__10. Measure the range of motion of the affected knee.

__11. Assess the strength of the athlete's hip abductors.

__12. Ask the athlete to perform toe raises.

__13. Perform a pivot shift test on the involved knee.

Section B

After evaluating the athlete's knee, you suspect the athlete has injured his anterior cruciate ligament. What steps would you take at this time? (Please select and prioritize your choices.)

__14. Issue crutches to the athlete and instruct him in toe-touch weightbearing.

__15. Wrap the athlete's knee in ice and elevate his leg.

__16. Call the team physician.

__17. Apply McConnell taping to the injured knee.

__18. Instruct the athlete to use a heating pad on his knee when he is at rest at home.

__19. Order a functional brace for use during activity.

__20. Apply ultrasound (pulsed) to the injured knee.

Section C

The team physician comes to the training room and, after examining the athlete, agrees with your assessment and recommends the athlete have an MRI to confirm the physical findings. Until the severity of the injury is known, he asks you to instruct the athlete in the appropriate treatments for home. (Please select and prioritize your choices.)

__21. Instruct the athlete in knee and hip active range of motion exercises as tolerated.

__22. Have the athlete apply ice to the knee every few hours to minimize swelling.

__23. Tell the athlete to wean himself from the crutches to a cane over the next 24 hours.

__24. Work on proprioception by having the athlete practice balancing on the unaffected leg twice a day.

__25. Instruct the athlete to perform isometric quadriceps and hamstring exercises.

__26. Give the athlete a TENS unit for home use.

__27. Have the athlete practice going up and down stairs and jog as normally as possible.

PROBLEM XV

Opening Scene

A football player comes to you requesting help in improving his general lower body strength and overall conditioning.

Section A

What suggestions would you make in assisting this athlete in a preseason training program? (Please select and prioritize your choices.)

__1. Give the athlete anabolic steroids.

__2. Instruct the athlete in a general flexibility program.

__3. Have the athlete run up and down the stadium stairs in pads.

__4. Monitor the athlete's respiratory rate while at rest.

__5. Incorporate warm-up and cool-down periods.

__6. Make the exercises sport-specific.

__7. Have the athlete participate in other sports, such as basketball or tennis.

__8. Have the athlete perform progressive-resistance lower extremity exercises 3 days a week.

__9. Put the athlete on a red meat and legume diet.

__10. Mix the training schedule to keep it interesting.

__11. Keep the training schedule intense and emphasize training for long periods of time (eg, 3 to 4 hours).

__12. Progress the conditioning program gradually as the athlete improves his tolerance for work.

__13. Help the athlete adjust to working in the heat.

Section B

As the football season begins, the athlete continues to seek your advice to keep him fit and healthy. What types of things might you emphasize to keep him in condition during the season? (Please select and prioritize your choices.)

__14. Have the athlete run 2 miles three times a week.

__15. Continue strength training exercises for the lower body.

__16. Make sure the athlete takes 2 to 3 days off a week so he gets adequate rest.

__17. Monitor the athlete's blood pressure on a daily basis.

__18. Have the athlete perform plyometric activities for power.

__19. Establish a maintenance-conditioning program to be performed on a regular basis.

__20. Put the athlete on a clear liquid diet.

__21. Have the athlete participate in a cross-training program.

__22. Give the athlete a tennis ball so he can work on grip strengthening.

__23. Encourage the athlete to take a class in Judo.

Section C

What types of activities might you suggest the athlete participate in as part of an off-season program? (Please select and prioritize your choices.)

__24. Continue a general flexibility program.

__25. Have the athlete participate in a cross-training program.

__26. Have the athlete jog four to five times a week.

__27. Have the athlete eat a high-calorie diet to build up muscle strength.

__28. Have the athlete meet with a sport psychologist to learn visual imagery.

__29. No physical activity. This is the period during which the athlete should rest and recover.

__30. Give the athlete time during his training schedule to participate in nonathletic events.

__31. Have the athlete take up another sport to stay in shape.

PROBLEM XVI

Opening Scene

An ice hockey player slams head first into the boards during practice. He is lying face down on the ice and is not moving. You have witnessed this event and no other players are involved.

Section A

How will you begin your initial evaluation of this athlete's condition? (Please select and prioritize your choices.)

__1. Perform a secondary survey of the athlete's entire body.

__2. With assistance, roll the athlete onto his back while maintaining the head and neck in neutral.

__3. Remove the athlete's helmet.

__4. Perform a primary survey.

__5. Establish the level of consciousness.

__6. Begin chest compressions.

__7. Have the coach get a vacu-splint.

__8. Ask the other players what happened during the last play.

__9. Sit the athlete up so he can breathe.

Section B

You have determined the athlete is unconscious and is not breathing, but he has a pulse. What are your next steps in treating this athlete? (Please select and prioritize your choices.)

__10. Perform a secondary survey.

__11. Have the coach call for an ambulance.

__12. Vigorously shake the athlete to try and get a response.

__13. Take the athlete's blood pressure.

__14. Cut off the face mask.

__15. Log-roll the athlete onto his side.

__16. Check the athlete for a positive Romberg's sign.

__17. Perform abdominal thrusts to clear the airway.

__18. Begin artificial respiration.

__19. Establish if the athlete is in cardiac arrest.

__20. Remove the athlete's mouthguard.

__21. Use a jaw-thrust to open the athlete's airway.

Section C

The EMS team has arrived. The athlete begins breathing again and becomes responsive. He states he cannot feel anything. With this information, what will be your next actions? (Please select and prioritize your choices.)

__22. Perform a secondary survey.

__23. Continue to monitor breathing, pulse, and blood pressure.

__24. Tell the athlete not to worry, that he should feel something soon, and it is a temporary problem.

__25. With assistance, secure the athlete onto a spine board while maintaining the head and neck in neutral.

__26. Call your team doctor.

__27. Check pupillary response with a penlight.

__28. Argue with the EMS team about whether or not the athlete's helmet should be removed.

__29. Tell the coach you will be at the emergency room and you will be in touch with him later.

__30. Fill out an incident report to document what happened.

Section D

After practice, you go to the hospital to check on the athlete's condition. The emergency room physician informs you the athlete will probably be a C5,6 quadriplegic. With this information available, what would you do next? (Please select and prioritize your choices.)

__31. Check on the athlete to see how he is doing.

__32. Call the team physician to inform him what has happened.

__33. Contact the athlete's parents.

__34. Tell the athlete sometimes doctors make mistakes and not to give up hope.

__35. Check your liability insurance.

__36. Call the local newspaper to give them the story.

__37. Return to school and inform the coach.

__38. With the coaching staff, inform the team what has happened.

__39. Have the emergency room physician contact your athletic director.

PROBLEM XVII

Opening Scene

A wrestler stops by the training room after practice complaining of chronic low back pain which increases a few hours to a day after a workout. He states he has had this pain before and has seen an orthopedic surgeon who had diagnosed him with a chronic low back strain. The athlete denies having any radicular signs and states the pain is localized to the lumbar area.

Section A

With the information that is available to you, what would your initial evaluation include? (Please select and prioritize your choices.)

__ 1. Observe the athlete's posture in standing.

__ 2. Ask the athlete to describe his pain.

__ 3. Check the range of motion of both knees.

__ 4. Perform a Scour test of the right hip.

__ 5. Palpate the lumbar erector spinae.

__ 6. Observe the low back for signs of atrophy.

__ 7. Palpate the posterior superior iliac spine (PSIS) bilaterally.

__ 8. Check the athlete for genu varum.

__ 9. Check the athlete for a leg-length discrepancy.

__10. Have the athlete do a partial squat.

__11. Evaluate the range of motion of the lumbar spine.

__12. Measure hip abduction with a goniometer.

__13. Check the flexibility of the hamstrings and hip flexors.

Section B

Your findings from the initial evaluation are consistent with a chronic lumbar strain. The athlete does not appear to be in severe pain but does seem uncomfortable with active lumbar movement. Which of the following modalities would be appropriate to decrease this athlete's pain? (Please select and prioritize your choices.)

__14. Friction massage.

__15. Ice packs.

__16. Warm whirlpool treatments (full body).

__17. Ultrasound.

__18. Iontophoresis.

__19. Ice massage.

__20. Chiropractic treatments.

__21. TENS therapy.

__22. Moist heat packs.

__23. Short-wave diathermy.

__24. Stationary bicycling.

__25. Functional electric stimulation.

__26. Cervical traction.

__27. Paraffin bath.

__28. Effleurage.

__29. Neoprene lumbar support.

Section C

Regarding the initial phases (I and II) of the rehabilitation program, which of the following exercises would be most appropriate? (Please select and prioritize your choices.)

__30. Active trunk extensions in prone.

__31. Gentle active-assisted low back stretching.

__32. Resisted knee extensions.

__33. Passive hamstring stretching.

__34. Active posterior pelvic tilts.

__35. Passive iliopsoas stretching.

__36. PNF exercises to the hip and lower extremity.

__37. Lower trunk rotations in supine.

Section D

Regarding the later phases (III and IV) of the rehabilitation program, which of the following exercises would be most appropriate? (Please select and prioritize your choices.)

__38. PNF exercises to the trunk.

__39. Resistive abdominal strengthening.

__40. Resistive cervical strengthening.

__41. Resistive prone hip extension.

__42. Achilles' stretching exercises.

__43. Groin stretching exercises.

__44. Shoulder press.

__45. Jogging.

__46. Swimming.

__47. Resistive bridging exercises.

__48. Trunk extensions in prone.

PROBLEM XVIII

Opening Scene

One of your swimmers comes to your office complaining of severe ear pain that is accompanied by intense itching and a mild discharge.

Section A

Upon examining the athlete's ear, you notice the ear canal is inflamed, and the athlete has partial hearing loss. Based on these findings, you determine the athlete has external otitis (swimmer's ear). What should you do to begin treatment of this condition? (Please select and prioritize your choices.)

__ 1. Dispense penicillin.

__ 2. Clear out the ear with a Q-tip soaked in epinephrine.

__ 3. Arrange for the athlete to see the team physician.

__ 4. Cover the ear with a sterile gauze pad.

__ 5. Advise the athlete to wear a hood in cold environments.

__ 6. Use a TENS unit for pain.

__ 7. Apply a moist heat pack to the affected ear.

__ 8. Allow the athlete to continue swimming as tolerated.

Section B

The team physician comes to the athletic training room, examines the athlete, and makes a diagnosis of external otitis. He dispenses an oral antibiotic and ear drops (3% boric acid and alcohol) to be administered daily. In addition to these treatments, you instruct the athlete in which of the following measures? (Please select and prioritize your choices.)

__ 9. Protect the athlete's ear while swimming with a plug of lamb's wool soaked with lanolin.

__10. Have the athlete wear a bathing cap when swimming.

__11. Have the athlete cross-train to prevent frustration from not swimming.

__12. Instruct the athlete to wear goggles while swimming.

__13. Instruct the athlete not to stick any object into his ears.

PROBLEM XIX

Opening Scene

You are covering a high school field hockey game when one of your players gets hit hard in the mouth with a stick. She comes running off the field with her hand covering her mouth. There is a copious amount of blood on her face and hands.

Section A

What steps would you take during your initial evaluation of this athlete? (Please select and prioritize your choices.)

__ 1. Rinse the athlete's mouth out with water.

__ 2. Clean the athlete's mouth out with a paper towel.

__ 3. Don gloves.

__4. Ask the athlete why she is crying.

__5. Ask the athlete if she was wearing a mouthguard.

__6. Review the school's liability insurance.

__7. Observe the mouth, lips, and surrounding structures for lacerations or abrasions.

__8. Palpate the mouth and surrounding structures for deformity.

__9. Ask an athletic training student to get a cervical collar.

__10. Have the athlete open and close her mouth.

Section B

During your initial evaluation, you observe the athlete is missing a front tooth. One of the athlete's teammates comes to the sidelines with the tooth in her hand. What actions would you take at this time? (Please select and prioritize your choices.)

__11. Ask the officials to stop the game.

__12. Have an athletic training student take the athlete to the school nurse.

__13. Discuss your findings with the athlete's parents.

__14. Call your team physician for guidance.

__15. Apply an ice pack to the mouth area.

__16. Apply a cotton plug between the lip and injured gum.

__17. Place the tooth in a container of sterile saline solution.

__18. Rinse the tooth off with water.

__19. Send the athlete with the tooth to a dentist in less than 30 minutes.

__20. Discard the tooth.

__21. Place the athlete in a side-lying position.

PROBLEM XX

Opening Scene

A wrestler comes to the athletic training room during his off-season and asks you to help him lose 15 pounds. This athlete had attempted to lose a significant amount of weight before and failed.

Section A

How would you advise the wrestler in his initial steps to lose the weight safely? (Please select and prioritize your choices.)

__1. Have the athlete consume a protein drink once a day in addition to his regular diet.

__2. Measure the athlete's percent body fat using calipers.

__3. Have the athlete read the American Heart Association Cookbook.

__4. Send the athlete to an acupuncturist.

__5. Have the athlete keep a log of what he eats on a daily basis.

__6. Monitor the athlete's weight loss progress once a week.

__7. Put the athlete on a fasting diet for 2 days.

__8. Make sure the athlete drinks eight glasses of water daily.

__9. Weigh the athlete prior to beginning his program.

__10. Have the athlete sit in a sauna.

__11. Monitor the athlete's exercise program.

__12. Assist the athlete in developing a balanced diet.

__13. Have the athlete wear a rubber suit while running.

__14. Put the athlete on a lower extremity strengthening program.

Section B

The athlete successfully loses the weight. How would you go about advising the athlete in maintaining his current weight? (Please select and prioritize your choices.)

__15. Continue to monitor the athlete's food intake via a log.

__16. Have the coach monitor the athlete's food intake.

__17. Have the athlete drink eight glasses of water a day.

__18. Have the athlete double his exercise session in duration.

__19. Have the athlete take laxatives.

__20. Refer the athlete to a sports nutritionist.

__21. Encourage the athlete to eat four to six small balanced meals a day.

__22. Put the athlete on an upper body strength program.

PROBLEM XXI

Opening Scene

A wide receiver gets a hard hit from the front while catching a football and lands hard on his right leg. He is lying on his back and is in severe pain. You immediately observe that his injured lower extremity is in a flexed, adducted, and internally rotated position.

Section A

How will you begin to evaluate the severity and nature of this injury? (Please select and prioritize your choices.)

___ 1. Immediately straighten the leg and splint it in neutral.

___ 2. Check the athlete's vital signs.

___ 3. Immediately cut away the athlete's pant leg.

___ 4. Perform a Lachman's test.

___ 5. Remove the face mask.

___ 6. Ask the athlete where his pain is located.

___ 7. Sit the athlete upright.

___ 8. Test bilateral lower extremity sensation.

___ 9. Move the athlete off the playing field.

___10. Elevate both legs.

___11. Have the coach call for an ambulance.

___12. Check the rest of the athlete's body for other injuries.

___13. Ask the athlete what happened.

___14. Tell the athlete not to move.

___15. Palpate the rest of the right lower extremity for any deformities.

Section B

You have ruled out a knee injury and suspect the athlete has sustained a traumatic right hip dislocation. With this information how would you proceed? (Please select and prioritize your choices.)

___16. Call the athlete's parents.

___17. Check the athlete for symptoms of shock.

___18. Allow the competition to continue.

___19. Keep the area clear of players.

___20. Get the athlete up on crutches.

___21. Apply a Vaccusplint to the entire lower extremity.

___22. Put an ice pack on the right thigh and groin.

___23. Give the athlete aspirin for pain.

___24. Check the hip for crepitus.

___25. Ask the athlete if he can actively extend his right leg.

___26. Palpate the popliteal and dorsalis pedis pulses.

___27. Keep the athlete calm, and encourage him not to move.

Section C

The ambulance has arrived with the EMS team, and the athlete is going to be transported to the emergency room of the local hospital. What are your final steps before he leaves with the paramedics? (Please select and prioritize your choices.)

___28. Call ahead to the emergency room to make arrangements for his arrival.

___29. Allow the athlete to drink some Gatorade.

___30. Have a coach follow the athlete to the hospital.

___31. Reassure the athlete that he will be taken care of before he departs.

___32. Take the athlete's helmet off.

___33. Move the athlete onto a spine board.

___34. Fill out an injury report.

___35. Call the athlete's parents to let them know what has happened.

___36. Contact the athletic director to give him a verbal report.

Problem XXII

Opening Scene

As the second half of a high school basketball game begins, you are returning to the court when you find one of the referees kneeling down. He states that he is nauseous, and he is sweating profusely. He also tells you that he has "a heavy pressure in his chest."

Section A

How will you begin your initial evaluation of the referee's condition? (Please select and prioritize your choices.)

___ 1. Ask the referee what happened.

___ 2. Send someone for an ACE.

___ 3. Tell the referee "not to worry about it"; and that "he's just a little out of shape".

___ 4. Have the referee remove his shirt.

___ 5. Ask the other referee to stop the game.

___ 6. Check the referee's vital signs.

___ 7. Ask the referee if he is taking any medications.

___ 8. Administer nitroglycerine.

___ 9. Walk the referee to the men's locker room.

___10. Ask the referee if he has ever experienced this before.

___11. Ask the referee if he smokes.

___12. Ask the referee if he has pain going down the left arm.

Section B

Based on the above information, you suspect the referee might be having a myocardial infarction. How will you proceed at this time? (Please select and prioritize your choices.)

___13. Send someone for the team doctor.

___14. Send someone for the AED.

___15. Lie the referee on his back.

___16. Inform the referee that he is having a heart attack.

___17. Call the referee's wife to inform her that her husband is having a heart attack and you are "sending for a squad."

___18. Put ice on the back of the referee's neck.

___19. Ask the referee to cough.

___20. Ask the referee is he is short of breath.

___21. Check the capillary refill of the fingers and toes.

___22. Try to put the referee at ease; speak to him with confidence, and let him know what you are doing to keep him calm.

___23. Activate the EMS.

Section C

The referee suddenly clutches his chest and collapses onto the court. What would your next actions be? (Please select and prioritize your choices.)

___24. Check the referee for responsiveness.

___25. Look for a doctor in the stands.

___26. Conduct a primary survey.

___27. Scream at the referee to "wake-up!"

___28. Place the referee on a spine board with assistance from the coaches.

___29. Check for facial droop.

___30. Apply the AED.

___31. Perform abdominal thrusts.

___32. Begin CPR until the AED arrives.

___33. Roll the referee onto his right side.

Section D

The referee responds to the use of the AED. He is breathing on his own and has a palpable carotid pulse. The paramedics have just arrived at the field house and are preparing to take him to the hospital. What actions would you take after the referee leaves the school? (Please select and prioritize your choices.)

___34. Contact the local newspaper to inform them of the incident so they have the correct information.

___35. Fill out an incident report.

___36. Contact your athletic director.

___37. Follow the ambulance to the hospital.

___38. Return to the basketball game as play resumes.

PROBLEM XXIII

Opening Scene

You are covering a soccer game on a cold day when you notice one of your players is having difficulty breathing about 7 minutes into the game. He comes off the field coughing and complaining of "chest tightness."

Section A

How will you begin your initial evaluation of this player's condition? (Please select and prioritize your choices.)

___1. Ask if the athlete is a diabetic.

___2. Ask the athlete if this has ever happened to him before.

___3. Give the athlete Immodium.

___4. Lie the athlete in supine, and flex his knees to his chest.

___5. Ask the athlete if he has an inhaler.

___6. Talk with the athlete to keep him calm.

___7. Tell the coach you are going to send the athlete to the team doctor.

Section B

You suspect that the athlete has EIB. What would your next steps be when caring for this athlete? (Please select and prioritize your choices.)

___8. Have the athlete breathe slowly through the nose.

___9. Check the athlete's pulse rate.

___10. Have the athlete breathe into a paper bag.

___11. Have the athlete take two puffs of a short-acting inhaler.

___12. Have the athlete slow to a less intense pace by performing a slow jog and/or stretch on the sidelines.

___13. Give the athlete a warm drink like tea or hot chocolate.

___14. Have the athlete sit down to rest.

___15. Tell the coach you are taking the athlete out of the game.

___16. Monitor the athlete's symptoms until they subside, and continue to monitor the athlete for up to 12 hours after exercise.

PROBLEM XXIV

Opening Scene

A football player comes to the athletic training room complaining of severe low back pain that is radiating down his right leg. He is very guarded and is slightly forward flexed at the waist. He states that he was lifting in the weight room and his pain started after he lowered a dumbbell to the floor.

Section A

Your initial evaluation of this problem would include which of the following actions? (Please select and prioritize your choices.)

__ 1. Use iontophoresis on the athlete's back.

__ 2. Put a moist heat pack on the athlete's back.

__ 3. Palpate the lumbar erector spinae, SI areas, and both PSIS for tenderness.

__ 4. Observe the athlete's trunk to see if there is a "lateral shift" present.

__ 5. Perform an Apley's compression test.

__ 6. Perform a "Slump" test.

__ 7. Ask the athlete how far the pain is felt down his leg.

__ 8. Ask the athlete if he has a history of low back problems.

__ 9. Give the athlete a back massage.

__ 10. Lie the athlete in supine with his knees in full flexion.

Section B

The athlete reports significant increasing pain down his leg to the level of his foot when he tries to bend forward. You suspect the athlete has a lumbar herniated nucleus propulsus. What steps would you take at this time to treat this athlete? (Please select and prioritize your choices.)

__11. Have the athlete lie in prone.

__12. Teach the athlete a series of Williams' Flexion exercises.

__13. Tape the athlete's lower back for support.

__14. Give the athlete a muscle relaxant like Flexeril.

__15. Call the team physician, and suggest he order a MRI.

__16. Send the athlete to a chiropractor.

__17. Teach the athlete how to perform prone press-ups.

__18. Place an ice pack on the athlete's back after exercise.

Section C

After a couple of days of treatment, the athlete's radicular signs begin to centralize. What recommendations would you make to this athlete to prevent another episode of lumbar pain? (Please select and prioritize your choices.)

__19. Keep his quadratus lumborum flexible.

__20. Avoid lifting heavy objects.

__21. Make sure he is using proper body mechanics while lifting.

__22. Maintain good hamstring flexibility.

__23. Take Advil on a regular basis before playing football.

__24. Make sure he bends at the waist when lifting.

__25. When sitting for prolonged periods of time, make sure he sits with his pelvis posteriorly rotated.

__26. Have the athlete perform standing extensions when moving from a seated to a standing position.

Problem XXV

Opening Scene

You have been assigned to the medical tent located at the finish line of a half-marathon. As one of the runners crosses the line, you notice he appears somewhat ashen in color and is looking confused. As you escort him to the tent, you notice that his skin is cool and clammy to the touch.

Section A

How will you begin your initial evaluation of this athlete's condition? (Please select and prioritize your choices.)

__1. Immediately administer an IV of glucose and water.

__2. Ask the athlete what medications he is taking.

__3. While maintaining the athlete's privacy with a light blanket/sheet, obtain a core temperature measurement.

__4. Take the athlete's blood pressure and pulse rate.

__5. Perform a cranial nerve check.

__6. Check the athlete for a positive Homan's sign.

__7. Check the athlete's fingernails for good capillary refill.

__8. Ask the athlete's name, the date, and where they are right now.

Section B

Based on your initial evaluation, you determine the athlete is experiencing an episode of heat exhaustion. How would you proceed in treating this athlete? (Please select and prioritize your choices.)

__9. Have the athlete rebreathe into a paper bag.

__10. Move the athlete into a cool area.

__11 Place the athlete in supine and elevate his feet.

__12. Give the athlete a massage to relax him.

__13. Restrict the athlete's fluid intake for at least 1 to 2 hours.

__14. Continue to monitor the athlete's vital signs.

__15. Cover the athlete with a cotton blanket

__16. Cool the athlete by sponging or toweling him with cold water, by use of a fan, or by placing ice packs around the neck, and in the axilla and/or groin area.

__17. Advise the athlete not to run again until he is cleared by a doctor.

Problem XXVI

Opening Scene

You are covering a collegiate women's lacrosse game when you observe two players collide as they try to catch a ball in the air. One of the players is struck by her opponent's stick in the side of the chest. She falls to the ground and is in obvious pain. She is clutching her right side.

Section A

How will you begin to evaluate the severity of this injury? (Please select and prioritize your choices.)

__1. Observe the athlete for cyanosis.

__2. Immediately move the athlete off the field.

__3. Ask the athlete to move her fingers and toes.

__4. Ask the athlete to cough a couple of times to check respiratory competency.

__5. Perform a primary survey.

__6. Perform an Adson's maneuver.

__7. Perform an upper quarter screen.

__8. Look for coughing up of blood.

__9. Palpate the thorax for point tenderness and crepitus.

Section B

You are able to assist the athlete to the sidelines. She complains of significant pain during inspiration and continues to try to splint her chest with her arms. After a few minutes, you notice her lips look cyanotic. What steps would you take at this time to treat this athlete? (Please select and prioritize your choices.)

__10. Record the rate and depth of respirations.

__11. Monitor vital signs.

__12. Tightly and continuously wrap the chest with an elastic bandage.

__13. Use a vapocoolant spray such as Flouromethane to reduce spasm.

__14. Apply a sling and swathe, using the athlete's arm as a splint and support with the forearm supported across the chest.

__15. Observe the rib cage for any areas of deformity.

__16. Check the athlete's shoulder for active range of motion to make sure there is no injury to the scapula.

__17. Perform an Allen's test.

__18. Perform a Phalen's test.

__19. Activate the EMS.

__20. Apply a pad over the suspected fracture site.

__21. Refer the athlete to a physician as soon as possible.

Problem XXVII

Opening Scene

It is 1:00 pm and you are rehabilitating a volleyball player for a shoulder injury when you notice he is "slumping" in his chair as he is working on an upper body ergometer (UBE). When you ask him if he is all right, he responds slowly, and his speech appears to be slurred. You know this athlete is a Type I diabetic.

Section A

How will you begin to evaluate this athlete's condition? (Please select and prioritize your choices.)

__1. Ask if the athlete if he is having difficulty breathing.

__2. Observe for diaphoresis.

__3. Take the athlete's pulse rate.

__4. Ask the athlete when he last injected himself with insulin.

__5. Observe for facial drooping.

__6. Perform a cranial nerve assessment.

__7. Perform a Rhomberg's test.

__8. Bring the athlete into your office and gently approach him about substance abuse.

__9. Check for fruity smelling breath.

Section B

Based on your initial assessment, you determine the athlete is experiencing insulin shock. What would your next steps be in treating this athlete? (Please select and prioritize your choices.)

__10. Administer short-acting insulin.

__11. Have the athlete eat a protein bar.

__12. Lie the athlete in supine, and elevate his feet.

__13. Monitor vital signs.

__14. Give the athlete a drink with high levels of sugar.

__15. Keep the athlete warm with a blanket.

__16. Give the athlete a drink that is high in electrolytes.

Section C

The athlete recovers well after drinking some orange juice that is mixed with added sugar. What advice would you provide the athlete with to prevent further episodes of hypoglycemia? (Please select and prioritize your choices.)

__17. Advise the athlete to consume sufficient carbohydrates prior to exercising.

__18. Remind the athlete to inject himself with high dosages of insulin on a regular basis before exercising to avoid "crashing" during periods of intense activity.

__19. Make sure he knows to inject himself in the muscles that will not be very active during a particular sporting event.

__20. Advise the athlete to keep small amounts of candy with him in case he feels the symptoms of hypoglycemia occurring.

__21. Tell the athlete to attend a diabetic support group.

PRACTICAL PRACTICE SAMPLE QUESTIONS

Chapter 5

You will need two partners and a stopwatch or wristwatch to practice for this section of the exam. One partner will play the role of the model, and the other partner will be the examiner. Have the partner who is playing the examiner read through a few of the questions to him- or herself first and collect any necessary items to complete the tasks on which you intend to work. For example, if you are required to tape a knee, you will need the appropriate selection of supplies. Try to avoid having your partners "help" you by giving you hints, either verbally or nonverbally, along the way. The idea is for you to become confident in your skills and speed of execution. Go over any mistakes you have made after you have totally completed this practice section.

Each task will be assigned a specific time limitation. You must correctly perform 90% of the steps to pass each task, except for Problems X and XIV, which must be correctly demonstrated in full.

PROBLEM I

A soccer player mildly strains his right hip flexor during a game. The athlete needs his leg wrapped in an elastic bandage to make him more comfortable prior to returning to play. You have 2 minutes to perform this task.

A. Is the athlete positioned in standing with the involved leg slightly flexed and internally rotated?
    Yes ___   No ___
B. Was a double 6-inch elastic wrap selected?
    Yes ___   No ___

C. Was the elastic wrap started at the upper part of the inner thigh and brought around to the posterior aspect of the thigh?
    Yes ___   No___
D. Was the wrap anchored onto the opposite iliac crest?
    Yes ___   No ___
E. Does the wrap prevent excessive hip extension?
    Yes ___   No ___
    Passing score = 4 questions correctly answered

PROBLEM II

An athlete comes to the athletic training room after undergoing an arthroplasty of his left shoulder. Using a goniometer, measure the range of motion of shoulder flexion (normal active range of motion is 0 to 180 degrees). Please report your measurement to the examiner. (Note: The examiner should take the initial reading.) You have 2 minutes to perform this task.

A. Is the athlete positioned in supine?
    Yes ___   No ___
B. Is the axis of the goniometer aligned through the lateral aspect of the humeral head?
    Yes ___   No ___
C. Is the stationary arm of the goniometer aligned parallel to the trunk?
    Yes ___   No ___
D. Is the movable arm aligned parallel to the humeral shaft, siting the lateral epicondyle?
    Yes ___   No ___

E. Is the athletic trainer's recording within 5 degrees of the examiner's reading?

Yes ___   No ___

Passing score = 4 questions correctly answered

PROBLEM III

This next task is to test your palpation skills. With a skin-marker or small pieces of athletic tape, place a mark on the following anatomical landmarks of the lower extremity. You have 2 minutes to perform this task.

A. The anterior talofibular ligament.

(Correct?) Yes ___   No ___

B. Gerdy's tubercle.

(Correct?) Yes ___   No ___

C. The anterior superior iliac spine.

(Correct?) Yes ___   No ___

D. The popliteal fossa.

(Correct?) Yes ___   No ___

E. The quadriceps tendon.

(Correct?) Yes ___   No ___

F. The lateral collateral ligament of the knee.

(Correct?) Yes ___   No ___

G. The medial malleolus.

(Correct?) Yes ___   No ___

H. The deltoid ligament of the ankle.

(Correct?) Yes ___   No ___

I. The greater trochanter of the femur.

(Correct?) Yes ___   No ___

J. The medial border of the patella.

(Correct?) Yes ___   No ___

K. The lateral head of the gastrocnemius.

(Correct?) Yes ___   No ___

L. The first ray of the foot.

(Correct?) Yes ___   No ___

M. The navicular of the foot.

(Correct?) Yes ___   No ___

N. The base of the fifth metatarsal.

(Correct?) Yes ___   No ___

O. The tendon of the biceps femoris.

(Correct?) Yes ___   No ___

P. The fibular head.

(Correct?) Yes ___   No ___

Passing score = 14 questions correctly answered

PROBLEM IV

A gymnast reports to the athletic training room after sustaining a knee injury during practice. To test the integrity of the medial collateral ligament, you must perform a valgus stress test. Demonstrate this test just as you would on an injured athlete. You have 3 minutes to perform this test.

A. Is the athlete positioned in supine?

Yes ___   No ___

B. Is the involved leg extended?

Yes ___   No ___

C. Has the athletic trainer stabilized the distal limb with one hand?

Yes ___   No ___

D. Has the athletic trainer placed his or her other hand over the lateral joint line?

Yes ___   No ___

E. Has the athletic trainer applied adequate force in the appropriate direction with the knee in full extension?

Yes ___   No ___

F. Has the athletic trainer applied adequate force in the appropriate direction at 30 degrees of flexion?

Yes ___   No ___

G. Has the athletic trainer performed the valgus stress test bilaterally?

Yes___   No ___

Passing score = 6 questions correctly answered

PROBLEM V

A basketball player has been participating in a rehabilitation program for a hamstring strain. Prior to allowing the player to return to playing, the athletic trainer should test the strength of the hamstrings to be sure they are of equal strength to the uninvolved side and are pain free to resistance. Demonstrate a manual muscle test for the hamstrings just as you would on an athlete. You have 2 minutes to perform this task.

A. Is the athlete positioned in prone?

Yes ___   No ___

B. Did the athletic trainer have the athlete first move the limb actively from full knee extension to full knee flexion?

Yes ___   No ___

C. Has the athletic trainer stabilized the posterior thigh with one hand?

Yes ___   No ___

D. Has the athletic trainer placed his or her hand on the posterior aspect of the distal lower leg?

Yes ___   No ___

E. Was the proper force applied to resist knee flexion (in neutral)?

Yes ___   No ___

F. Did the athletic trainer position the lower leg in internal rotation to resist the medial hamstrings?

Yes ___   No ___

G. Did the athletic trainer position the lower leg in external rotation to resist the lateral hamstrings?

Yes ___   No ___

Passing score = 6 questions correctly answered

PROBLEM VI

This task will require you to properly fit a football helmet on a player. Proceed through all the steps, verbalizing each step to the examiner until the fitting process is complete. Inform the examiner when you are done. You have 3 minutes to perform this task.

A. Did the athletic trainer verbalize he or she would wet the player's hair to simulate playing conditions and ensure a proper fit?
Yes ___   No ___

B. Did the athletic trainer apply the helmet from the back to the front and check to make sure the helmet fits snugly with no gaps between the pads and the head or face?
Yes ___   No ___

C. Did the athletic trainer check to see if the helmet covers the base of the skull?
Yes ___   No ___

D. With the chin strap in place, did the athletic trainer pull down on the face mask to make sure the helmet did not move?
Yes ___   No ___

E. Did the athletic trainer push down on the helmet to make sure there is no movement?
Yes ___   No ___

F. Did the athletic trainer attempt to rock the helmet back and forth to check for any movement?
Yes ___   No ___

G. Did the athletic trainer attempt to rotate the helmet to check for any movement?
Yes ___   No ___

H. Did the athletic trainer check to see if the front edge of the helmet is no less than two finger widths above the eyebrows?
Yes ___   No ___

I. Did the athletic trainer check to see if the jaw pads fit snugly against the face?
Yes ___   No ___

J. Did the athletic trainer check to see if the face mask was three finger widths from the nose?
Yes ___   No ___

K. Did the athletic trainer check to see that the ear holes were aligned?
Yes ___   No ___

L. Did the athletic trainer check to make sure the chin strap was properly adjusted?
Yes ___   No ___

Passing score = 11 questions correctly answered

PROBLEM VII

A lacrosse player is recovering from Achilles' tendinitis of the right lower leg. This athlete will need to be taped to prevent aggravating the area during play. Demonstrate the proper technique to tape the Achilles' tendon. You will have 3 minutes to perform this task.

A. Is the athlete positioned in prone with the ankle in slight plantar flexion over the edge of the table?
Yes ___   No ___

B. Did the athletic trainer verbalize that tape adherent would be applied to the lower leg (after shaving it if necessary)?
Yes ___   No ___

C. Has the athletic trainer applied underwrap to the lower third of the calf area?
Yes ___   No ___

D. Has the athletic trainer applied anchor strips one third of the way up the calf and around the forefoot?
Yes ___   No ___

E. Has the athletic trainer applied a 3-inch elastic strip from forefoot to the anchor strip on the calf?
Yes ___   No ___

F. Has the athletic trainer applied a second 3 inch-elastic strip on top of the first, splitting it down the middle lengthwise and wrapping the two pieces anteriorly around the leg?
Yes ___   No ___

G. Did the athletic trainer close the tape job with elastic strips around the calf and the ball of the foot?
Yes ___   No ___

H. Does the tape job adequately prevent excessive dorsiflexion of the foot?
Yes ___   No ___

Passing score = 7 questions correctly answered

PROBLEM VIII

A football player has injured his ankle during a game. After having the ankle wrapped for support, crutches are issued. Demonstrate how to properly fit and walk with crutches in nonweightbearing. You have 3 minutes to perform this task.

A. Are the tips of the crutches approximately 6 inches from the lateral aspect of the shoe and approximately 2 inches in front of the toe during fitting?
Yes ___   No ___

B. Are the crutch handles in a position so the elbows are bent to approximately 30 degrees?
Yes ___   No ___

C. Are the tops of the crutches approximately two finger widths from the top of the axilla?
Yes ___   No ___

D. Did the athletic trainer review a tripod gait in which both crutches are moved forward approximately 12 inches and the athlete swings through the stationary crutches with the affected foot elevated?
Yes ___   No ___

Passing score = 3 questions correctly answered

PROBLEM IX

A football player comes to the sidelines after making a tackle. He is complaining of some neck discomfort and tingling sensations down his left arm. As part of the athletic trainer's initial assessment, an upper quarter screen is performed. Please demonstrate how to assess the motor function of the upper quarter and verbalize each level as it is evaluated. You have 2 minutes to perform this task.

A. (C3,4) Did the athletic trainer resist shoulder shrugs?

Yes ___   No ___

B. (C4,5) Did the athletic trainer resist shoulder abduction?

Yes ___   No ___

C. (C5,6) Did the athletic trainer resist elbow flexion and wrist extension?

Yes ___   No ___

D. (C6,7) Did the athletic trainer resist elbow extension and wrist flexion?

Yes ___   No ___

E. (C8,T1) Did the athletic trainer resist finger adduction and grip strength?

Yes ___   No ___

Passing score = 4 questions correctly answered

PROBLEM X

A baseball player comes into the training room following a practice complaining that his shoulder clicks and occasionally feels like it is slipping when he throws hard. To test the integrity of the glenohumeral joint, the athletic trainer performs an apprehension test. Demonstrate this test just as you would on an injured athlete. You have 2 minutes to perform this task.

A. Has the athletic trainer placed the athlete in sitting or supine?

Yes ___   No ___

B. Did the athletic trainer position the shoulder in 90 degrees of abduction with the elbow flexed to 90 degrees?

Yes ___   No ___

C. Did the athletic trainer gently externally rotate the shoulder until the athlete demonstrates apprehension (facial grimace or the athlete requests the trainer to stop the motion)?

Yes ___   No ___

Passing score = 3 questions correctly answered

PROBLEM XI

A gymnast has a subacute left biceps strain. This athlete will need to be taped before participating in her next meet. Demonstrate the proper technique to tape the elbow to prevent hyperextension. You will have 3 minutes to perform this task.

A. Did the athletic trainer verbalize that tape adherent would be applied to the elbow area?

Yes ___   No ___

B. Has the athletic trainer positioned the athlete with the elbow in 90 degrees of flexion?

Yes ___   No ___

C. Has the athletic trainer applied underwrap to the affected area?

Yes ___   No ___

D. Has the athletic trainer placed anchor strips with elastic tape at the midupper arm and midforearm areas?

Yes ___   No ___

E. Did the athletic trainer apply a checkrein made out of fanned 1.5-inch white tape or 2-inch or 3-inch elastic tape vertically down the anterior portion of the arm?

Yes ___   No ___

F. Did the athletic trainer apply additional anchor strips above and below the checkrein to secure it?

Yes ___   No ___

G. Did the athletic trainer apply a final wrap with elastic tape to close the tape job?

Yes ___   No ___

Passing score = 6 questions correctly answered

PROBLEM XII

A field hockey player comes into the athletic training room with a large abrasion (4 inch x 4 inch) on the lateral side of her thigh. Demonstrate the proper procedure to care for this wound. You will have 3 minutes to perform this task.

A. Did the athletic trainer verbalize or demonstrate good hand washing techniques?

Yes ___   No ___

B. Did the athletic trainer don protective gloves?

Yes ___   No ___

C. Has the athletic trainer cleansed the wound thoroughly with soap and water or hydrogen peroxide?

Yes ___   No ___

D. Has the athletic trainer applied an antiseptic to the wound?

Yes ___   No ___

E. If medication is applied, has the athletic trainer placed the ointment or cream on the pad or dressing (ie, not directly on the wound)?

Yes ___   No ___

F. Has the athletic trainer secured the dressing in place with an elastic wrap or tape?

Yes ___   No ___

G. Did the athletic trainer verbalize that the contaminated gloves would be disposed of in a biohazard bag?

Yes ___   No ___

Passing score = 6 questions correctly answered

PROBLEM XIII

A volleyball player limps into the athletic training room after twisting her ankle on the court during a practice drill. An inversion sprain is suspected. To test the integrity of the ankle joint, an anterior drawer test is performed. Please demonstrate this test just as you would on an injured athlete. You have 2 minutes to perform this task.

A. Is the athlete positioned in supine or sitting on the edge of a treatment table with the feet relaxed and hanging freely over the edge of the table?
    Yes ___   No ___
B. Has the athletic trainer stabilized the lower tibia with one hand?
    Yes ___   No ___
C. Did the athletic trainer grasp the calcaneus with the other hand?
    Yes ___   No ___
D. Did the athletic trainer attempt to move the calcaneus anteriorly with adequate force?
    Yes ___   No ___
E. Did the athletic trainer verbalize that a clunking feeling at the endpoint of the movement is a positive finding?
    Yes ___   No ___
    Passing score = 4 questions correctly answered

PROBLEM XIV

A baseball player reports having pain along the ball of his right foot while walking and running. It has now progressed to the point where he is limping slightly. To decrease his pain while he is being treated for the inflammation, a metatarsal pad is applied for use during activity. Please demonstrate the proper technique to apply a metatarsal pad to this athlete's foot. You have 2 minutes to perform this task.

A. Is the athlete positioned in supine or sitting with the plantar surface of the affected foot turned upward?
    Yes ___   No ___
B. Has the athletic trainer placed a 2- to 2.5-inch oval approximately 0.125- to 0.25-inch thick felt metatarsal pad just behind the metatarsal heads?
    Yes ___   No ___
C. Did the athletic trainer secure the pad with loosely applied elastic tape?
    Yes ___   No ___
    Passing score = 3 questions correctly answered

PROBLEM XV

During a poorly executed dismount, a gymnast lands on his shoulder. After an initial assessment of the injury,

the athletic trainer suspects a potentially serious shoulder injury. To make the athlete more comfortable and for protection, the athletic trainer applies a cloth triangular bandage as a cervical arm sling. Please demonstrate how a cervical arm sling is properly applied. You will have 2 minutes to perform this task.

A. Is the athlete positioned in standing with his or her arm in approximately 70 degrees of elbow flexion?
    Yes ___   No ___
B. Has the athletic trainer positioned the triangular bandage under the injured arm so that the apex is facing the elbow joint?
    Yes ___   No ___
C. Has the athletic trainer brought the superior corner up over the shoulder of the injured arm?
    Yes ___   No ___
D. Has the athletic trainer brought the inferior corner up over the shoulder of the uninjured side, tying it in a knot to the opposite corner behind the neck?
    Yes ___   No ___
E. Has the athletic trainer brought the apex of the triangle forward and secured it with a safety pin?
    Yes ___   No ___
    Passing score = 4 questions correctly answered

PROBLEM XVI

A baseball player mildly sprains his left ankle during a game. Following treatment, he is able to return to the next scheduled game but requires his ankle to be taped prior to playing. Please demonstrate the proper technique to tape an ankle to prevent a second inversion sprain. You will have 3 minutes to perform this task.

A. Are the athlete's foot and ankle positioned in maximal dorsiflexion and eversion?
    Yes ___   No ___
B. Did the athletic trainer verbalize that he or she would apply tape adherent and underwrap prior to taping?
    Yes ___   No ___
C. Has the athletic trainer applied anchor strips around the lower third of the calf at the musculotendinous junction of the gastrocnemius?
    Yes ___   No ___
D. Has the athletic trainer applied anchor strips loosely around the foot over the base of the fifth metatarsal?
    Yes ___   No ___
E. Has the athletic trainer applied stirrup strips?
    Yes ___   No ___
F. Has the athletic trainer applied horizontal strips continually up the leg in either a basket weave form or as continual support?
    Yes ___   No ___

G. Has the athletic trainer applied double heel locks (with a figure-eight strip) for additional support?

Yes ___   No ___

H. Upon inspecting the tape job, are there any gaps visible?

Yes ___   No ___

I. Does the model feel the tape prevents active inversion of the ankle?

Yes ___   No ___

J. Upon removing the tape, are there any noticeable wrinkles that could cause blisters?

Yes ___   No ___

Passing score = 9 questions correctly answered

Problem XVII

Two football players collide on the field while scrambling for a fumble. One player appears dazed as he walks off the field to the sideline. During the athletic trainer's assessment, the cranial nerves are checked. Please demonstrate how each nerve, numbers I through XII, are evaluated. You have 3 minutes to perform this task.

A. (CN I—Olfactory) Did the athletic trainer ask the athlete to smell something with his or her eyes closed?

Yes ___   No ___

B. (CN II—Optic) Did the athletic trainer ask the athlete if he or she can see his or her fingers in his or her periphery?

Yes ___   No ___

C. (CN III—Oculomotor) Did the athletic trainer ask the athlete to track his or her finger up and down and side to side?

Yes ___   No ___

D. (CN IV—Trochlear) Did the athletic trainer ask the athlete to track his or her finger up and down and side to side (same test as CN III)?

Yes ___   No ___

E. (CN V—Trigeminal) Did the athletic trainer check the sensation of the face (bilaterally)?

Yes ___   No ___

F. (CN VI—Abducens) Did the athletic trainer ask the athlete to track his or her finger side to side (similar test as CN III)?

Yes ___   No ___

G. (CN VII—Facial) Did the athletic trainer ask the athlete to frown or smile?

Yes ___   No ___

H. (CN VIII—Acoustic) Did the athletic trainer check the athlete's hearing (eg, with a watch or a tuning fork)?

Yes ___   No ___

I. (CN IX—Glossopharyngeal) Did the athletic trainer ask the athlete to swallow?

Yes ___   No ___

J. (CN X—Vagus) Did the athletic trainer ask the athlete to say "ah"?

Yes ___   No ___

K. (CN XI—Spinal accessory) Did the athletic trainer ask the athlete to shrug his or her shoulders?

Yes ___   No ___

L. (CN XII—Hypoglossal) Did the athletic trainer ask the athlete to stick his or her tongue out?

Yes ___   No ___

Passing score = 11 questions correctly answered

Problem XVIII

An athlete is brought to the athletic training room by his coach and a teammate. His right knee is positioned in slight flexion, and a small effusion is noted. To test the integrity of the anterior cruciate ligament, a Lachman's test is performed. Please demonstrate this test as you would on an injured athlete. You have 2 minutes to perform this test.

A. Is the athlete positioned in supine?

Yes ___   No ___

B. Is the athlete's knee positioned in 30 degrees or less of flexion?

Yes ___   No ___

C. Has the athletic trainer stabilized the distal femur with one hand?

Yes ___   No ___

D. Has the athletic trainer grasped the proximal tibia with the other hand, attempting to move the tibia anteriorly on the femur?

Yes ___   No ___

E. Has the athletic trainer applied adequate force in the appropriate direction?

Yes ___   No ___

Passing score = 4 questions correctly answered

Problem XIX

An athlete has been undergoing therapy after a significant ankle sprain. Using a goniometer, measure the range of motion of plantar flexion of the ankle (normal active range of motion is 0 to 40 degrees). Please verbalize your measurement to the examiner. The examiner should take the initial reading. You have 2 minutes to complete this task.

A. Is the athlete positioned in sitting with his or her foot hanging freely?

Yes ___   No ___

B. Is the axis of the goniometer centered over the lateral malleolus?
Yes ___   No ___
C. Is the stationary arm of the goniometer aligned with the fibular shaft, siting the fibular head?
Yes ___   No ___
D. Is the movable arm of the goniometer aligned parallel to the plantar aspect of the calcaneus?
Yes ___   No ___
E. Is the athletic trainer's recording within 5 degrees of the examiner's reading?
Yes ___   No ___
Passing score = 4 questions correctly answered

PROBLEM XX

This task will require you to properly fit football shoulder pads on a player. Proceed through all the steps, verbalizing each step to the examiner until the fitting process is complete. Inform the examiner when you are done. You will have 3 minutes to perform this task.
A. Did the athletic trainer verbalize he or she would measure the width of the shoulders to determine the proper size of the shoulder pads?
Yes ___   No ___
B. Did the athletic trainer check to make sure that the inside shoulder pad covers the tip of the shoulder and is in line with the lateral aspect of the shoulder?
Yes ___   No ___
C. Did the athletic trainer check to make sure that the epaulets and cups cover the deltoid muscle(s)?
Yes ___   No ___
D. Did the athletic trainer check to make sure that the athlete can raise his or her arms overhead without the pads sliding back and forth?
Yes ___   No ___
E. Did the athletic trainer check the straps located under the arms to make sure the pads are not free to move?
Yes ___   No ___
Passing score = 4 questions correctly answered

PROBLEM XXI

You are covering an ice hockey game when a player comes to you complaining that he "pulled a muscle in his inner thigh" as he was skating. Once you have gotten him into the locker room, you find that he has most discomfort when he tries to cross his leg over the other one at the knee. You suspect an injury to the sartorius muscle. Demonstrate a manual muscle test for the sartorius muscle as you would on an athlete. You have 2 minutes to perform this task.

A. Is the athlete positioned in sitting?
Yes ___   No ___
B. Did the athletic trainer have the athlete first move the limb actively into full hip flexion, abduction, and external rotation with the knee in a flexed position?
Yes ___   No ___
C. Has the athletic trainer placed his or her hand on the distal/lateral aspect of the thigh just above the knee joint?
Yes ___   No ___
D. Has the athletic trainer placed his or her other hand on the posterior/medial aspect of the lower leg just above the ankle joint?
Yes ___   No ___
E. Has the athletic trainer applied adequate force on the distal/lateral thigh to resist hip flexion and abduction?
Yes ___   No ___
F. Has the athletic trainer applied adequate force on the posterior/medial aspect of the lower leg to resist hip external rotation and knee flexion?
Yes ___   No ___
G. Did the athletic trainer perform this manual muscle test bilaterally?
Yes ___   No ___
Passing score = 6 questions correctly answered

PROBLEM XXII

A rower reports to his athletic trainer that during practice, he felt a sharp pain on the left side of his lower back that is now radiating into his left buttock and posterior thigh to just above the knee. To test for possible neurological involvement, a slump test should be performed. Demonstrate this test just as you would on an injured athlete. You have 3 minutes to perform this test.
A. Is the athlete positioned in sitting with the legs supported, hips in neutral (ie, no rotation, abduction/adduction), and with his hands behind his back?
Yes ___   No ___
B. Did the athletic trainer ask the athlete to "slump" back into full thoracic/lumbar flexion while keeping the chin in neutral?
Yes ___   No ___
C. Has the athletic trainer then applied overpressure while maintaining thoracic and lumbar flexion?
Yes ___   No ___
D. Has the athletic trainer asked the athlete to fully flex his cervical spine (ie, chin to chest)?
Yes ___   No ___
E. While maintaining this position with overpressure, has the athletic trainer asked the athlete to actively extend his knee while dorsiflexion of the foot is maintained?
Yes ___   No ___

F.   Has the athletic trainer repeated the test with the other leg and with both legs together?
     Yes ___   No ___

G.   If the athlete reported that he was unable to fully extend his knee because of pain, did the athletic trainer release the overpressure to the cervical spine and have the athlete extend his neck to see if the symptoms were relieved?
     Yes ___   No ___

Passing score = 6 questions correctly answered

PROBLEM XXIII

An athlete comes to the athletic training room eight weeks post Colle's fracture of the left wrist. His wrist movements continue to appear somewhat limited because of the immobilization. Using a goniometer, measure the range of motion of wrist radial deviation (normal active range of motion is 15 degrees). Please report your measurement to the examiner. (Note: The examiner should take the initial reading.) You have 2 minutes to perform this task.

A.   Is the athlete positioned in sitting with the left forearm pronated and resting on a tabletop with the elbow flexed to 90 degrees?
     Yes ___   No ___

B.   Is the wrist neutrally positioned among radial deviation/ulnar deviation, flexion, and extension, and are the fingers loosely extended?
     Yes ___   No ___

C.   Is the axis of the goniometer positioned over the capitate bone?
     Yes ___   No ___

D.   Is the stationary arm of the goniometer aligned along the forearm siting the lateral epicondyle of the elbow?
     Yes ___   No ___

E.   Is the movable arm aligned along the shaft of the third metacarpal?
     Yes ___   No ___

F.   Is the wrist in the correct position of radial deviation at the end of the movement?
     Yes ___   No ___

G.   Is the athletic trainer's recording within 5 degrees of the examiner's reading?
     Yes ___   No ___

Passing score = 6 questions correctly answered

PROBLEM XXIV

A lacrosse player has been participating in a rehabilitation program for an injury to the gluteus minimus and/or the tensor fasciae latae muscle(s). Using a goniometer, measure the range of motion of hip internal rotation (normal active range of motion is 0 to 45 degrees). Please report your reading to the examiner. (Note: The examiner should take the initial reading.) You have 2 minutes to perform this task.

A.   Is the athlete positioned in sitting at the edge of a table top?
     Yes ___   No ___

B.   Is the axis of the goniometer aligned over the mid-patellar surface?
     Yes ___   No ___

C.   Is the stationary arm of the goniometer aligned perpendicular to the floor?
     Yes ___   No ___

D.   Did the athletic trainer palpate a point midway between the two malleoli of the ankle as the site for the movable arm?
     Yes ___   No ___

E.   Is the hip in the correct position of internal rotation at the end of the movement?
     Yes ___   No ___

F.   Is the athletic trainer's recording within 5 degrees of the examiner's reading?
     Yes ___   No ___

Passing score = 5 questions correctly answered

PROBLEM XXV

A baseball pitcher complains he is having diffuse left elbow pain after prolonged periods of throwing. While evaluating his elbow, the athletic trainer notices that the athlete is not able to actively fully extend his left elbow because of a tight bicep muscle. Demonstrate how to stretch the bicep using a PNF stretching technique known as "hold-relax." You have 2 minutes to perform this task.

A.   Is the athlete positioned in a seated or supine position?
     Yes ___   No ___

B.   Has the athletic trainer asked the athlete to actively move the elbow into maximal extension and hold this position?
     Yes ___   No ___

C.   Did the athletic trainer isometrically resist elbow flexion for 10 seconds?
     Yes ___   No ___

D.   Did the athletic trainer ask the athlete to relax for ten seconds and then move the elbow into the new range of extension?
     Yes ___   No ___

Passing score = 3 questions correctly answered

PROBLEM XXVI

A tennis player reports that he has "lost power" while hitting overhead shots. When observing his thoracic area, the athletic trainer notices that his right scapula is "winging" (movement of the vertebral border of the scapula away from the thorax). Demonstrate a manual muscle test for the serratus anterior as you would perform on an athlete. You have 2 minutes to perform this task.

A.   Is the athlete positioned in supine?
        Yes ____   No ____
B.   Is the upper extremity positioned in 90 degrees of shoulder flexion and slight abduction?
        Yes ____   No ____
C.   Does the athletic trainer have one hand on the athlete's forearm and the other on his elbow?
        Yes ____   No ____
D.   Has the athletic trainer applied adequate force in a downward/inward direction toward the table?
        Yes ____   No ____

Passing score = 3 questions correctly answered

Please note that the answer to all questions in this chapter is "Yes."

WHAT TO DO IF YOU DO NOT PASS THE FIRST TIME

There will always be a few candidates who do not pass the examination. If you find yourself in this position, do not panic. It is important to identify factors that may have led to mistakes.

Although it is understandable to feel sad, frustrated, or angry, it is best not to dwell too long on what cannot be changed; focus your energy on the next examination being offered. The BOC certification examination is offered up to five times a year at various sites across the country. You should allow yourself another 3 to 6 months (depending on your employment situation) to prepare and pass the next exam. You may retake the exam as many times as you want as long as it is within 1 year of the date of your last attempt at passing the examination.

It is very important that you reregister as soon as you are ready. Your Emergency Cardiac Care CPR certification must be current and all of your academic coursework within the semester must be complete when you send in your application. Do not forget to send the application fee. You are allowed to select the site at which you would prefer to take the exam. Be sure you are aware of the application deadline; do not forget to mark your calendar!

The BOC recommends that if you fail the certification examination that you review your results with your endorsing athletic trainer so that he or she can counsel you regarding taking additional coursework or participating in further fieldwork to help you build your skills. This is a good piece of advice, given that your supervising athletic trainer should know you the best and can provide valuable guidance. In addition, a list of references that are used to develop the BOC certification examination can

be found on the BOC website at www.bocatc.org/become atc/CERT/EXAM/. These books may help you with your studies for your next attempt.

If for any reason you feel that you may have a disability or handicap that may have affected your performance during the examination, you may request that the BOC modify the certification procedures to accommodate your disability. Make sure that you send your request for this accommodation in writing to the BOC well in advance of the application deadline so special arrangements can be made.

It might benefit you to take a course on stress management techniques (eg, meditation or visualization) to help you reduce your anxiety while studying. It helps to talk things out with friends, coworkers, or your professors, but they may be limited in their ability to provide you with the tools needed to improve your coping skills. If you are finding you are having significant difficulty dealing with not passing the examination or your anxiety level is not manageable, we suggest you seek professional counseling. In general, try to maintain a positive attitude as you study and get yourself reorganized. Keep in mind that you will have a better idea of how the examination is presented because you have already been through it once.

It is also important to notify your employer (if it is relevant) of the status of your examination results. If you are honest and up front, he or she may be more understanding of your situation. Remember that you may not practice as a certified athletic trainer or refer to yourself as an athletic trainer until you pass the certification examination, and to do so will put both you and your employer in jeopardy of a malpractice suit.

If you are determined to be a certified athletic trainer badly enough, you will pass this examination. As mentioned before, give yourself the appropriate time to heal and then pull yourself up by the bootstraps and reorganize your approach. Critically examine your strengths and weaknesses and dig in for the long haul. Remember, the word "quit" is never in a true athletic trainer's vocabulary.

SAMPLE STUDY CALENDAR AND DAILY LOG

Sun	Mon	Tues	Wed	Thurs	Fri	Sat
	1 Make hotel reservations	2 Review	3 Written	4	5	6
7	8	9 Review	10 Written	11 Simulation	12	13
14	15	16	17 Review	18 Practical	19	20
21 Check route to site	22	23	24	25	26	27 Arrive at hotel
28 Exam day	29	30	31			

Figure 1. Sample study calendar.

Hour	Thurs, May 7	Fri, May 8	Sat, May 9
6:00 to 7:00 am			
7:00 to 8:00 am	breakfast	breakfast	breakfast
8:00 to 9:00 am	anatomy (UE)	practice emergency procedures with Tim, Mike, Bob	practice evaluations
9:00 to 10:00 am	anatomy (UE)		shoulder, knee, ankle
10:00 to 11:00 am	ankle/UE taping	practice emergency procedures with Tim, Mike, Bob	shoulder, knee, ankle
11:00 am to 12:00 pm	knee taping		shoulder, knee, ankle
12:00 to 1:00 pm	lunch	lunch	lunch
1:00 to 2:00 pm	nutrition	anatomy (LE)	anatomy (back/neck)
2:00 to 3:00 pm	run	anatomy (LE)	anatomy (back/neck)
3:00 to 4:00 pm	kinesiology/biomechanics	health care administration	psychology
4:00 to 5:00 pm	kinesiology/biomechanics	professional responsibility/ development	human physiology
5:00 to 6:00 pm	physics	swim at pool	biking with Sue
6:00 to 7:00 pm	dinner	dinner	dinner
7:00 to 8:00 pm	rehabilitation/ therapeutic exercise	athletic training evaluation	exercise physiology
8:00 to 9:00 pm	rehabilitation/ therapeutic exercise	athletic training evaluation	movie
9:00 to 10:00 pm	rehabilitation/ therapeutic exercise	athletic training evaluation	movie
10:00 to 11:00 pm			

Figure 2. Sample daily log.

Answer Key—
Written Examination
Sample Questions

Athletic Training Domains

Prevention

1. D) A sphygmomanometer is an instrument used to indirectly determine arterial blood pressure.
2. B) The Q-angle is taken by first drawing an imaginary line from the anterior superior iliac spine, down the thigh, and through the midpoint of the patella. A second line is drawn down the midline of the anterior thigh to the tibial tubercle. The angle created by the intersection of the two lines is then recorded. An angle greater than 20 degrees is abnormal, causing excessive genu valgus. Excessive genu valgus may lead to patellar problems in the athlete.
3. D) Shortening the stride during running may actually decrease the incidence of an overuse syndrome. Overstriding may result in a hamstring pull or knee pain.
4. C) Numbness or tingling in either or both hands in cold weather is symptomatic of Raynaud's syndrome, which is bilateral episodic spasms of the digital blood vessels. The cause is usually idiopathic.
5. E) Significant height, an arm span that is greater than the individual's height, pectus carinatum or excavatum, a high-arched palate, and myopia are all signs of Marfan syndrome.
6. C) Vital capacity is defined as the maximum amount of air that can be expired after a maximum inspiration.
7. D) Myopia is nearsightedness.
8. D) The liver participates in the metabolism of carbohydrates; detoxifies the blood of metabolic by-products; and produces albumin, clotting factors, and plasma transport proteins.
9. D) Measuring the maximal O_2 consumption during exercise is a good way to determine the athlete's ability to adapt to increased metabolic demands. Adequate pulmonary diffusion, appropriate vascular adaptation, and good physical condition of the active musculature all contribute to the athlete's ability to maintain homeostasis during exercise.
10. D) Skin-fold measurements for estimating body fat are routinely taken from the biceps, triceps, suprailiac, and subscapular areas.
11. E) The ability to dissipate heat by evaporation is severely limited in a hot, humid environment because evaporation cannot occur unless volumes of dry air are available to absorb the water vapor given off.
12. E) Running short distances stimulates the breakdown of phosphocreatine into phosphorus and creatinine in the muscle and glycogen and glucose to breakdown into lactic acid, allowing the muscles to work for short durations of time.
13. C) Power = force x distance. It is the intensity at which a muscle is able to perform work.
14. C) As a result of prolonged training and conditioning, the heart may increase in size to meet the increased demands.
15. B) The formula for calculating target heart rate is $220 - 25$ (athlete's age) $= 195$ x $80\% = 156$ BPM.

16. D) It takes between 15 and 30 minutes of a warm-up period to prepare the body for athletic competition. This warm-up period varies with each athlete and may have to be extended with an older athlete.

17. D) The average amount of calories an athlete expends in a day is between 2200 and 4400 calories.

18. A) These percentages are according to USDA guidelines.

19. E) Because specific types of food and timing of the pre-event meal are significant to performance, it is important that the coach, athlete, and athletic trainer are all involved in its proper planning.

20. B) It takes a minimum of 3 to 4 hours for food to digest. Fats take as long as 5 hours to leave the stomach. Proteins take as long as 3 hours and carbohydrates take approximately 2 hours to pass into the upper small intestine.

21. C) It is crucial that an athlete stay properly hydrated to maintain homeostasis and proper cardiac function. Average water needs for an adult are approximately 1 mL/Kcal burned. This equals approximately 2.4 liters for a 2400 Kcal energy output. Since the body does not conserve water well, it must be frequently replenished, especially while competing.

22. D) Female athletes who do not menstruate on a regular basis or those who vigorously exercise may eventually sustain severe bone loss, and osteoporosis may result. A calcium supplement of 1500 mg/day may effectively reduce the bone loss in the total skeleton and reduce the need for estrogen therapy.

23. A) The idea behind a carbohydrate-loading program is to increase the storage of glycogen in the muscles to improve performance in the endurance athlete. The athlete should consume a meal that is high in carbohydrates, such as pasta, and only lightly exercise the day before competition.

24. C) As per universal precautions, the athletic trainer should always wear gloves when treating a bleeding athlete.

25. A) To avoid the effects of jet lag, athletes should adjust all training, eating, and sleeping schedules to the local time in which they are competing.

26. C) The athletes may play in this type of heat as long as they take at least a 10-minute break every hour and change t-shirts when they are wet to allow for adequate evaporation.

27. C) Pediculosis is an infestation of body lice and is usually spread by close sexual contact.

28. E) When fitting an athlete for protective equipment, the athlete's skill level, size, sport position, physical development, and strength should be considered.

29. A) The helmet should not move if tilted, rotated, or turned side to side. The athletic trainer should push down on the crown of the helmet and check to see that the jaw pads and chin strap fit correctly.

30. D) An athlete with renal disease, uncontrolled hypertension, or an acute infection would be disqualified from athletic competition.

31. B) The coach, equipment manager, athlete, and athletic trainer should all be involved in the selection and maintenance of the athlete's protective equipment.

32. E) NOCSAE stands for the National Operating Committee on Standards of Athletic Equipment.

33. A) The two major categories that football helmets may fall into are the air- or fluid-filled helmet and the padded helmet.

34. A) Maximum protection is provided by a mouthpiece when it is made of a flexible, resilient material and is form-fitted to the teeth and upper jaw.

35. B) The epaulets and cups of properly fitting shoulder pads should cover the deltoids.

36. D) A flak jacket is a piece of protective equipment designed to protect the thoracic area after a rib injury.

37. D) ASTM is responsible for setting the standards for eye protection for racquet sports.

38. D) Palm protectors for gymnastics are not considered an NCAA-mandated piece of equipment.

39. A) Research has shown that increasing vitamin B_6 intake may increase the synthesis of serotonin, thus decreasing the emotional disturbances related to premenstrual syndrome.

40. B) Red meat and pork are the best sources of dietary iron.

41. B) Sodas contain caffeine, which is a dehydrating substance. This would not be an appropriate drink when trying to maintain adequate hydration during exercise.

42. E) Vitamin A in large doses consumed over a prolonged period of time may lead to toxic symptoms and death in extreme cases.

43. A) An athlete may sustain a stress fracture of the bone if he or she is subjected to a few high loads (eg, jumping on a hard floor) or many small loads (eg, jogging long distances).

44. C) Most schools are not prepared to have a bloodwork station at a preparticipation examination, nor is it necessary or cost-effective for most schools to do so.

45. E) The most common cause of an indirect sports death is heat stroke (ie, no direct trauma is sustained by the athlete).

46. B) It is the responsibility of the manufacturers or distributors of recreational sports equipment to report any defective or potentially dangerous products to the Consumer Product Safety Commission.

47. A) Tanner's five stages of assessment is an assessment tool used to document the maturity of an athlete's secondary sexual characteristics.

48. C) During the final checkout following a preparticipation physical examination, the athletic trainer and team physician should review each examination for final approval to participate.

49. E) The individual athlete is the only person who can decide whether or not to participate in a sport according to the Americans with Disabilities Act.

50. E) Significantly overweight individuals who have large muscle mass are much more susceptible to heat stroke than small-framed, lightweight individuals.

51. C) It is prudent to advise the athlete to place a damp towel between his or her skin and the ice pack to prevent a cryotherapy injury.

52. D) The spread of impetigo can be decreased by having the athlete avoid sharing towels and clothing with other individuals.

53. A) Furosemide (Lasix) is a potent diuretic and is banned by the IOC.

54. D) It is wise to suggest to this athlete that he trim his toenails by cutting them straight across. He should do this on a weekly basis.

55. A) When advising an athlete about the proper construction of a running shoe, the athlete should make sure that the midsole is somewhat soft but does not flatten out easily under pressure, the forefoot area has good flexibility, the shoe is of good quality, and the heel counter is strong and fits well around the foot.

56. B) Antihistamines have a sedative side effect; therefore, it is advisable that the athlete avoid taking them during the day.

57. D) A well-balanced diet will provide the required vitamins and minerals to keep the athlete healthy.

58. E) Shin guards are a necessary piece of protective equipment to dissipate the force from a direct blow to the anterior leg.

59. B) Wind and wet weather may increase the possibility of hypothermia while exercising in very cold weather conditions.

60. C) Cooper's ligaments are the suspensory ligaments of the breast and should be supported during exercise.

61. E) A fleshy, pink hue of the distal extremity is a normal finding.

62. C) Abuse of anabolic steroids will cause a reduction in body fat in the female.

63. A) It is important to maintain good hydration on long flights that cross numerous time zones.

64. A) Chronic use of chewing tobacco can cause leukoplakia (ie, the development of white patches on the mucous membranes of the mouth and cheek); mouth and throat cancer; bad breath; gum disease; tooth, bone, and enamel loss; cavities; and stained teeth.

65. C) The athlete should be advised to concentrate on strengthening his ankles rather than relying on prophylactic taping.

66. A) An antioxidant is a nutrient that may be found in high amounts in fruits and vegetables and may protect the cells in the body from the detrimental effects of naturally occurring agents, such as oxygen.

67. C) Hyperextension of the wrist when hitting a backhand shot in tennis is a primary cause of lateral epicondylitis.

68. A) Those athletes who weigh more than 220 lbs should avoid high volume, high intensity plyometric exercises because greater weight increases the compressive forces on joints during plyometric exercises, predisposing these joints to injury.

69. C) Free-weight exercises requiring the bar to pass over the face, move over the head, be positioned on the back, or racked at the front of the shoulders require one or more spotters.

70. C) Keratoderma is the hypertrophy of the stratum corneum of the epidermis, which occurs most frequently on the palms of the hands and soles of the feet. Keratoderma is also known as a callus and can be prevented by wearing two pairs of socks and properly fitting shoes; applying a lubricant to the skin to prevent friction; and protecting the palms of the hands with special gloves, tape, or moleskin.

71. B) UTIs may be avoided with adequate hydration, practicing sanitary bowel and bladder habits, washing the genital area before intercourse, emptying the bladder after intercourse, and removing contraceptive devices after intercourse.

72. A) According to NCAA guidelines, a period of 7 to 10 days should be allowed for acclimatization to prevent heat illness.

73. E) The number of servings should be according to the athlete's height and weight.

74. A) At the secondary school level, educational items that involve the athletic training student should include the education/training of the universal precautions and first aid for wounds, education regarding the risks of transmissions/infection from the athletes for which they care, education on the availability of HIV testing, education on the availability of HBV vaccinations and testing, and the education of parents/guardians regarding the students' risk of infection.

75. B) The American College of Sports Medicine (ACSM) recommends that when performing flexibility exercises, a stretch should be held 10 to 30 seconds—only as long as it is comfortable—to obtain optimal results.

76. D) To rectify low blood glucose levels, more free fatty acids are mobilized from adipose tissue than the liver can metabolize, resulting in ketosis. These excess ketone bodies are released into the urine and during respiration, resulting in low blood pH levels.

77. C) Increased muscle capillary density is a morphological change that occurs during resistance training. It is not a neural change.

78. C) Storage and the inventory of athletic uniforms/equipment are not a facilities maintenance task.

79. A) The use of multiple adapters and extension cords may cause a serious electrical hazard in the athletic training room and should never be used.

80. B) The physician or physician's assistant are the only personnel qualified to examine the athlete for adenopathy, abnormalities of the genitalia, and hernias.

81. C) The "flash-to-bang" method is a means by which an athletic trainer can estimate how far away lightning is occurring.

82. D) Athletes who live/play in urban or industrial areas should practice in the late afternoon after rush hour when the pollution level is at its lowest point.

83. A) A rubberized, padded cup has an elevated heel, which can compress downward so that the heel never actually makes contact with the interior of the shoe. The other heel cup is a rigid plastic cup. It fits snugly and does not allow the fat tissue to flatten, thus protecting the heel.

84. D) The Achilles' tendon tape job is used to restrict the amount of dorsiflexion at the ankle.

85. C) Wearing layers of lightweight clothing is recommended for the prevention of cold-related injuries.

86. B) The athlete should alternate pairs of shoes every day to help prevent fungal skin infections.

87. D) Water alone cannot kill an infectious microorganism. Water can be mixed with bleach (10:1), and this will disinfect soiled surfaces. There are also a number of commercial products that will disinfect soiled surfaces.

88. B) The secondary stage of disease prevention focuses on early detection of an illness or disease and preventing or reversing progression of the disease.

89. E) Medications, age, and conditioning level of the athlete are all predisposing conditions to heat illness.

90. E) Constant pain, insomnia, malaise, and fatigue are all considered red flags that should alert the athletic trainer to certain pathologies.

91. B) Immobilization of muscles causes a decrease in muscle tension produced.

92. E) Malaria is transmitted through blood/body fluids.

93. A) Isokinetic exercise is a type of exercise that involves a muscle contraction in which the length of the muscle is changing while the contraction is performed at a constant velocity.

94. B) A shoe with shorter and more cleats is better because the foot does not become fixed to the surface and the shoe still allows controlled running and cutting.

95. A) Ballistic stretching is not recommended.

96. E) To prevent hypothermia, the athlete should replace wet clothing with dry clothing, perform warm-up exercises, and wear warm clothing.

97. C) Sixty-five percent of heat produced by the body during exercise is lost by evaporation.

98. D) Heat is lost in the warm, vascular areas of the head and neck, which may account for 50% of heat loss from the body.

99. A) SPF 5 means an individual can be exposed to ultraviolet light five times longer than without having the sunscreen on before his or her skin turns red.

100. E) Seizures are not a primary sign of dehydration.

101. E) Shoe sharing between athletes may spread tinea pedis.

102. D) A headband will not prevent internal ear damage from loud noises.

103. A) An athlete should have a spotter when lifting at all times to prevent weight-training injuries.

104. B) Weather is not an intrinsic factor of injury.

105. E) Russian stimulation prevents atrophy by contracting the muscles.

106. A) The D2 flexion pattern involves external rotation with flexion and abduction. The D2 extension pattern involves internal rotation with extension and adduction across the anterior aspect of the body.

107. C) Symptoms of bulimia include binge eating followed by self-induced vomiting.

108. E) Enlargement of the spleen is usually a complication caused by mononucleosis.

109. B) The entire sternum should be covered for the shoulder pads to be legal.

110. C) This is irrelevant because as soon as a person suspects infection, he or she should cease work and be tested.

111. E) Calcium increases the density of bone, which decreases the risk of osteoporosis.

112. E) An anorexic athlete will not gain weight during the off-season because of abnormal eating habits.

113. A) Ballistic stretching involves a bouncing motion during stretching and should be discouraged in favor of a static stretch.

114. C) Stretching should be performed bilaterally.

115. E) Stretching, wearing proper footwear, and proprioceptive and strength training may prevent injuries to the lower leg.

116. D) Minimizing the effects of microtrauma; maintaining cardiovascular and lower extremity conditioning; and facilitating good communication among the athlete, athletic trainer, coach, and physician will help a throwing athlete prevent injuries while training.

117. C) Tertiary prevention is the prevention of a chronic or debilitating illness or injury through appropriate care and rehabilitation.

118. E) Periodization is the concept of dividing the annual training plan into smaller segments, phases, or cycles.

119. D) Extrinsic risk factors are those factors that are independent of the individual's physical makeup. Intrinsic risk factors are inherent in the physical makeup of the individual.

120. E) The overload principle states that muscle strength, power, endurance, and hypertrophy increase only when muscles perform workloads greater than those loads previously encountered.

121. A) An athlete with mononucleosis will present with an enlarged spleen, which is susceptible to rupture while playing a sport.

122. B) If sent back to play after receiving a concussion, the athlete could sustain another head injury, causing his or her brain to swell even more and possibly causing death. This is known as second impact syndrome.

123. E) Removing the shoulder pads and helmet or moving the athlete before completely assessing the injury can cause a greater spinal injury.

124. D) If the athletic trainer suspects shoulder dislocation, it is important to check the neurovascular status of the upper extremity, including the dermatomes and myotomes.

125. A) Shoulder pads protect the superior and lateral aspect of the shoulder. This prevents injury to the AC joint.

Recognition, Evaluation, and Assessment

1. E) Thompson's sign involves squeezing the gastrocnemius-soleus complex while the athlete lies prone on a table. The foot should plantar flex when the common muscle belly of these muscles is squeezed. An absence of plantar flexion upon squeezing is a positive test, indicative of a possible Achilles' tendon rupture.

2. B) The radial nerve innervates the extensor carpi radialis longus, extensor carpi radialis brevis, extensor carpi ulnaris, and extensor digitorum of the wrist, which when acting together, extend the wrist.

3. D) The most common type of ankle sprain is an inversion sprain. The primary mechanism of injury is a plantar flexion/inversion movement, which usually affects the anterior talofibular ligament first. As the sprain increases in severity, other ligaments around the ankle become involved, such as the calcaneofibular or tibiofibular ligaments.

4. C) A "burner" is a nerve injury commonly caused when the head is forced to one side while the opposite shoulder is depressed. It usually affects the upper trunk of the brachial plexus. A pinched nerve syndrome may also be caused by a nerve root entrapment, subluxed cervical facets, a bulging intervertebral disc, or a combination of lesions (nerve root entrapment and traction injury).

5. A) A sag sign is positive for a torn posterior cruciate ligament when the tibial plateau sags posteriorly as the athlete is lying supine and the knee is flexed to 45 degrees, causing a sulcus just inferior to the inferior border of the patella of the affected leg.

6. A) An athletic trainer's initial evaluation of an injury should begin the moment the injury is witnessed or upon initial contact with the athlete or another individual who might have witnessed the injury.

7. E) The Glasgow Coma Scale is used to determine an individual's level of consciousness or degree of coma. The three indicators of consciousness used are the stimulus needed to elicit eye opening, type of verbal response, and type of motor response.

8. C) The L5 nerve root innervates the extensor hallucis longus muscle.

9. E) A positive Phalen's test is indicative of carpal tunnel syndrome. The athlete is asked to stand with the dorsal aspect of both hands in full contact so both wrists are maximally flexed for 1 minute. A complaint of numbness and tingling in the medial nerve distribution of the fingers is a positive test.

10. C) Trendelenburg's test is used to test for gluteus medius weakness of the hip. The athlete is asked to stand on one leg for approximately 10 seconds and then switch to the other leg. If the pelvis on the unsupported side drops noticeably lower than the pelvis on the supported side, it is a positive finding (ie, weakness of the gluteus medius on the supported side).

11. D) The varus stress test is used to test the integrity of the lateral collateral ligament of the knee. The athlete is asked to lie supine with the knee in full extension. The athletic trainer places his or her hand distally on the lateral ankle and the other hand proximally on the knee medially. With the ankle stabilized, a varus force is applied with the proximal hand. Lateral joint pain and/or increased varus movement with an absent or poor endpoint when compared to the uninvolved side are positive findings for a torn lateral collateral ligament.

12. B) A positive drop-arm sign is indicative of rotator cuff pathology. The athlete is asked to stand as the athletic trainer passively abducts the athlete's arm to 90 degrees and then instructs the athlete to slowly lower his or her arm to the side. If the athlete has significant pain with the movement or is unable to control the adduction of the arm during testing, the sign is positive.

13. B) The golfer's elbow test is used to identify inflammation in the area of the medial epicondyle. The athlete is asked to flex both the elbow and wrist with the forearm fully supinated. The athlete is then asked to fully extend the elbow. If the athlete complains of pain over the medial epicondyle during testing, the findings are considered positive.

14. D) A sign is an objective entity, one that can be measured, felt, seen, smelled, or heard. A symptom, such as dizziness, is subjective in nature. Symptoms can only be experienced by the individual who is affected by the ailment or injury.

15. D) Tactile information alone will not provide the athletic trainer with enough information to adequately assess the athlete's functional status. It is crucial that a well-planned, comprehensive evaluation is performed to assess all aspects of the athlete's condition prior to treatment.

16. E) The extensor pollicis longus of the thumb is innervated by the C8 nerve root.

17. D) A positive clunk test is indicative of a possible glenoid labrum tear. The athlete is asked to lie supine. The athletic trainer places his or her proximal hand on the posterior aspect of the involved shoulder and the other hand distally on the humerus. As the athletic trainer passively abducts and externally rotates the subject's arm overhead, an anterior force is applied to the humerus as he or she circumducts the humeral head in the glenoid fossa. A clunking or grinding sensation is a positive finding.

18. D) Recurrent anterior subluxation of the shoulder most frequently occurs with repetitive throwing motions, primarily during the cocking and follow-through phases. With constant repetition, the anterior capsule and labrum may stretch or tear, allowing the humeral head to slip anteriorly.

19. B) A pneumothorax occurs when there is the presence of air within the chest cavity in the pleural space but outside the lung. In an intact chest, a pneumothorax can occur if a fractured rib has lacerated a lung or spontaneously if the athlete has a congenitally weakened area on the surface of the lung, which may rupture without antecedent trauma. Sudden chest pain and difficulty breathing as the lung collapses are major signs of a spontaneous pneumothorax.

20. A) The posterior tibial and dorsalis pedis pulses should always be palpated after an acute knee injury to ensure the peripheral circulation of the involved limb is intact.

21. E) An injury to the peroneal nerve of the lower leg will result in foot drop. The common peroneal nerve innervates the peroneus longus muscle, the superficial peroneal nerve innervates the peroneus brevis muscle, and the deep peroneal nerve innervates the peroneus tertius muscle of the lateral aspect of the lower leg and foot.

22. B) A type V Salter-Harris epiphyseal fracture is a crush injury to the epiphysis.

23. C) Cranial nerve VII is the facial nerve. It supplies both sensation and motor control to the facial muscles.

24. B) The latissimus dorsi muscle is innervated by the thoracodorsal nerve.

25. D) A second-degree burn is also known as a partial thickness burn and appears as a bright red area with blisters.

26. A) The medial and lateral pectoral nerves innervate the pectoralis major muscle, which flexes, adducts, and internally rotates the upper arm.

27. D) Spondylolysis occurs when there is a defect in the pars interarticularis. A "Scottie dog" sign is a radiographic finding of spondylolysis. On an oblique view of the lumbosacral spine, there is an outline that looks like a Scottish terrier. The defect in the pars interarticularis appears as the collar on the neck of the Scottie dog.

28. C) The levator palpebrae superioris muscle elevates the eyelid.

29. D) Vision is controlled by the occipital lobe of the brain.

30. E) Jaundice is a symptom of liver disease that causes the skin to appear yellow in color. It occurs when bile cannot be made or excreted normally.

31. A) A Bankart lesion is an injury to the anterior capsule of the shoulder with an associated tear of the glenoid labrum.

32. B) Pronation and supination of the forearm take place in the horizontal plane.

33. A) An aura is a sensation that occurs just prior to a seizure. It may last for a few seconds and appears as a smell, sound, or specific feeling. It acts as a warning to the athlete and generally takes the same form every time it occurs.

34. E) Signs of inflammation include redness (rubor), pain (dolor), warmth (calor), and swelling (tumor).

35. A) Exercise may cause a temporary increase in blood pressure, while a change in posture may raise or lower the pressure.

36. B) Type I diabetes is also known as juvenile-onset diabetes or insulin-dependent diabetes, and it usually has its onset prior to age 25. It is not usually associated with obesity.

37. C) Symptoms of mononucleosis include tender lymph nodes, fever, sore throat, and a stiff neck. Low back pain is not a characteristic symptom of this illness.

38. D) Candida is a yeast infection that causes vaginitis.

39. D) Osteoporosis rarely occurs in an obese individual. Obesity is not considered a risk factor for the disease.

40. C) The normal leukocyte (white blood cell) count is between 4000 and 10,000 cu mm.

41. C) The AIDS virus attacks the T-helper lymphocytes of the body's immune system, leaving the individual vulnerable to infection.

42. B) EIA stands for exercise-induced asthma.

43. C) The athlete will hike the hip to allow his or her foot to clear the floor during the swing phase of gait.

44. E) Crutches widen the base of support. This allows for the line of gravity to fall within the base of support, increasing stability.

45. E) Anorexia nervosa is an eating disorder that is most commonly seen in adolescent females. The athlete consumes a progressively diminishing amount of food until she is malnourished, and there is a weight loss of 25% of the original weight. Because of an intense fear of becoming obese, the athlete will not maintain normal body weight for her height and age, even when emaciated. It is a sign of a significant underlying psychological problem.

46. E) There are five emotional phases an athlete may experience after a significant injury or loss. These phases include denial, anger, bargaining, depression, and acceptance. These reactions are normal when faced with a serious injury or illness, and the athletic trainer should allow the athlete a chance to work through each stage without interference.

47. D) Symptoms of overtraining include emotional lability, loss of appetite, decreased concentration, decreased motivation to participate in practices and competitions, chronic fatigue, indigestion, and changes in bowel and sleeping patterns. An athlete who experiences staleness should be temporarily removed from activity and allowed time to rest and relax to stimulate renewed interest and motivation to play.

48. E) Signs of depression include loss of appetite, insomnia, fatigue, and a feeling of hopelessness.

49. C) An obsessive-compulsive athlete may perform ritualistic behaviors, such as cleaning his equipment after each game, and repeat specific behaviors obsessively, such as hand washing numerous times after touching a dirty uniform or money.

50. A) An athlete might be prone to injury for a number of reasons, some of which are physical and some of which are psychological. Physical factors include poor strength and endurance, inflexibility or hypermobility, and poor coordination. Emotional factors include depression, family or school problems, or anxiety.

51. A) Dehydration causes a decrease in blood volume, which results in lowered cardiac filling pressure and stroke volume. The heart rate increases to compensate for these adverse effects.

52. B) This meal is high in fat and protein and will take a long time to pass through the digestive tract.

53. A) Consuming a simple sugar prior to an event will stimulate the pancreas to produce high levels of insulin, which in turn will cause a sudden reduction in blood glucose.

54. D) Vitamin C is found in high concentrations in green vegetables, fruits, and citrus.

55. C) Tetracycline should be taken 2 to 3 hours after meals to avoid the possibility of the drug binding to either iron or calcium.

56. D) The healthy range for percent body fat for the female athlete is between 13% and 18%.

57. E) Water loss of 2% to 3% total body weight will begin to adversely affect athletic performance. Loss of 4% to 5% total body weight or greater are life-threatening percentages.

58. C) Tylenol (acetaminophen) has analgesic and antipyretic properties but is not an anti-inflammatory drug.

59. B) Ultram is a centrally acting analgesic drug used to control moderate to severe pain.

60. B) Tinactin is an antifungal medication, which is supplied as an aerosol powder, cream, powder, or solution and is indicated for treatment of tinea pedis (athlete's foot) or tinea cruris (jock itch).

61. B) To determine if there is a fracture of the jaw, it is appropriate for the athletic trainer to have the athlete bite down and observe for any malocclusion, ask the athlete to open and close his mouth and observe for movement asymmetry, and palpate the jaw for any deformities.

62. A) The liver is located in the upper right quadrant and may be injured with blunt trauma to that area of the abdomen.

63. C) A second-degree concussion presents with blurring of vision or unconsciousness lasting from 20 seconds to 5 minutes, complaints of headache with associated amnesia, and the athlete appears confused and often disoriented. (Note: This is according to the Cantu scale).

64. C) Cauliflower ear is an injury to the pinna of the ear caused by continuous friction or direct trauma to the auricle, which results in bleeding into the soft tissue of the ear. It is characterized by localized perichondrial swelling, discomfort, and deformity of the outer ear.

65. C) If an athlete has increased protein in the urine (most commonly diagnosed by urinalysis during a preparticipation medical exam), it may indicate renal or urinary tract pathology.

66. E) Because stress fractures of the bone can be so small, a typical x-ray will often miss the injury. A bone scan involves injection of a radioactive substance into a vein, which is absorbed by bone. A scanner is used to detect abnormal levels of uptake or hot spots in the bone, indicating a stress fracture or abnormal lesion.

67. D) The cornea, which is the clear surface covering the front of the eye, is most often injured by a foreign body, causing a corneal abrasion.

68. D) Measuring the amount of motion available at a joint will provide the athletic trainer with no significant information regarding the neurovascular status of the injured limb.

69. E) Anaphylactic shock is caused by a severe allergic reaction to a foreign protein or drug. There is a contraction of smooth muscle fibers and increased capillary permeability, causing dyspnea, cyanosis, convulsions, unconsciousness, and, if untreated, death.

70. C) Endorphins are polypeptides that are produced in the brain and produce analgesia by binding to the opiate receptor sites of pain perception in the body.

71. C) The classical mechanism of injury for an anterior shoulder dislocation is forceful shoulder abduction with external rotation.

72. B) Insomnia, shortness of breath with exertion, headache, fatigue, tachycardia, bradycardia, confusion, and edema are all symptoms of acute mountain sickness.

73. E) A manual muscle grade of 2/5 is also known as a poor muscle grade and is defined as completing full range of motion in a gravity-eliminated position. A grade of 3/5, or fair, is defined as completion of full range of motion against gravity, and a grade of 1/5 is a trace grade, in which the examiner observes or palpates contractile activity in the muscle, but no movement is present.

74. C) The scouring test is used to test for hip joint pathologies, such as arthritis, osteochondral defects; avascular necrosis, and acetabular defects.

75. A) To test the strength of the piriformis, the athlete should be sitting. The lower leg is resisted as the athlete attempts to externally rotate the hip.

76. B) Average range of motion for elbow flexion is 0 to 135 degrees.

77. B) The biceps femoris is tested with the athlete lying in the prone position. Knee flexion is then resisted with the tibia in full external rotation.

78. A) The SI nerve root innervates the posterior tibialis, plantaris, peroneus longus, and peroneus brevis muscles, which act to plantar flex the ankle and foot.

79. A) To test the function of the rhomboid major, the athletic trainer should ask the athlete to retract his or her scapula.

80. C) The biceps brachii muscle originates on the supraglenoid tubercle of the scapula (long head) and the apex of the coracoid process (short head). It inserts into the tuberosity of the radius. It functions to supinate the forearm, flex the elbow, and flex the shoulder.

81. A) Hip abduction occurs in the frontal plane.

82. E) The gastrocnemius muscle plantar flexes the foot and flexes the knee.

83. B) The flexor pollicis longus originates on the radius, adjacent interosseous membrane, and coronoid process of the ulna and inserts on the distal phalanx of the thumb. Its primary action is flexion of the thumb.

84. D) Movements of the eyes are controlled by the oculomotor nerve—cranial nerve III.

85. D) The rectus femoris muscle flexes the hip and extends the knee when it contracts.

86. B) The gluteus maximus externally rotates the hip.

87. B) Nerve roots C6, C7, and C8 represent the sensory dermatomes of the hand (from radial to thumb sides, respectively).

88. E) The serratus anterior muscle functions to protract the scapula and stabilize it against the rib cage.

89. C) The quadratus lumborum originates on the iliac crest, the lumbar vertebrae, and lumbodorsal fascia and inserts onto the 12th rib and the transverse processes of upper lumbar vertebrae. It functions to laterally flex the trunk.

90. C) The supinator muscle of the forearm is innervated by the radial nerve.

91. B) The extensor digitorum longus extends the toes.

92. E) Food passes from the stomach through the duodenum and mixes with the secretions from the pancreas and liver before continuing into the jejunum and ileum.

93. C) The median nerve passes though the carpal tunnel at the wrist.

94. C) The ileum is part of the lower small intestine.

95. C) The femoral nerve innervates the pectineus muscle, and the obturator innervates the adductor longus, magnus, brevis, and gracilis.

96. B) The abductor digiti minimi abducts the fifth finger.

97. D) The sternocleidomastoid flexes and rotates the head.

98. C) The tibial nerve innervates the gastrocnemius, flexor hallucis longus, and biceps femoris musculature.

99. D) Cranial nerve II is the optic nerve (vision), cranial nerve I is the olfactory nerve (smell), and cranial nerve XII (hypoglossal) is the nerve responsible for movement of the tongue.

100. A) To test the gluteus medius in an antigravity position against resistance, the athlete must be side lying with the affected limb on top.

101. E) The average range of motion of the knee is 0 to 135 degrees.

102. D) True leg length discrepancy is measured between the anterior superior iliac spine to the medial malleolus of the ankle.

103. C) To test the hip flexor musculature, the athlete should be sitting. The athletic trainer then applies a force down onto the anterior aspect of the thigh as the athlete resists the movement.

104. B) To test the deltoids, the athlete's shoulder should be positioned to 90 degrees.

105. C) Scoliosis is a lateral curvature of the spine with rotation of the vertebrae around its long axis. The ribs may become prominent on the convex side of the curve (rib hump) as the vertebral bodies rotate toward the convex side and the spinous processes rotate toward the concave side of the curve.

106. C) If there is an injury to the long thoracic nerve, which innervates the serratus anterior muscle, the scapula cannot be protracted, and it will result in winging, which is a prominence of the vertebral border of the scapula.

107. B) The average range of VO_2 max for the average college athlete is 45 to 60 mL/kg/min.

108. E) Measuring the heart rate during submaximal stress testing is used to indirectly determine the VO_2 max. It is known that heart rate rises linearly with increasing workloads.

109. D) The oxygen consumed by the athlete during the recovery phase of exercise replenishes the oxygen levels in the tissue fluids, increases the myoglobin in the muscles to preactivity levels, and restores the venous oxyhemoglobin to pre-exercise levels.

110. D) Progressive pulse rate test, the Harvard step test, and the Cooper 12-minute run-walk test are all classified as submaximal stress tests.

111. A) A goniometer is the instrument most commonly used for measuring joint range of motion in the clinical setting. A goniometer may come in a variety of shapes and sizes and may be made of metal or plastic.

112. C) Periostitis, myositis, tendinitis, or a combination of conditions may cause tenderness and pain with induration and swelling of the pretibial musculature of the athlete's lower leg. They may be classified as anterior or posteromedial "shin splints," depending on which group of structures are involved.

113. C) A positive Speed's test may suggest bicipital tendinitis. The athlete is asked to stand or sit with the involved shoulder flexed to 90 degrees and the elbow fully extended with the forearm supinated. The athletic trainer should have his or her distal hand on the volar aspect of the forearm and the proximal hand palpating the bicipital groove. As the athletic trainer resists shoulder flexion, it should be noted if there is tenderness or pain over the biceps tendon.

114. B) A physician is the only person who can legally diagnose a medical condition or problem.

115. A) A positive talar tilt test is indicative of a torn calcaneofibular ligament. The athlete is asked to lie on his or her uninvolved side with the involved foot and ankle over the edge of the table and the knee flexed to 90 degrees. The athletic trainer's proximal hand stabilizes the tibia as the distal hand grasps the talus. As the ankle is initially placed in neutral, the examiner then tilts the talus into an adducted position. If the range of motion in the adducted position of the involved ankle is greater than the uninvolved, the findings are considered positive.

116. D) Whether or not the athlete has medical insurance should not be an immediate concern of the athletic trainer during the history-taking portion of the initial evaluation. Only those pieces of information that assist the athletic trainer in developing a course of action or treatment plan for the athlete should be considered pertinent.

117. C) The L4 nerve root innervates the rectus femoris muscle and the vastus medialis, intermedius, and lateralis muscles, all of which extend the knee.

118. C) A positive Neer's test is indicative of shoulder impingement of the supraspinatus tendon or the tendon of the long head of the biceps.

119. A) A positive finding, such as a palpable clunk or shift with 20 to 30 degrees of knee flexion, is indicative of an anterolateral instability of the knee, secondary to a torn anterior cruciate ligament or torn posterolateral capsule of the knee.

120. B) Spearing occurs when a football player uses the top of his head as a ram, making contact with an opponent. The force is transmitted axially through the cervical spine, causing injury. Most cervical spine injuries result from forced hyperflexion, often with a combined rotation movement.

121. D) The most common mechanism of injury for an anterior shoulder dislocation is shoulder abduction and external rotation.

122. D) Glenohumeral instability allows increased movement of the humeral head within the glenoid fossa, which in turn may lead to microscopic damage to the tissues that lie beneath the coracoacromial arch. Resultant edema and microhemorrhage cause a reduction in the joint space and impingement, most commonly of the supraspinatus tendon.

123. C) Plantar fasciitis is an inflammation of the plantar fascia of the foot. It has a variety of possible causes but is commonly due to one or all of the following: pronated feet; poor footwear, leading to decreased shock absorption; and/or tight plantar fascia, Achilles', and hamstrings. A metatarsal pad would only be indicated if the athlete also had a diagnosis of metatarsalgia (ie, inflammation in the area of the metatarsal heads).

124. A) Because of the constant purging, the athlete is vulnerable to an electrolyte imbalance and dehydration. Hypokalemia (potassium deficiency) may result from chronic vomiting or laxative/diuretic abuse, causing muscle fatigue, weakness, kidney damage, or an arrhythmia.

125. B) Hypoesthesia is dulled sensation to touch.

126. A) Diabetic coma, which results from severely elevated blood sugar levels, results in the athlete feeling drowsy and having an acetone-smelling or fruity breath. The skin may be flushed and dry, the respirations deep, and the thirst intense. This is caused by inadequate insulin intake (ie, insulin-dependent athlete). Although diabetic coma rarely occurs in an active athlete, it can result from a mismanaged insulin schedule, severe infection, or poor diet.

127. E) McMurray's test is used to test the knee for a tear in the medial or lateral meniscus with the athlete lying in supine. The knee is fully flexed, and the tibia is externally rotated with a valgus force and extended, or internally rotated with a varus force and extended. A palpable "click" is indicative of a positive test.

128. A) Impetigo is a skin infection caused by staphylococcal bacteria. It is prevalent in wrestlers because of their close contact with other athletes. The bacteria can be carried under the nails and in the nose, infecting open skin wounds or abrasions. The lesion looks similar to herpes simplex lesions—a superficial ulcer with a yellow crust. The skin around the lesion appears normal. Treatment consists of local cleansing with soap and water and oral antibiotics.

129. A) Altered vital signs, such as a rapid pulse; decreased blood pressure; ashen skin color; rapid, shallow respirations; and rebound tenderness are all signs of shock, indicating a significant internal injury.

130. D) The primary movements of the pectoralis major are shoulder adduction, flexion, and internal rotation. If the pectoralis muscle is torn, the athlete will experience pain and weakness with resistance to these movements, as well as pain to palpation of the injured area.

131. D) Signs of pulmonary edema include acute dyspnea, cough, headache, and weakness. These symptoms can occur in athletes who train in high altitudes.

132. D) Most often a "pop" is associated with an anterior cruciate ligament injury and less frequently with a subluxed patella.

133. C) A Colles' fracture is a fracture of the distal radius and tip of the lunate. This usually occurs as a result of a fall on an outstretched arm and hand.

134. B) The Alien test is used to test the integrity of the radial and ulnar arteries of the hand. It is performed by first having the athlete pump his or her hand by repetitively making a fist. The athlete then maintains the fist while the examiner compresses the radial artery with his or her thumb and the ulnar artery with his or her finger. As the athlete relaxes his or her hand, the radial artery is released, followed by the ulnar artery. If there is a delay in flushing of the radial or ulnar sides of the hand or fingers, there may be an occlusion of the radial or ulnar artery, respectively.

135. B) The lunate is the most frequently dislocated carpal bone, which occurs from a fall on an outstretched hand. This in turn opens the space between the proximal and distal carpal bones, and the lunate dislocates to the palmar side of the wrist.

136. A) When the tibia is stabilized in an externally rotated position and a strong valgus force is applied, the medial collateral ligament, medial meniscus, and anterior cruciate ligament are vulnerable to injury.

137. A) Nerve root compression is most appropriately evaluated by electromyography or by a nerve conduction velocity test.

138. B) A papule may be described as a solid, well-defined pink/red elevated area on the skin. A wart is an infection of the skin caused by the Papilloma virus. The lesions are raised flesh-colored or pink papules with a rough surface that tend to grow inward into the foot, causing pain while walking.

139. E) The C5 dermatome is located over the area of the middle deltoid.

140. B) In order to expose the anterior deltoid to resistance in an antigravity position, the shoulder must be in 90 degrees abduction and in full external rotation. The forearm must be in full supination.

141. D) The most common symptom of lumbar discogenic injury is a sharp, radiating pain down one or both legs. This is caused by a bulging or herniated disc impinging on a nerve root in the lumbar spine.

142. D) An avulsion of the ischial tuberosity will cause local acute pain deep in the proximal thigh/distal buttock area.

143. D) The iliotibial band moves back and forth over the lateral epicondyle of the femur as the knee is flexed and extended. If the iliotibial band is too tight or it overrides and rubs on the lateral epicondyle during downhill running, the bursa between the iliotibial band and epicondyle becomes inflamed. Pain is elicited as the knee is brought into about 30 degrees of flexion. A popping sensation is not a consistent finding with this syndrome.

144. B) The contact phase of the running gait consists of foot strike, midsupport, and take-off. The swing phase includes the follow-through, forward swing, and foot descent. One foot is in contact with the ground during the contact phase, and the leg and foot freely move through the air during the swing phase.

145. B) The tibia internally rotates during midsupport, following pronation of the subtalar joint.

146. B) To check the vascular integrity of the hand after an acute elbow dislocation, it is important to assess the presence and quality of the radial pulse and check for good capillary refill of the nailbeds of the fingers.

147. B) The cardinal symptoms of an extradural hemorrhage include a lucid interval usually lasting for a few minutes up to a couple of hours, followed by a period of lethargy, which may precede a seizure and coma. This is a true medical emergency, and the athlete must receive treatment immediately in order to survive.

148. C) Concussions are classified according to the length of time of unconsciousness and the severity of the signs and symptoms of head trauma.

149. B) Pain with resisted hip adduction and hip flexion with diffuse tenderness and ecchymosis of the medial thigh is indicative of a strain of the groin area.

150. C) With a rupture of the rectus femoris muscle, a large bulge is seen in the upper thigh, and there is pain along the entire muscle belly. Extension is limited because of the inability to contract the rest of the quadriceps musculature.

151. C) Burning pain with tenderness to palpation over the lateral epicondyle of the femur is associated with iliotibial band syndrome. If the iliotibial band is too tight, it will rub over this area during running, causing localized inflammation. Ober's test is appropriate for a tight iliotibial band.

152. E) The quadriceps musculature is innervated by the femoral nerve, which originates at the L2, L3, and L4 nerve levels.

153. A) The spinal accessory nerve innervates the upper trapezius muscle. If it is injured, the athlete will not be able to perform a shoulder shrug.

154. A) The pes anserinus (sartorius, gracilis, semitendinosus) flexes the knee and will weakly internally rotate the tibia.

155. D) Heat exhaustion is characterized by profuse sweating, cool and clammy skin, rapid pulse, a mildly elevated rectal temperature (approximately 102°F), and hyperventilation.

156. C) A CBC is a test that assesses the red and white blood cell count, hemoglobin and hematocrit levels, and platelet count.

157. E) A -3/5 muscle denotes an incomplete movement against gravity.

158. D) Mallet finger is caused by a blow to the tip of the finger by a thrown ball, which jams the finger and results in an avulsion of the extensor tendon from its insertion.

159. E) Decreased sensation over the dorsum of the foot, inability to dorsiflex the great toe/ankle, and a diminished patellar reflex are suspect of L5 nerve root irritation or injury.

160. A) Active range of motion is used to determine the athlete's willingness to move.

Immediate Care

1. D) Naproxen is the generic form of the brand name drug Naprosyn, which is an NSAID. Naproxen does not come in a topical form and is delivered orally.

2. D) Aristocort, Kenalog, and Topicort are all corticosteroids that are used to treat the inflammation and pruritic manifestations of psoriasis. Betadine is a topical microbicide agent used for skin and wound infections.

3. E) Butisol is a barbiturate used as a sedative in the treatment of insomnia.

4. B) Xanax is a medication used to treat anxiety and panic disorders.

5. B) Penicillin inhibits the metabolism of bacteria.

6. A) Acute compartment syndrome is a condition in which soft tissue pressure is increased and the viability of the muscles and nerves of the anterior lower leg are jeopardized. This condition may progress from an initial hematoma, usually resulting from a blow to the anterolateral side of the leg, to total foot drop as a result of injury to the peroneal nerve.

7. D) It is appropriate during the acute stages of a quadriceps contusion to apply ice to the injured area and put the knee into a slight amount of passive

flexion to maintain the flexibility of the quadriceps muscle.

8. C) With deep frostbite, there should be rapid rewarming of the body part in warm water between 100°F to 110°F. Rewarming of the body part should continue until it is deep red/bluish in color.

9. A) An athlete should be immediately referred to a dentist if a tooth has been knocked out, if a tooth has been displaced 2 mm or more, or when a crown is fractured and the tooth is still alive.

10. C) When a male athlete sustains a direct blow to the genitalia, the testicular area may go into spasm. It is best to have the athlete lie supine and flex his knees to his chest until the pain subsides and then apply an ice pack to the scrotal area.

11. B) When performing two-person CPR, the correct compression-to-breath ratio is 15 compressions to 2 breaths 15:2.

12. D) Shock after a severe injury can result from hemorrhage or stagnation of blood.

13. B) An athlete who has a known diagnosis of mononucleosis is vulnerable to a possible spleen injury/rupture if the athlete returns to a sport too soon. The athlete may resume light activity after 3 weeks from the onset of the illness if the spleen is not enlarged or painful, the athlete's liver function studies are normal, no fever is present, and any other complications are resolved.

14. D) Romberg's sign is the inability to balance the body when the eyes are shut and the feet are together. It is a sign of sensory ataxia.

15. D) In this case, it is known the athlete is unconscious from a blow to the head and neck, not from aspirating an object or debris. It is only necessary to perform a finger sweep if the athletic trainer cannot ventilate the athlete and an object that is blocking the passage of air is visible in the mouth.

16. A) The proper position for the fist that is resting on the athlete's body is on the abdomen between the xyphoid process and the umbilicus.

17. A) When treating for an impaled object, always leave the object in place and apply a bulky bandage around it to control bleeding and to stabilize the object.

18. B) During a seizure, it is best to keep the area around the athlete clear of objects or spectators and protect the athlete's head and body from further injury. It is important to turn the athlete on his or her side so if he or she vomits, he or she will not aspirate. A prolonged seizure is a serious medical situation, and it is prudent to call for additional medical support.

19. C) Brain damage is most likely to occur if the brain is deprived of oxygen for approximately 4 to 6 minutes.

20. A) The carotid pulse is palpated in the groove between the larynx and sternocleidomastoid muscle.

21. C) The sternum must be depressed 1.5 to 2 inches for compressions to be effective in an average-sized adult during CPR.

22. C) Heat stroke is considered a medical emergency. Heat stroke results in severe hyperthermia with the failure of the thermoregulatory system and dysfunction of the central nervous system. This condition does not spontaneously reverse its course, and the athlete may die without immediate medical attention.

23. D) Signs of an acute tension pneumothorax include tracheal deviation, distended neck veins, unilateral absence of breath sounds, and cyanosis.

24. E) Flank pain, difficulty/inability to void, and hematuria are all signs of kidney, bladder, or urethra injury.

25. E) During emergency care of the unconscious athlete, the athletic trainer should make sure the athlete's airway is clear and he or she is breathing normally.

26. D) The most devastating cervical injuries sustained in athletic participation occur from cervical hyperflexion and axial compression.

27. A) The athlete will complain of severe lower right abdominal pain with acute appendicitis and will complain of tenderness to the same area with palpation.

28. D) When transporting an athlete with a suspected spinal cord injury, a spine board should be used to stabilize the athlete during transport and additional medical support should be employed.

29. E) The elbow should be slightly flexed to approximately 30 degrees, which places the hand at hip level.

30. D) CPR should not be stopped until the athletic trainer is too exhausted to continue, spontaneous breathing and circulation have resumed, or another responsible party continues CPR in place of the athletic trainer.

31. C) Reflex pain experienced in the left shoulder and upper arm after a severe blow to the abdomen, resulting in a ruptured spleen, is known as Kehr's sign.

32. A) Although total immobilization of the ribs is not possible, a rib belt or rib taping may help minimize movement and make the athlete more comfortable.

33. C) Athletic taping and bandaging serves many functions, including supporting or immobilizing an injured body part, protecting wounds from further injury or infection, holding protective equipment in place, and controlling hemorrhage.

34. C) Continuous taping around a limb may result in compromised circulation.

35. B) The compression to breath ratio during one-person CPR is 15:2.

36. A) Applying pressure will minimize the bleeding. Keep the area clean with sterile saline or hydrogen peroxide; apply Steri-Strips for temporary closure, and use ice and a compressive dressing to minimize further bleeding. Refer the athlete to the physician for sutures, if necessary.

37. D) Placing the tooth in a moist cloth and encouraging immediate implantation is the only means by which to save the tooth. Tooth reimplantation after 24 hours has a poor success rate.

38. E) During an emergency, important information the athletic trainer should provide to the emergency personnel includes the type of emergency, the type of injury that is suspected, the current status of the athlete, the type of care currently being given to the athlete, and the exact location of the emergency (including landmarks).

39. D) With a suspected fracture of the knee joint or of the surrounding area, the splint should stabilize all the lower limb joints and one side of the trunk.

40. E) Mast cells and platelets release histamine and serotonin during the reaction phase of an acute injury.

41. C) During the initial phases following a soft tissue injury, there is transitory vasoconstriction followed by vasodilatation and increased permeability, causing redness and swelling of the area.

42. D) The bone marrow contains immature stem cells that differentiate into red and white blood cells and platelets.

43. C) When an athlete is injured, he or she may react strongly to pain and become very fearful of the possibility of being disabled. During this time, the athlete may display signs of overreacting by becoming argumentative or sarcastic. It is important that the athletic trainer provides emotional support and allows the athlete to express his or her emotions. It is best to be reassuring and divert the athlete's attention away from the injury.

44. E) Vitamin K contributes to blood clotting because it imparts a calcium binding ability to certain blood proteins, such as prothrombin.

45. A) RICE stands for rest, ice, compression, and elevation.

46. D) A potentiating drug is one that is used to increase the effect of another drug.

47. B) Athletes should avoid standing near tall objects, such as trees or telephone poles, which may attract a lightning strike.

48. A) Tinea pedis (athlete's foot) is caused by a fungus infection. The athletic trainer should advise the athlete to keep his feet clean and dry and wear clean socks on a daily basis.

49. B) Pulling the tick off the skin can leave the tick's head still embedded in the skin. Covering the tick's body with mineral oil or nail polish remover will cause the tick to remove its head from the skin.

50. E) The primary adverse side effect of the NSAID group is gastrointestinal discomfort.

51. B) Common side effects of antibiotic therapy are abdominal cramping, diarrhea, nausea, and vomiting.

52. E) Aspirin is administered in 325-mg tablets.

53. B) Side effects of oral contraceptives include nausea and vomiting, fluid retention, amenorrhea, and a feeling of sluggishness.

54. C) A female may develop a condition known as hirsutism, which is the excessive growth of hair in unusual places, with the ingestion of testosterone.

55. C) Otitis externa is a bacterial or fungal infection of the outer ear canal that is characterized by severe ear pain, hearing difficulty, drainage from the ear canal, swelling of the canal, and occasional dizziness. Prevention includes avoiding prolonged exposure to water (eg, swimming/showering) and keeping the ear dry after water activities with acetic acid or a similar drying agent.

56. B) The helmet should be left in place unless the face mask cannot be removed to gain access to the airway, OR if with the face mask is removed, ventilation still cannot be provided, OR if the helmet and chin straps do not hold the head secure, OR if the helmet prevents immobilization for transport in an appropriate position.

57. C) Because rust can develop on the screws and t-bolts of a helmet or the screw can be damaged during a rescue, the effectiveness of a screwdriver has been determined to be limited and unreliable.

58. D) An athlete with congenital or acquired spinal stenosis is more likely to develop paralysis after a fracture dislocation because the spinal canal is already too small for the spinal cord.

59. C) The athlete may be immobilized on a standard spine board, a vacuum mattress, a scoop stretcher (otherwise known as a split litter), or the Miller full-body splint.

60. D) Histamine is given off by blood platelets, basophilic leukocytes, and mast cells during the beginning of the inflammatory process, causing arterial dilation and capillary permeability.

61. B) Dysplasia is the abnormal development of tissue.

62. A) Poor blood supply and poor immobilization are two conditions that interfere with fracture healing.

63. A) Epinephrine is a sympathomimetic drug that may be delivered via an injective device, such as an Epipen, to halt an anaphylactic reaction.

64. D) Tagamet (cimetidine) and Zantac (ranitidine) are both examples of histamine-2 blockers, which reduce stomach acid output by blocking the action of histamine cells in the stomach.

65. E) Before administering an NSAID, the athletic trainer must determine if the athlete is allergic to aspirin because a cross reaction may occur in athletes allergic to aspirin.

66. E) Manual conveyance is a method by which an injured athlete is transported a greater distance than he or she is able to walk with ease. The most convenient carry is performed by two athletic trainers.

67. C) The average respiratory rate for an adult is 12 to 15 breaths/min.

68. A) The bell of the stethoscope should be placed over the brachial artery during auscultation.

69. B) During orthostatic syncope, the rapid perfusion of the limbs decreases the blood supply to the brain, which will cause a loss of consciousness. Orthostatic syncope occurs during a rapid change in postural positioning.

70. C) Fatty foods may exacerbate gallbladder pathology.

71. D) A seizure that lasts over 5 minutes, a primary seizure, and a seizure that does not fit into the athlete's pattern of previous seizures are all indications for physician referral.

72. E) TID means three times a day.

73. A) When there is a suspected spinal cord injury and the decision is made to remove the helmet and shoulder pads, they should be removed simultaneously to avoid cervical hyperextension.

74. A) The interassociation task force recommends that no fewer than four-plus persons lift an athlete suspected of having a spinal cord injury.

75. E) An otoscope is an instrument used to visually examine the ear canal and tympanic membrane.

76. B) The primary reason an athletic trainer would perform pulmonary auscultation is to identify potential abnormal breath sounds that would indicate a pathological condition.

77. E) Dysuria, an urgency to urinate, decreased urine volume, nocturia, back pain, pyuria, or hematuria all indicate the athlete has cystitis, which is a bladder infection.

78. C) These are symptoms of a rhinovirus infection, which causes the common cold. Supporting the immune system with fluids, rest, and good nutrition will help to limit the duration of the infection. It is best to limit the athlete's activities until the fever subsides and slowly increase exercise as tolerated.

79. A) Itchy skin on the feet and toes is not a medical emergency requiring immediate referral to a physician.

80. C) A hard-shell pad would be an appropriate choice when the goal is to completely cover an injured area (such as a contusion) and prevent further harm.

81. A) The brace should be adaptable to a variety of anatomic shapes and sizes. Not all prophylactic braces need to be custom-molded to achieve this goal.

82. D) A running shoe should have a sole that is made of a carbon-based material for greater durability.

83. D) The rigid orthotic device is the most expensive and difficult orthotic device to fit and has the highest degree of complications.

84. E) An AED, or automated external defibrillator, is used when an unconscious victim has no pulse.

85. D) Avoidance is one of the most frequent methods utilized by managers, but it resolves nothing. The conflict will occur again if the athletic trainer is not proactive in seeking a resolution.

86. E) Abnormal pain associated with a burning sensation that gets worse when the athlete lies supine or consumes caffeine, spicy food, or alcohol is highly indicative of esophageal reflux or peptic ulcer.

87. A) A sudden onset of chest pain, dyspnea, hemoptysis, and cyanosis is highly suspect for a pneumothorax.

88. E) Diarrhea, vomiting, and abdominal cramping that occurs within 6 hours of eating is highly indicative of food poisoning.

89. B) Each quadrant of the abdomen should be auscultated for at least 2 to 3 minutes before deciding bowel sounds are absent.

90. C) Cold urticaria is an allergic reaction to cold exposure. If left unrecognized, it may lead to a systemic anaphylactic response.

91. D) The athletic trainer should not provide psychological counseling unless he or she is qualified to do so.

92. C) When using iontophoresis, the athletic trainer should be aware of possible skin irritation and chemical burns caused by ion flux during treatment.

93. A) An athlete with an abdominal injury should never be given anything to eat or drink because it increases the risks of surgery if an operative procedure becomes necessary and it may make the athlete's symptoms worse.

94. B) Confusion, dizziness, apprehension, and diaphoresis are all signs of insulin shock. Any diabetic athlete who does not respond favorably within 2 to 3 minutes of receiving sugar should be transported immediately to the hospital.

95. B) The point at which the first sounds of the pulse are heard through the stethoscope is the systolic pressure.

96. D) A relationship between the athletic trainer and the athlete built on trust and mutual respect is

essential to the athlete's psychological and physical well-being.

97. A) An athlete that shows undue concern over minor injuries, but the concern is self-limiting, should not be referred for professional psychological counseling.

98. E) Deficits such as tinnitus, decreased hearing, or deafness may suggest involvement of the vestibulocochlear nerve.

99. C) The initial dose of Tylenol (acetaminophen) is two tablets, 325 mg each. The dose may be repeated every 4 hours, PRN.

100. A) The initial dose of Advil (ibuprofen) is one to two tablets, 200 mg each. The dose may be repeated every 6 hours, PRN. Do not exceed six tablets in a 24-hour period without consulting with a physician. (Note: This medication should not be administered to an athlete who is less than 12 years old regardless of parental consent.)

101. B) The initial dose of Pepcid AC (famotidine) is one 10-mg tablet to be taken with water up to two times a day. Do not administer more than two tablets in a 24-hour period.

102. B) Constipation may occur secondary to poor hydration or decreased fiber intake. It is recommended that the athlete increase his fluid intake and increase his consumption of foods high in fiber.

103. C) Nonsteroidal anti-inflammatory analgesics, skeletal muscle relaxants, and anti-inflammatory steroids (glucocorticoids) all have complementary/synergistic effects to cryotherapy treatments.

104. D) Systemic vasoconstrictors may decrease perfusion of the peripheral tissues.

105. A) The three most common sites for avulsion fractures and apophysitis in the pelvic region are the ischial tuberosity and the hamstring attachment, the anterior inferior iliac spine and rectus femoris attachment, and the anterior superior iliac spine and the attachment of the sartorius.

106. D) A shin contusion that is poorly managed can lead to osteomyelitis, which results in the destruction and deterioration of the bone.

107. E) A metatarsal bar is used for the treatment of metatarsalgia and sesamoiditis.

108. E) The median, radial, and ulnar nerves and the neurovascular status of the brachial artery should be evaluated pre- and post-reduction of a dislocated elbow.

109. B) A Bennett's fracture occurs at the carpometacarpal joint of the thumb. It is structurally unstable and the athlete should be referred to an orthopedic surgeon.

110. E) Anxiety caused by fear may in turn lead to hyperventilation. An increased breathing rate results in the athlete rapidly blowing off carbon dioxide, which causes respiratory alkalosis, which is manifested by peripheral numbness, tingling, and light-headedness.

111. D) The muscle spasm has an end feel that is an abrupt, firm, springy resistance to motion. This is caused by the protective muscle spasm.

112. A) Checking for sensations of numbness, tingling, or burning is a component of a secondary survey.

113. C) Immediately transport the athlete to an emergency care facility for intravenous glucose administration. This is necessary to avoid possible brain damage or death.

114. A) Referred symptoms occur distally from the site of injury.

115. B) Restlessness is not a sign/symptom of postconcussion syndrome. The athlete will show signs of fatigue.

116. D) Tinel's sign identifies ulnar nerve compression or transmission interference at the elbow.

117. C) During anaphylactic shock, blood pressure drops very quickly as the blood pools into the expanded capillaries.

118. B) A contusion is a closed wound (ie, an injury of the soft tissue beneath the skin).

119. C) Heat stroke is a condition of rapidly rising internal body temperature that occurs when the body's mechanisms for the release of heat are overwhelmed.

120. E) The dorsal pedal pulse should always be assessed when dealing with injuries to the lower extremity.

121. E) Psychogenic shock is commonly referred to as fainting and is caused by a temporary dilation of blood vessels that reduces the normal amount of blood in the brain.

122. B) When a minor is injured and it is a life-threatening situation, the athletic trainer may provide emergency care even if the parents have not given written consent. This is known as implied consent.

123. C) A sign of heat stroke is hot and relatively dry skin.

124. D) Slow and weak pulse is not a sign of a diabetic coma.

125. A) The brachial and femoral arteries are the two most common sites to apply direct pressure to control severe bleeding of an upper or lower extremity.

126. B) Septic shock is the result of a widely disseminated infection of the body.

127. D) Slow and weak pulse is not a sign of hypovolemic shock.

128. C) Brain cells begin to die after the brain has been deprived of oxygen between 4 to 6 minutes.

129. D) Noisy respiration, such as wheezing or gurgling, is a sign of inadequate ventilation.

130. C) Gaining access to the airway is the only reason a football helmet should be removed before a spinal injury has been ruled out.

131. E) The xyphoid process is the bony prominence most commonly chipped during CPR.
132. B) Heat exhaustion causes a person to sweat profusely and become dizzy and nauseated. Also, their blood pressure (BP) drops during heat exhaustion.
133. D) It is not wise to give food or fluids to an athlete who is in shock because of the possibility of aspiration.
134. D) An athlete with a skull fracture may have a bony deformity, Battle's sign, "raccoon" eyes, and tenderness of the hard palate.
135. A) Apply direct pressure to the wound.
136. B) Hold in-line stabilization decreases any chance of increasing the severity of the injury.
137. D) Immobilization is initiated before rehabilitation begins.
138. A) When ice is applied during the initial care of an acute injury, there is a decrease in local metabolism.
139. B) Afferent pathways carry impulses toward the central nervous system.
140. E) Friction massage is a type of deep massage.
141. D) To determine if an athlete is breathing, the athletic trainer should LOOK for the rise and fall of the chest, LISTEN for the breath sounds, and FEEL for breathing.
142. C) Dilated pupils are a sign of shock, hemorrhage, or cardiac arrest.
143. B) An athlete's blood pressure will be low if he or she is in shock.
144. A) Signs of frostbite include blotchy white to yellow-gray skin.
145. D) An athlete suspected of having heat exhaustion should be administered cool fluids, unnecessary clothing should be removed, and he or she should be moved to a cool place.

Treatment, Rehabilitation, and Reconditioning

1. D) An extension lag exists when the athlete cannot fully extend his or her knee.
2. D) A hand dynamometer is a simple tool used to objectively assess the functional strength of the hand and forearm.
3. A) Tissue healing begins with a cellular response, which is associated with vascular changes, followed by phase II, or regeneration, of both soft tissue and bone. The third phase is known as remodeling, in which there is an increased organization of extracellular matrix and decreased synthetic activity.
4. E) It may take up to 1 year before soft tissue remodeling is complete.
5. A) The primary location of adenosine triphosphate (ATP) in skeletal muscle is the sarcomere.
6. C) Golgi tendon organs (GTOs) are sensory receptors found in the muscle tendons that monitor the tension generated in a muscle during contraction.
7. A) A neurapraxia is the demyelination of the axon sheath of a nerve fiber. This condition will cause a failure of the nerve to conduct impulses, causing a conduction block. It is usually reversible.
8. D) Osteoclasts are cells that reabsorb bone during growth.
9. A) Cell division for new cartilage growth does not occur in the adult.
10. D) The athlete will experience the feelings of cold, followed by burning, then aching, and finally numbness.
11. D) A warm whirlpool is a superficial heater. It will only heat the superficial tissues.
12. E) Fibroblasts become active during the regeneration phase of the inflammatory response to begin building collagen.
13. A) Shivering is a method by which the body generates heat.
14. B) External force created by a muscle depends on the velocity of the muscle shortening (as the speed of shortening increases, the force decreases), the angle of the pull of the muscle (ie, when the muscle pulls at right angles to the bone it's moving, the muscular force will be optimal), and the length of the muscle (the tension developed with a contraction is greatest if the muscle is at its maximum resting length to start).
15. D) Proprioception is the awareness of movement, changes of equilibrium, and posture of the body and its segments. The "control center" for proprioceptive awareness in the brain is located in the cerebellum.
16. A) A static stretch requires that the athlete stretch the muscle and hold the position to prevent a muscle injury, which may occur with ballistic stretching.
17. A) The cardiovascular and respiratory systems must work together to meet the oxygen demands of the skeletal musculature during exercise. If the demand is not met by increasing the respiratory rate, the cardiac output must increase to increase the delivery of the red blood cells from the lungs to the heart to the muscles.
18. E) Visualization, also known as therapeutic imagery, incorporates the mental rehearsal of a positive rehabilitative experience followed by full recovery. It is a psychological tool used to enhance physical healing after an injury.
19. A) For rehabilitation of an injury to be successful, the athletic trainer must establish a good rapport

with the athlete so that the athlete is comfortable and there is a mutual environment of trust.

20. C) An attention-seeking athlete generally will not accept responsibility for him- or herself and enjoys being dependent upon other individuals. As a result, the athlete is demanding and is not satisfied with the amount of time other athletes receive, always wanting more time and attention by the athletic trainer taking care of him or her. This type of athlete is very draining to the health care staff and requires specific boundaries so the staff is not burned out by the athlete.

21. D) In order to lose 1 to 2 pounds a week, an athlete must reduce his or her daily caloric intake by 500 to 1000 calories a day.

22. E) Cryotherapy is used as an anesthetic and to prevent or decrease the inflammatory process.

23. C) Eddy currents are heat-producing currents that are administered by means of an induction coil or condenser plate of a short-wave diathermy unit. It uses a magnetic field to create these currents within the tissues.

24. D) A monophasic spike waveform delivered in pairs is used with HVPGs.

25. B) Because a moist heat pack is a form of superficial heat, it does not increase the muscle tissue temperature.

26. A) The negative pole or cathode will cause local vasodilatation under the pad, tissue softening, irritation, and edema reduction.

27. B) Inflammation of a body part is an indication for the use of cryotherapy.

28. B) Single-leg hopping would be an appropriate functional skill in assessing the athlete's readiness for play after an ankle injury. Lifting tolerance is not a skill.

29. A) Normal range of motion of a joint must be restored before and concurrently with strengthening exercises during rehabilitation. Limb endurance and proprioception follow in the later phases of treatment.

30. C) Slow-reversal-hold-relax is a PNF stretching technique.

31. D) The hip is moving into a pattern of flexion, adduction, and external rotation during a Dl flexion pattern.

32. A) The proper timing sequence for a D2 extension pattern of the upper extremity is shoulder extension followed by forearm pronation and finger flexion.

33. A) Grade I joint mobilization is appropriate for decreasing pain and spasm.

34. A) An inferior humeral glide is the proper glide to employ when trying to restore or increase shoulder abduction.

35. B) Isokinetic training is generation of a muscular force with observable joint movement that occurs at a constant speed with variable external resistance.

36. D) Cupping, hacking, and pinching are all methods of tapotement.

37. E) Effleurage is a superficial or deep stroking technique used to produce relaxation.

38. C) Proprioception is the awareness of posture, positioning, and movement as the limb is moved through space.

39. E) The quadriceps must contract eccentrically to allow for deceleration of the body in downhill running.

40. D) Postseason conditioning should focus on identifying and emphasizing specific areas of the conditioning components the athlete needs to improve upon.

41. B) During the acute phase of an ankle injury, some form of cryotherapy should be initiated. The water temperature should be set at 55°F to 65°F (cold) to prevent swelling.

42. B) The girth measurements of the involved leg do not have to be exactly equal before returning the athlete to full activity, as slight differences are normal.

43. C) Restoration of normal proprioception of the affected limb is the most commonly forgotten component of the rehabilitation program.

44. C) Isometric strengthening exercises are the safest exercises to initiate immediately postoperatively, as there is no joint movement initiated during muscular contraction.

45. B) Jumper's knee is an overuse syndrome of the extensor mechanism of the knee. There is injury to the proximal pole of the patella, as it is subjected to the repetitive traction pull of the quadriceps musculature. The quadriceps muscle should be strengthened during rehabilitation to prevent further injury.

46. B) Trochanteric bursitis can be caused or aggravated by a tight tensor fascia latae muscle.

47. D) A tight Achilles' tendon can cause early heel-off or excessive pronation in order to allow the lower leg to move over the foot during running.

48. D) The coach's opinion concerning when the athlete should return to play should not influence the athletic trainer's professional judgment in designing a rehabilitation program and following prudent guidelines for care.

49. A) Range of motion and strength of the shoulder girdle is intimately related to the function of the cervical area.

50. A) The proper sequence for rehabilitating a grade II ankle sprain includes RICE (rest, ice, compression, elevation), stretching exercises, isometric exercises,

proprioceptive exercises, and isotonic strengthening exercises.

51. A) Rehabilitation should begin as soon as possible after an injury with the initiation of modalities for pain relief (ie, RICE).

52. E) The first set of 10 repetitions is with a weight that is 50% of the weight that will be lifted in set three when utilizing the DAPRE technique of progressive resistive exercise.

53. C) With a diagnosis of patellofemoral pain syndrome, chondromalacia patellae, or subluxing patella, it is important to strengthen the quadriceps with an emphasis on the vastus medialis obliques muscle (VMO) and the hip adductors in order to improve the tracking of the patella.

54. D) Stretching the anterior chest wall (especially the pectoralis muscles) and strengthening the mid-thoracic musculature (especially the rhomboids and middle trapezius) improve posture and decrease pressure on the structures of the thoracic outlet.

55. E) Williams' flexion exercises encourage a position of lumbar flexion, which opens the vertebral foramina, taking the pressure off the nerve root.

56. A) The athlete's body is in a stable, static position while using a recumbent stationary bicycle and does not need to rely on proprioception to perform this activity.

57. C) Scapular musculature should be strengthened first to promote stability before the distal musculature is strengthened to provide mobility.

58. E) Hamstring strengthening should be initiated early in anterior cruciate reconstruction rehabilitation because the hamstrings are the main secondary stabilizers for the anterior cruciate ligament.

59. D) An isotonic knee extension machine is not a closed-chain exercise because the feet are not in contact with any surface.

60. B) Lateral epicondylitis is an overuse syndrome of the wrist extensors. Once the inflammatory process is under control, strengthening the wrist extensors will help prevent a reoccurrence of the problem.

61. B) McKenzie extension exercises are appropriate for treating a lumbar herniated disc, as they encourage the mechanical movement of the disc anteriorly away from the nerve root.

62. B) When performing an abdominal crunch (sit-up), the athlete should cross his arms across his chest, tuck in his chin, bend his knees, inhale, and then exhale as he pulls his torso up toward his knees.

63. C) A rehabilitative brace might be used postoperatively or during rehabilitation after an acute injury.

64. E) Running on a treadmill would most closely relate to the type of activity a soccer player would participate in during his or her sport.

65. A) Mechanical traction is not indicated for treatment of acute sprains and strains.

66. C) The anterior deltoid, triceps, pectoralis major, and latissimus dorsi are all active while performing a bench press.

67. C) The quadriceps, hamstrings, the erector spinae, and the gluteus maximus are all active when performing a full squat with weights.

68. D) The trapezius, pectoralis major, serratus anterior, and triceps musculature are all active when performing a seated military press.

69. B) A grade III joint mobilization is a large amplitude movement throughout the full available range of motion of the joint.

70. A) The SAID principle stands for Specific Adaptation to Imposed Demands.

71. E) A wall is an immovable object and may be used for an isometric exercise. During isotonic exercise, there is a fixed resistance with variable speed of movement.

72. A) Ballistic stretching places high, intermittent demands on the muscle, possibly exceeding its physiological limitations, leading to a muscle tear.

73. C) Plyometric training involves loading a muscle eccentrically prior to performing a powerful concentric contraction. This places the muscle in a fully stretched position just prior to contraction-enhancing explosiveness, which is important in a sport such as volleyball.

74. B) Having the athlete stand on the injured limb on a mini-trampoline enhances proprioception by making the athlete react to a slightly unleveled surface. The goal is to have the athlete maintain this position without wobbling or losing his or her balance.

75. D) Because eccentric muscle strengthening requires high muscle tension to be generated, exercising the quadriceps eccentrically is initiated in the later stages of the rehabilitation.

76. A) Full knee extension exercises (from 90-degree knee flexion to 0-degree extension) should be avoided in the early stages of anterior cruciate reconstruction rehabilitation because of the high shearing forces placed on the tibia by the contracting quadriceps.

77. C) Partial sit-ups assist in strengthening the abdominals, and trunk extension exercises (with or without resistance) strengthen the erector spinae musculature.

78. B) Any finding that the athletic trainer observes, palpates, or measures is recorded under the objective (O) section of a SOAP note.

79. C) Bracing for structural scoliosis may be effective up to approximately age 18. After this age, the

epiphyseal plates close and external devices for correction do not work well.

80. E) Ultrasound is based on the reverse piezoelectric effect.

81. E) Ultrasound waves cannot be transmitted through air. Ultrasound energy must be transmitted through a coupling medium, such as water or a lotion.

82. B) Convection is a method of heating by which heat is transferred from the source to the recipient by means of movement of the heating medium (eg, air or water).

83. D) The duty cycle is that time in which sound waves are being emitted during one pulse period.

84. A) A moist heat pack is considered a superficial heater.

85. B) Conventional TENS uses a frequency in the 50 to 100 pulses per second (PPS) range with a phase duration of 2 to 50 μseconds.

86. A) Galvanic burns are the most serious adverse reaction to iontophoresis and are caused by the galvanic current itself.

87. C) The temperature of a paraffin bath should be maintained between 126°F and 130°F to keep it in a molten state.

88. B) Ultrasound converts high-frequency sound energy into heat energy as it penetrates the tissue.

89. D) Ultrasound waves are reflected by bone and absorbed by muscle.

90. B) Inflammation, hemorrhage, infection, and phlebitis are all contraindications for massage.

91. D) Diathermy is used to increase local circulation, reduce spasms, and decrease pain after a musculotendinous injury.

92. A) Scar tissue may be reduced with the use of pulsed ultrasound.

93. B) The inverse square law states that the intensity of radiation from a light source varies inversely to the square of the distance from the source.

94. D) Phonophoresis is the delivery of medication via sound waves, and iontophoresis is the delivery of medication via direct electric current.

95. A) The primary indication for cervical traction is to reduce muscle pain and spasm.

96. E) The proper referral for an athlete with an eating disorder would be to a psychologist or psychiatrist because of the complex nature of the condition. It should be recognized by the athletic trainer that anorexia nervosa or bulimia is not just a simple nutritional problem but an underlying psychological problem.

97. D) Symptoms of gonorrhea in a male include a tingling sensation in the urethra followed by a greenish-yellow discharge of pus with painful urination. The athlete should be instructed to refrain from all sexual activity until he is treated.

98. C) It is important that the athletic trainer educate the athlete about the treatment process, as it will decrease his anxiety.

99. A) It is proper to have the athlete breathe in deeply at the beginning of the lift and forcefully exhale at the end of the lift.

100. B) Constant pressure on the axilla may cause crutch or "Saturday night" palsy, which is temporary or permanent numbness in the upper extremities and hands.

101. C) It is important to assess the athlete's training schedule and diet to make sure he or she is not overtraining and eating a poor diet. Both may affect an athlete's performance level.

102. E) To prevent reinjury during the rehabilitation of a soft tissue injury, it is important that the athlete not experience pain during active movement.

103. A) Larsen-Johansson disease is an apophysitis at the inferior pole of the patella and is characterized by swelling, pain, and point tenderness at the site. It usually occurs during adolescence. Isotonic exercise is not appropriate for this particular condition, as it may increase the symptoms by causing too much stress on the affected area.

104. D) It is important that the athlete be advised as to when to take his or her medication and with which foods/drugs it should not be combined.

105. B) It is appropriate for the athletic trainer to encourage the athlete to express her feelings and needs.

106. D) Heavy strength training work-outs should be limited to off-season and preseason periods.

107. B) Scheuermann's disease is a degeneration of the vertebral epiphyseal endplates, which may cause the intervertebral disc to herniate. An increased kyphotic curve is seen in an athlete with this condition. Extension and postural exercises may help reduce the symptoms of backache in the early phases of the disease.

108. A) It is important to emphasize the importance of good hip flexor, lumbar paraspinal, and hamstring flexibility during the rehabilitation of a lumbar strain to prevent reinjury.

109. B) It is best to sleep in a sidelying position with the knees bent slightly to avoid pressure on the low back area.

110. E) It is wise for the athletic trainer to advise and consult with the team strength-and-conditioning coach regarding the development of a reconditioning program postinjury.

111. A) Empathy and humor are important qualities that an athletic trainer should possess when counseling an athlete that is in a state of distress.

112. C) The athlete may feel a burning sensation during an ultrasound treatment if the intensity is set too

high, not enough coupling medium is being used, or if the transducer head is moving too slow.

113. B) Pain that occurs at a site distant to damaged tissue and does not follow the course of a nerve is known as referred pain.

114. B) Continuous and pulsed diathermy are used to decrease pain and muscle spasm. Diathermy is contraindicated for use with acute inflammation and joint effusion, pregnancy, and open wounds.

115. A) When a convex surface moves on a concave surface during joint mobilization, the roll and glide occur in opposite directions.

116. C) Cervical traction is indicated with a cervical disc herniation.

117. B) Muscle energy techniques are methods used to stretch tight muscles by having the athlete contract a muscle against a counterforce in a specific position.

118. C) DOMS normally occurs 24 to 72 hours postexercise.

119. A) Reduced submaximal heart rate does occur as a result of aerobic endurance training, but it is a cardiovascular adaptation, not a respiratory adaptation.

120. D) The latissimus dorsi, teres major, middle trapezius, and rhomboids are all involved when performing a seated row exercise.

121. D) The flexor carpi radialis and flexor carpi ulnaris are the primary muscles involved in performing a wrist curl.

122. B) Proprioceptors are specialized sensory receptors that are sensitive to changes in pressure or tension within a joint, muscle, or tendon. They are responsible for relaying information regarding muscle dynamics to the central nervous system.

123. E) Goal setting is the most effective motivator for compliance to rehabilitation of an athletic injury.

124. A) A major disadvantage of isometric exercise is that it can produce a spike in systolic blood pressure, which can lead to a potentially life-threatening cardiovascular accident.

125. C) The knee-jerk reflex (which is a monosynaptic stretch reflex) is a simple example of muscle spindle activity.

126. B) Passive insufficiency of a muscle occurs when the length of a muscle prevents full range of motion at the joint or joints over which the muscle crosses.

127. C) An exercise designed to improve balance must incorporate a multisensory approach.

128. C) An athlete who presents with posterior instability of the glenohumeral joint should avoid a combined position of internal rotation, horizontal adduction, and flexion.

129. D) The length of a rehabilitation program is irrelevant in regards to the development of a functional progression sequence.

130. A) Closed kinetic chain exercises of the upper extremity are used primarily for strengthening and improving proprioception and neuromuscular control of the muscles that stabilize the shoulder girdle.

131. B) The general adaptation syndrome (GAS) consists of three stages: the alarm stage, the resistance stage, and the exhaustion stage.

132. D) An ice bath (or ice immersion) is a mixture of ice and water with a temperature range of 50°F to 60°F in which a body part, most typically the fingers or toes, is immersed. It is used to decrease pain and edema.

133. A) One method of decreasing skin-electrode resistance when performing an electrotherapy treatment is to moisten the electrodes with water.

134. D) 99.9% of ultrasound energy is reflected when it is met with air.

135. C) The stimulation point placement of electrodes is most commonly used with brief-intense TENS.

136. A) Goal setting is important when developing a treatment program because it identifies outcomes, establishes timeliness of the treatment program, and measures the effectiveness of the treatment protocol.

137. E) There should be no metal in the immediate treatment area when using short wave diathermy.

138. B) Dexamethasone and lidocaine are commonly combined when utilizing iontophoresis.

139. E) Ultrasound units should be calibrated at least once a year to ensure their safe use.

140. E) The athlete is presenting with a carbuncle, which is a bacterial (staphylococci) infection often resulting as a complication of folliculitis.

141. A) Herpes simplex is caused by a viral strain that is associated with skin and mucous membrane infection. Herpes simplex labialis is most commonly known as a cold sore.

142. E) Pediculosis (ie, lice) is an infestation by the louse and is most effectively treated with a parasiticide.

143. A) An infection caused by tetanus bacillus may occur secondary to a deep puncture wound.

144. C) Adaptations in skeletal muscle that occur as a result of resistance training, such as increases in strength and muscle mass, may begin to reverse in 48 hours.

145. B) Circuit training is an effective technique for improving strength and flexibility.

146. D) Computerized parts will significantly drive up the cost of the bike and do not ensure superior results.

147. C) Treading water is not a necessary skill for participating in an aquatic therapy program. Many types

of buoyant devices may be used to keep the athlete afloat.

148. D) Decongestants are vasoconstrictors increasing the possibility of heatstroke. Antihistamines decrease the peripheral sweating, and diuretics limit cutaneous vasodilatation.

149. E) An athlete's heart rate will gradually rise as the intensity of the exercise rises and will plateau at a given level in approximately 2 to 3 minutes.

150. B) The efferent/motor response to neural/sensory information is known as neuromuscular control.

151. D) A fracture that fails to heal spontaneously within a normal time frame is known as a nonunion fracture.

152. D) The thermal effects of ultrasound may increase edema.

153. A) Iontophoresis results in the movement of ions into the body through the use of an electrical current.

154. E) Petrissage is the method of massage that involves lifting and kneading the skin, subcutaneous tissue, and muscle with the fingers or hand.

155. B) Loss of function is a cardinal sign of inflammation.

156. C) Raynaud's phenomenon is a vascular reaction to cold that results in a white, red, or blue discoloration of the extremities. The fingers and toes are the first to be affected.

157. C) The heat of the water causes vasodilatation and creates an outward filtration of fluid into the tissues. When combined with the dependent position of the body part, a warm whirlpool will cause an increase in edema.

158. A) Graves' disease is the most common form of hyperthyroidism.

159. E) Dyspnea is air hunger marked by labored or difficult breathing.

160. B) Neurapraxia is a stretch injury to a nerve resulting in transient symptoms of paresthesia and weakness.

161. A) The pes anserinus muscle group is formed by the semitendinosus, gracilis, and sartorius muscles.

162. C) Stress is the internal reaction or resistance of tissue to an external load.

163. D) Clonic cramps/spasms are an involuntary muscle contraction characterized by alternate contraction and relaxation in rapid succession.

164. C) Myofascial release is a term that refers to a group of techniques used for the purpose of relieving soft tissue from the abnormal grip of tight fascia.

165. B) Half-life is the rate at which a drug disappears from the body through metabolism, excretion, or both.

166. B) Circuit training is a type of training that employs a series of stations consisting of various combinations of weight training, flexibility, calisthenics, and brief aerobic exercise.

167. E) Diaphoresis means sweating.

168. B) Mechanoreceptors are found in ligaments, musculotendinous junctions, capsules, menisci, and fat pads. They are not found in the brain.

169. D) Cognitive function may be affected by dehydration, malnutrition, abnormal body temperature, or medication.

170. E) Polydipsia means excessive thirst.

171. D) Strengthening exercises generally follow a progression from isometric, to isotonic, to isokinetic, to plyometric.

172. D) Isotonic exercises for external rotation of the glenohumeral joint focus on the infraspinatus, teres minor, and posterior deltoid muscles.

173. C) Injury or disease of the pancreas creates pain in the upper left quadrant of the abdomen.

174. B) A Morion's neuroma is most commonly located between the third and fourth metatarsals.

175. B) An excessive valgus force would cause tension on the medial collateral ligament, resulting in a sprain or tear.

176. A) The female athletic triad describes the simultaneous presence of an eating disorder, amenorrhea, and osteoporosis.

177. E) Neer's test is performed to assess for shoulder impingement.

178. B) Cryostretch involves the use of ice or a cold spray prior to stretching a body part.

179. C) Ultrasound would increase blood flow to the area and should not be used when an acute hemorrhage is present.

180. A) Functional braces are used after rehabilitation to prevent recurrent injury but maintain range of motion (ROM).

181. B) Russian stimulation deeply penetrates the muscle and causes an intense contraction of the muscle.

182. B) Protective spasm of the muscular abdominal wall is known as rigidity.

183. A) Black, tar-like stools are indicative of upper gastrointestinal (GI) bleeding.

184. D) An ice pack can decrease the mean skin temperature 3.4°C during a 15-minute application.

185. C) A dry, nonproductive cough is most often caused by allergies to environmental irritants.

186. B) Rehabilitation or a reconditioning program is developed with the main goal of returning the athlete to his or her previous functional level.

187. D) Archimedes discovered the principle of buoyancy, which states that when a body is wholly or partially immersed in a fluid at rest, the body experiences an upward thrust equal to that of the fluid it displaced.

188. A) Interferential current is not a classification of electric stimulation.
189. C) Electrical stimulation (ie, TENS) is used to control labor pains.
190. B) Coulomb's law states that like charges repel each other, but unlike charges attract to each other.
191. C) Ice massage should never be applied to anesthetized skin because of the loss of sensation to the area.
192. B) Low intensity stimulators deliver current at very low frequencies (1 PPS) and are of subsensory intensity.
193. C) Galvanic current is uninterrupted direct current.
194. D) Intensity is the amount of power given off by the ultrasound unit during treatment.
195. C) Treatment temperature ranges of fluidotherapy are usually between 100°F to 113°F.
196. B) The D2 flexion pattern works the abductors, flexors, and external rotators of the hip.
197. E) The rhomboids retract, rotate, and stabilize the scapula during the throwing motion.
198. D) McKenzie extension exercises are used for degenerative disk disease and postural dysfunction.
199. D) The biceps and triceps stabilize the rotator cuff. The rotator cuff consists of the supraspinatus, infraspinatus, teres minor, and subscapularis muscles, which all must be strengthened during rehabilitation.
200. C) During static stretching, the muscle is placed in a position of maximum stretch and held without bouncing or movement.
201. E) Plyometric exercise helps develop eccentric control during dynamic movements.
202. D) An evaluation of the injured area should be performed before proceeding with any treatment.
203. E) A positive posterior drawer test is indicative of a posterior cruciate ligament tear.
204. C) The medial condyle of the femur is one structure of the knee that should be palpated during the evaluation of a knee injury.
205. B) The athletic trainer should take a thorough history of the injury prior to proceeding with the rest of the evaluation.
206. B) Cartilage has limited ability to heal because it has limited or no direct blood supply.
207. A) The shoulder rarely dislocates in the superior direction because the acromion process is in the way.

Organization and Administration

1. D) Permission-to-treat forms, preparticipation physical examination forms, and release forms for athletes with increased risks should be completed and given to the athletic trainer prior to the first team practice.
2. B) A policy is a broad statement of intended action developed by those who are empowered to govern the operation of an organization. A procedure outlines a specific strategy for members of an organization to follow when following a policy.
3. E) The floor of an athletic training room should not be made of wood because of the possibility of it splintering or warping.
4. C) It is prudent for the athletic trainer to maintain some form of documentation on a daily basis.
5. D) An athlete's medical records may not be released to any individual or organization without written permission from the athlete or his or her guardian or parent.
6. C) The athletic trainer is legally responsible for the athlete's health care. The athletic trainer is acting in place of the team physician in making decisions for the athlete's physical health unless there is a situation that is out of the boundaries of the athletic training practice act.
7. B) Focus charting is a method of documentation that lists information about an athlete's injury, the actions taken by the athletic trainer, and the response to the athletic trainer's action in a column form instead of a narrative or SOAP note format.
8. D) A physician's letter of agreement is an informal legal contract that outlines the physician's duties and responsibilities. This type of contract should specifically identify the physician as the individual who is ultimately responsible for the athlete's health care.
9. E) An athletic trainer in the nontraditional setting can be considered a manager. A manager functions as an organizer, director, and controller.
10. A) In this situation the school nurse becomes responsible because the athletic trainer has deferred the care at the principal's request.
11. D) The athletic trainer should follow OSHA guidelines in maintaining proper hygiene and sanitation in the athletic training room.
12. E) Commission on Accreditation of Rehabilitation Facilities (CARF) establishes standards of quality for organizations that provide rehabilitation services.
13. D) A well-written SOAP note should be legible and concise, include many objective measurements, express progress in terms of functional achievements and it should describe a clear plan of treatment.
14. B) Documentation such as the athletic trainer's treatment log or SOAP notes could be subpoenaed during a civil litigation suit.
15. D) Capitation is a fixed method of payment made to a provider per member over a specific period of time, regardless of the amount of services provided.

16. A) An HCFA-1500 form is a standard insurance claim form that is accepted by most insurance carriers. It must be filled out thoroughly for quick reimbursement to be obtained.

17. A) It is illegal for an athletic trainer to dispense a prescription drug to an athlete. Only those individuals who are legally licensed to prescribe or dispense prescription drugs may give an athlete a prescribed medication.

18. D) Maintaining accurate records for a high school athlete is the responsibility of the athletic trainer, school nurse, and team physician.

19. C) The WOTS-UP analysis (weaknesses, opportunities, threats, and strengths) is a technique that looks at the strengths and weaknesses of an athletic training program.

20. A) A gatekeeper is appointed by an insurance company to oversee the medical care given to an athlete and is usually a primary care physician.

21. E) The UCR (usual, customary, and reasonable) is a charge that represents the maximum amount of money that an insurance company will pay for a service.

22. A) The National Safety Council is responsible for drawing sports injuries data from numerous sources.

23. B) The Hockey Equipment Certification Council (HECC) sets standards to certify face masks that are used in ice hockey helmets.

24. E) Expendable supplies include items such as adhesive tape, gauze pads, Band-aids, and items that cannot be used again.

25. B) Security, fire safety, and management of emergency injuries must be taken into consideration when developing a risk management plan.

26. D) Bidding is a process in which competing vendors quote prices on specific pieces of equipment, and orders by the purchasing institution are usually placed with the lowest bidder.

27. D) A copayment is a percentage of the total amount the policy holder is required to pay for medical services rendered.

28. E) Any athletic trainer who is in the position to hire a new staff member is governed by federal laws that require all applicants receive equal consideration regardless of race, gender, nationality, or religion.

29. D) The athletic trainer's daily documentation should include any treatments administered and how they were implemented, rehabilitation progression, the athlete's current playing status, and a daily injury log.

30. D) Only the team physician has the authority to clear an injured athlete so he or she can return to play.

31. B) Only a licensed physician may diagnose an illness and is in charge of overseeing the treatment administered by the athletic trainer.

32. C) The fee-for-service model is a traditional reimbursement model by which the provider is paid on the amount of service provided to a patient, often leading to a higher total reimbursement for the provider.

33. D) The goals must be written in functional terms to ensure proper reimbursement.

34. A) The ICD-9 codes are used to identify a patient's diagnosis and are employed by private insurance companies as a method of standardizing the classification of an injury.

35. D) It would be unethical for the athletic trainer to manipulate his or her documentation for any form of personal financial gain.

36. B) Space requirements and traffic flow patterns must be addressed in the schematic drawings to ensure adequate space to function, grow, and enhance the movement of people from one section of the athletic training room to another.

37. A) If the equipment is based on complex technology, the department may be able to replace it before it becomes obsolete.

38. C) Only confidential information relating to a staff member's employment should be included in the personnel file. This would include performance evaluations, salary and promotion records, employee application information, and employee contracts.

39. C) Database software allows the athletic trainer to input, store, manipulate, and retrieve information with regard to athletic injury and treatment.

40. A) A "rider" is a supplementary clause to an insurance contract that covers the cost of conditions that extend beyond those associated with the standard policy.

41. C) Consulting a certified public accountant (CPA) or professional financial advisor would not be appropriate in this situation.

42. D) A qualified individual, such as another certified athletic trainer or coach, should accompany an injured athlete to the hospital if it becomes necessary. It would be inappropriate to give a student athlete this responsibility.

43. A) It is critical that the athletic trainer meet at least once a year with the local rescue squad and any individuals who may be involved in the event of an emergency to establish and practice procedures that will be utilized.

44. A) The biggest budgetary obstacle a high school athletic trainer faces is the lack of a room and special facilities to operate his or her program.

45. E) There are four types of supervisory models commonly used by athletic trainers: clinical, developmental, inspection, and production. Inspection and production are usually combined because they have

very few differences. Clinical supervision involves direct observation of the employee's work and the subsequent development of an action plan to improve any deficiencies in his or her performance. Developmental supervision involves participative management, in which the employees discuss common problems and develop solutions with their supervisors. Inspection-production supervision was originally developed and implemented in industrial settings. It emphasizes authoritative managerial efficiency. It relies on the strict observance of program policies and procedures and measures success through the measurement of input and output, which is not easily accomplished in the sports medicine setting. This model is the least utilized in athletic training.

46. C) Negotiation is one of the six steps in the purchasing process and is not a phase of budget planning.

47. C) Third-party reimbursement is the process by which health care practitioners are reimbursed by a policyholder's insurance company.

48. E) Managed care is a system that has set forth coordinated efforts to help reduce the costs of medical coverage. The goal of managed care is to provide appropriate service with cost control in mind.

49. A) The athletic trainer who is designing a new sports medicine facility should always be concerned with function/economy of space instead of aesthetics.

50. E) Capitation is not a type of insurance. Capitation refers to a form of reimbursement used by managed care organizations to determine the amount of money that is going to be paid to a provider for services for a member in a predetermined period of time.

51. A) Establishing an emergency plan should be one of the first tasks that an athletic trainer should perform when developing a new high school program.

52. B) Developing a mission statement is a priority when developing any place of business, such as a sports medicine center. A mission statement is a written expression of an organization's philosophy, purpose, and characteristics.

53. E) CPT stands for current procedural terminology.

54. C) Personalistic culture is a type of organizational culture characterized by autonomy in decision making and problem solving, allowing an individual to make decisions with little consultation of others.

55. E) Quality control is a negotiable point in sports medicine purchasing that should be done prior to the purchasing process to ensure you will be receiving the appropriate items.

56. D) Health maintenance organization, point-of-service, exclusive, and preferred provider organizations are all types of managed care organizations.

57. A) The athletic trainer is not required to have a treatment consent form signed by the athlete's parent or guardian if the athlete is 18 years of age or older.

58. B) The team physician takes the lead in making the decisions regarding the transport of an injured athlete.

59. C) The statute of limitations set forth by each individual state gives the athletic trainer the time frame in which one can file a claim.

60. C) The primary care physician makes the decision that a referral to a specialist is needed. The primary care physician acts as the gatekeeper.

61. C) Planning is defined as a decision-making process in which a course of action is determined in order to bring about a future state of affairs.

62. E) Bedfellows support a plan but are not trustworthy and may be manipulative in their dealings.

63. A) A procedure is an operational plan that provides specific guidelines and directions for an individual of the company or organization to follow.

64. B) An insurance "carrier" is a charge-based provider contracted by the federal government charged with reviewing Medicare claims made by physicians or other health care providers.

65. E) Personal power is the potential to influence others by virtue of personal characteristics and personality attributes.

66. C) There is no such thing as laissez-faire budgeting.

67. B) Primary coverage is defined as a type of health, medical, or accident insurance that begins to pay for covered expenses immediately after a deductible has been paid.

68. A) Medical records provide an accurate account of ongoing treatment, history, and background information pertinent to the athlete. They are valuable tools in providing health care to an athlete.

69. E) The P in SOAP means "plan of action." In this section one should incorporate long-term goals, short-term goals, and the plan of care.

70. B) The athletic trainer should adopt and communicate policies that limit the institution's financial obligations to those injuries that are covered by the school's insurance policy.

71. D) Medical insurance is a contract between a policyholder and an insurance company to reimburse a percentage of the cost of the policyholder's medical bills.

72. A) Confidentiality between the athlete and the athletic trainer cannot be broken by pressure from the media.

73. C) There is a lower initial cost with leasing equipment.

74. E) Collegial culture is a type of organizational culture characterized by consensus, teamwork, and participatory decision making.

75. C) There are 10 steps for recruiting and hiring sports medicine personnel. The following is the correct order:
    1. Request for position
    2. Position request approval
    3. Position vacancy notice
    4. Application collection
    5. Telephone interviews
    6. Reference checks
    7. On-site interview
    8. Recommendation and approval for hiring
    9. Offer of contract
    10. Hiring

76. A) Lump-sum budgeting is a method that allocates a fixed amount of money for an entire program without specifying how the money will be spent.

77. C) Zero-based budgeting is a model that requires justification for every budget line item without reference to previous spending patterns.

78. D) Negligence is a type of tort in which an athletic trainer fails to act as a reasonably prudent athletic trainer would act under the same circumstances.

79. B) Feasibility standards are performance evaluation standards intended to help foster practicality in the employee appraisal process.

80. B) The correct order in the staff selection process should be hiring, promotion, retention, performance evaluation, and demotion.

81. C) Program goals are procedures carried out in the inspection-production supervision.

82. E) An organization plan is ideally used in short periods of times. This allows the organizational plan to change as needed.

83. D) The equal employment operating chief (EEOC) deals with all employees regarding any concerns that they may have. Any issue or problems related to employment or employees should be dealt with by the EEOC.

84. B) The individual must provide you with some type of medical documentation from a physician or state agency. The record should state the disability and any accommodations that may be necessary.

85. C) The design/build concept allows the firm to make adjustments and decisions regarding the building. They are able to work within their own firm rather than having to deal with any other outside groups or entities.

86. B) Developing a traffic pattern chart is a vital step in determining space needs when designing a new facility.

87. C) Endowments are usually used for scholarly endeavors in the educational field. These endowments are to ensure the continuation of the program. Endowments can be used to create or support a professorship or provide scholarships for students.

88. B) Chronic overuse injuries can be included in a rider. This may cause the cost of the premium to go up, but the injury will be covered.

89. E) Most catastrophic insurance coverage begins covering after the first $25,000 is paid. It is up to the institution to alter the amount when the benefits of the policy take effect.

90. C) Secondary coverage begins when the individual's personal insurance or any other primary policy that may be in use has already paid.

91. A) The American Medical Association (AMA) set forth codes to help standardize the language used by medical professionals when billing. This made it easier for insurance companies to reimburse correctly. Most of the common procedural terminology (CPT) codes that would be used by athletic trainers can be found under the physical medicine codes.

92. D) Capital expenses include major costs, such as buildings and land. Small supplies, such as tape, ultrasound gel, and others used for treatment purposes, are direct costs, while office supplies are indirect costs. Staff salaries are not capital costs.

93. D) Changing/locker rooms for the athletes should not be included as a section of the athletic training room.

94. B) An adequately sized athletic training room should be approximately 1000 to 1200 square feet.

95. B) The electrical outlets should be approximately 4 to 5 feet above the floor of the training room with spring-loaded covers to prevent the possibility of electrical shock.

96. A) The athletic trainer should utilize a password to maintain confidentiality and security and to prevent unwanted individuals from gaining access to the database.

97. C) The face mask should be located three finger widths from the nose for a correct fit.

98. C) Thermomoldable plastics, such as Orthoplast, may be used as a hard protective covering for an injured area of the body, such as a dome covering for a quadriceps contusion.

99. C) The BOC identified the domains of athletic training as defined by the role delineation study.

100. D) The athletic trainer should keep accurate and up-to-date records in the athletic training room. This information should include items such as injury reports, injury evaluations and progress notes, daily treatment logs, and medical records.

101. E) Line-item budgeting is a method in which the athletic trainer must anticipate the expenditures for specific program functions, such as team physician services, supplies, and equipment repair.

102. D) Licensure is the most restrictive form of regulation for athletic training. Licensure limits the prac-

tice of athletic training to those individuals who have successfully met the minimal requirements set by a state licensing board.

103. C) A successful athletic trainer must be an individual who has a love for athletics and competition. He or she must be able to adapt to a variety of environments and deal with diverse personalities of those he or she comes into contact with on a daily basis. The athletic trainer must have a sense of humor and be able to empathize with an athlete who has been injured or is ill. Most importantly, the athletic trainer must be of the highest morals and integrity.

104. D) The school nurse's function in a high school sports medicine program is to act as a liaison between the athletic trainer and the school's health services program.

105. D) The NATA was developed in 1950 to establish practice guidelines and a code of ethics for the athletic training profession.

Professional Development and Responsibility

1. E) This behavior violates the NATA Code of Ethics, which, in part, states that "members shall not engage in conduct that constitutes a conflict of interest or that adversely reflects on the profession."

2. C) Physical therapists are trained in the rehabilitation of a diverse patient population. The athletic trainer has expertise in the prevention, treatment, and rehabilitation of the athletic and physically active populations.

3. A) Difficulty sleeping, feelings of anger or guilt, self-preoccupation, and constantly feeling tired are all signs of job burnout.

4. D) Organizing professional seminars and conferences, providing high quality care to the athlete, and publishing articles in professional journals are among the best means of educating the general public and other health care workers regarding the role of the athletic trainer.

5. A) The most important thing an athletic trainer should do is listen carefully to what the athlete has to say relating to the injury or problem.

6. E) According to the definition developed by the ACSM, sports medicine is a generic term that is multidisciplinary in nature.

7. A) The athletic trainer must be competent in classroom teaching methods and should incorporate multimedia and visual aids.

8. C) A tort may be a direct result of an act of omission or commission.

9. B) The athletic trainer should carry professional liability insurance and be familiar with the details of the policy.

10. A) Developmental supervision could be considered a "mentoring" approach in which the head athletic trainer facilitates his or her assistant's professional development while overseeing the day-to-day operations of the athletic training room.

11. D) AIDS is not a bacterial infection.

12. A) It is crucial that any infected individual, including an infected health care worker, not deny his or her condition and seek the proper medical care when it is appropriate.

13. E) In general, a plaintiff has between 1 and 3 years to file a negligence suit. This can vary from state to state.

14. D) The athletic trainer should carry professional liability insurance in case of a criminal suit.

15. A) Principle I (1.2) states, "Members shall be committed to providing competent care consistent with both the requirements and limitations of their profession."

16. C) The three types of state regulations that govern athletic training are certification, licensing, and registration.

17. D) It is illegal for an athletic trainer to prescribe and dispense prescription medications.

18. E) The athletic trainer working in a clinical setting is best suited to treat the physically active patient.

19. D) It is not a violation for a certified athletic trainer to function as a clinical athletic trainer in a sports medicine clinic as long as he or she practices within the confines of the individual state's practice acts.

20. C) According to the 2006 to 2011 continuing education guidelines, BOC examiner/models may receive up to 10 CEUs per year (two examinations per year).

21. B) Liability is the state of being legally responsible for the harm one causes another person.

22. A) The athletic trainer may be considered negligent if he or she failed to dry the floor if it was wet or warn the athlete that the floor was wet prior to him stepping out of the whirlpool.

23. D) Keeping an updated resume on file with the athletic director will have no impact on avoiding litigation. However, it is important for the athletic trainer to have a written job description on file.

24. B) Maintaining a 3.25 grade point average (GPA) is not a core requirement to attain certification as an athletic trainer.

25. D) The main reason for the "uncomfortable" relationship between athletic trainers and physical therapists has been the role confusion between the two groups regarding injury rehabilitation.

26. B) Principle 2.4 of the NATA Code of Ethics states, "Members shall avoid substance abuse and, when necessary, seek rehabilitation for chemical dependency."

27. A) Principle 1.1 of the NATA Code of Ethics states, "Members shall not discriminate against any legally protected class."

28. E) Recreational therapy is not a field that is related to sport and injury.

29. E) In June of 1991, the AMA recognized certified athletic trainers as "Allied Health Care Professionals."

30. C) Athletic training scope of practice parameters set by legislation fall into the following areas: definition of athletic training or athletic trainer, site of practice restrictions, modality use restrictions, definition of athlete restrictions/physically active individual, and the supervision of athletic trainers.

31. E) A primary care provider is an individual who is the direct provider of care. He or she is usually a physician specializing in internal medicine, pediatrics, or general practice. A physical therapist, orthopedic technician, and nurse are all secondary providers (ie, those who render services, equipment, or testing procedures that enable the physician to care for his or her patient).

32. A) Delaware and New Mexico are two states that license athletic training.

33. B) The practice of athletic training is restricted to the "traditional setting" in Hawaii and Nebraska. Athletic trainers may also practice as clinical athletic trainers (but are not limited to) in Arkansas, Indiana, Alabama, Ohio, Kentucky, and New York.

34. E) When taking a history during an initial evaluation, the athletic trainer should be functioning at the "analytical" level of listening. The analytical level of listening involves listening for very specific kinds of information.

35. A) Commitment to the job, a state of open-mindedness, and professional growth and are key elements of professionalism.

36. D) Continuing education units would not be awarded by the BOC for writing a medical or health-related column in a local newspaper or popular magazine.

37. A) The athletic trainer and team physician should be the only individuals with access to databases containing an athlete's medical records.

38. A) Occupational "burnout" is demonstrated by physical and emotional exhaustion and a negative attitude toward work. Signs of burnout include anger, guilt, insomnia, and self-preoccupation.

39. D) A biomechanist is an expert in analyzing human movement through the use of video and computer-enhanced digital analysis equipment.

40. C) A hallux valgus deformity is also known as a bunion. A podiatrist would be the most appropriate individual for the athletic trainer to consult with in the care of this athlete.

41. C) The medical practice act of each state is what governs the athletic trainer and makes him or her aware of what is permissible practice of a certified/licensed athletic trainer within that particular state.

42. E) Malpractice occurs when an athletic trainer has an adverse outcome from a patient treatment. An athletic trainer can be sued for malpractice when he or she is not in full compliance with protocols set forth by state law and practice acts.

43. D) The athletic trainer is not allowed to provide anyone, aside from the parent, with any information regarding the athlete. Keeping in mind that the athlete is still a minor, the parents/guardians must be consulted first regarding any information that is given out about the athlete's status.

44. D) Random selection provides for an equal probability that any subject within a given group or population will be chosen for testing.

45. B) By signing the assumption of risk form the athlete is made aware of the risks of athletic participation and the activities that he or she engages in freely without being forced to do so. These activities include competition, practice, and conditioning.

46. B) Assessing activity areas for safety, proper equipment maintenance, and documentation of treatments are all ways of reducing the risk of injury.

47. C) Ethics are defined as the rules, standards, and principles that dictate right conduct among members of a society or profession. Ethics are based on moral values.

48. A) Good documentation is a way for the athletic trainer to protect him- or herself from litigation.

49. A) Licensure is a form of state credentialing, established by statute and intended to protect the public, that regulates the practice by specifying who may practice and what duties they may perform.

50. C) This principle should read, "Members shall not engage in any form of conduct that constitutes a conflict of interest or that adversely reflects on the profession."

51. C) Assumption of risk is a legal defense that attempts to claim that an injured plaintiff understood the risk of an activity and freely chose to undertake the activity regardless of the hazards associated with it.

52. B) The insured's mother's maiden name is not necessary when obtaining insurance information for an athlete's medical records.

53. D) Socialism is not an approach to ethical decision making. Egoism involves athletic trainers' making decisions that result in the greatest benefit to themselves. Utilitarianism involves choosing a course of action that benefits the greatest number of people. Formalism is most likely to be followed by athletic trainers who see a clear professional duty that they believe should be implemented universally.
54. E) Sports medicine encompasses the fields of biomechanics, massage therapy, and sports psychology.
55. D) Nurses, sports psychologists, and social workers all work with the athletic trainer to ensure the health and safety of the athletes.
56. C) NATA does not have a guideline or position statement regarding eye safety in sports.
57. C) The physical therapist is not considered a member of the primary sports medicine team.
58. E) The NATA was formed in 1950.
59. B) The team physician is responsible for compiling medical histories and conducting physical examinations for each athlete on a team.
60. E) An athletic trainer may be employed in an industrial, high school, college/university, or hospital setting.
61. C) Delegation is not a form of state regulation.
62. A) CAATE is the accrediting body for athletic training educational programs.
63. B) Diagnosis of athletic injuries is not a domain of athletic training.
64. B) Athletic trainers are secondary decision makers, which are professionals responsible for delivering a program within an organization.
65. A) Negligence is defined as a situation in which an athletic trainer fails to act as a reasonably prudent athletic trainer would act under the same circumstances.
66. A) Going to meetings for athletic training is not only a great way to network, it is also required as part of the continuing education that helps athletic trainers stay up to date.
67. D) Documentation cannot protect an athletic trainer from an individual attempting to sue.
68. B) Licensure does prohibit anyone that is not licensed from performing the task of an athletic trainer under state law.
69. E) Ethics dictate the rules, principle of right, conduct, and standards to which members of a specific organization or society must adhere.
70. C) Exceptions to the rule of confidentiality are when there is clear and imminent danger to the client, clear and imminent danger to other persons, and when legal requirements demand that information be released.

71. B) Internal chart audits are a procedure during chart auditing; it is accomplished before the outcome assessment methods.
72. C) Input and output are not easily quantified in sports medicine clinics.
73. E) Omission is the failure to carry out your legal duty.
74. E) An ally is a person who is highly cooperative in a support plan.
75. C) Athletic directors, owners, staff, and coaches are all part of a major inside interest group.
76. D) A sports medicine program should provide the best possible health care, have good communication among members of its team, and good communication between the athletic trainer and parents to be successful.
77. E) The physician has the final say regarding the athlete's ability to play.
78. D) The athletic administrator's role should include the following: establish a positive chain of command for the sports medicine team, ensure that each member's credentials are proper, and that the appropriate personnel are hired for specific positions.

RELATED ATHLETIC TRAINING SUBJECT MATTER

Human Anatomy

1. E) Golfer's elbow and Little League elbow are overuse syndromes of the medial forearm flexor musculature, resulting in medial epicondylitis. This group of muscles originates on the medial epicondyle and crosses the volar aspect of the wrist. Injury occurs with repetitive valgus stresses at the elbow.
2. A) The olecranon process is located on the proximal end of the ulna and extends posteriorly, preventing hyperextension of the elbow.
3. A) The peroneus tertius muscle originates on the lower two thirds of the fibula and inserts on the tuberosity of the fifth metatarsal bone. It assists to dorsiflex the ankle.
4. A) The deltoid muscle of the upper arm is innervated by the axillary nerve.
5. C) The collateral ligaments are most taut in full knee extension and at 30-degree knee flexion.
6. E) Cranial nerve I is the olfactory nerve.
7. C) The muscles of the rotator cuff include the supraspinatus, infraspinatus, teres minor, and subscapularis.
8. A) The rectus femoris muscle originates on the anterior inferior iliac spine and inserts into the quadriceps tendon, which attaches to the upper

border of the patella. The patella is attached to the tibial tuberosity by the patellar tendon. Therefore, the rectus femoris flexes the hip and extends the knee.

9. D) The pes anserinus is described as a goose foot-shaped expansion of the tendons of the sartorius, gracilis, and semitendinosus.

10. A) The subscapularis muscle of the rotator cuff originates on the subscapular fossa and inserts into the lesser tubercle of the humerus.

11. D) The gluteus maximus muscle originates on the upper portion of the ilium, sacrum, and coccyx and inserts on the gluteal tuberosity of the femur and the fascia latae. Its primary actions are to extend and externally rotate the hip.

12. E) The C7 nerve root innervates the triceps muscle, which extends the elbow.

13. A) Cranial nerve VIII, the vestibulocochlear or acoustic nerve, is responsible for hearing and equilibrium.

14. B) Movements of the tongue are controlled by the hypoglossal nerve (ie, cranial nerve XII).

15. A) Continuous pressure on the palm that irritates the deep branch of the ulnar nerve just distal to the canal of Guyon will cause weakness in the muscles of the hand that are innervated by the ulnar nerve.

16. C) The scaphoid bone of the wrist is palpated just distal to the styloid process of the radius.

17. D) The extensor carpi ulnaris is innervated by the radial nerve.

18. D) The hip joint is a diarthrotic or ball and socket joint.

19. B) Knee flexion and extension occur in the sagittal plane around a coronal axis.

20. A) An impacted fracture is a fracture in which one part of the bone telescopes on the other part of the bone.

21. A) A uniaxial diarthrodial joint is a synovial joint that is characterized by hyaline cartilage that covers the articulating surfaces and a synovial membrane that lines the interior of the joint. It moves in one plane only around a single axis.

22. E) The biceps femoris is one of the hamstring muscles and is active in hip extension.

23. A) Because of the angulation of the articulating surfaces of the facets of the thoracic vertebrae, movement is greatest in lateral flexion.

24. B) The peroneal nerve, artery, and muscle groups comprise the lateral compartment of the lower leg.

25. A) A Baker's cyst is a localized accumulation of fluid in the popliteal fossa of the knee. It may represent a true bursitis or synovial herniation through the posterior capsule.

26. B) The shoulder girdle is comprised of the sternoclavicular, acromioclavicular, glenohumeral, and scapulothoracic joints.

27. A) The coracoclavicular ligaments consist of the trapezoid and conoid ligaments and connect the coracoid process of the scapula to the inferior surface of the clavicle.

28. E) A mortise joint is a joint in which there is a groove or slot into or through which another bone fits or passes (eg, the talus sits between the distal ends of the tibia and fibula).

29. A) The ulnar nerve and artery run through the tunnel of Guyon, which is located in the wrist. It is formed by the volar carpal ligament, the pisohamate ligament (which is an extension of the flexor carpi ulnaris), the hook of the hamate, the transverse carpal ligament laterally, and the pisohamate ligament and pisiform bone medially.

30. A) The muscle most prominently involved with lateral epicondylitis is the extensor carpi radialis brevis.

31. D) The multifidi are small muscles located in the back, which extend and rotate the vertebral column.

32. C) The psoas major originates on the transverse processes of the lumbar vertebrae and inserts on the lesser trochanter of the femur. It acts to flex and internally rotate the hip.

33. D) The vastus lateralis originates on the lateral aspect of the femur and inserts into the common tendon of the quadriceps muscle.

34. D) The anatomical snuff-box is located along the dorsoradial aspect of the thumb and is bordered by the extensor pollicis brevis, abductor pollicis longus, and extensor pollicis longus tendons.

35. B) The superior vena cava carries deoxygenated blood from the head and upper body back to the heart.

36. E) Gas exchange of oxygen and carbon dioxide occurs at the alveoli.

37. E) The peroneal artery originates off the posterior tibial artery below the popliteal fossa in the proximal posterior lower leg.

38. C) The odontoid process, or dens, is a projection off the second cervical vertebra that acts as a pivot point for rotation of the atlas.

39. B) The cuneiform is one of the tarsal bones of the foot.

40. D) The plantar fascia is located on the sole of the foot.

41. A) The origin of the sternocleidomastoid muscle is on the superior/medial portion of the clavicle and the manubrium and inserts into the mastoid process.

42. B) The erector spinae is a large muscle group, comprised of the iliocostalis, longissimus, and the spinalis, that acts as the primary extensor of the trunk.

43. A) The femoral artery, vein, and nerve pass through the femoral triangle.

44. C) The axillary artery is a continuation of the subclavian artery beyond the first rib in the axilla.

45. D) The peroneus brevis assists to plantar flex and pronate the foot.

46. B) The cochlea is an osseous structure of the inner ear.

47. D) The dermatome for the C3,4 nerve roots is over the superior aspect of the shoulders and posterior neck area.

48. E) The spleen is located in the upper left abdominal quadrant below the diaphragm.

49. A) Little finger abduction is controlled by the abductor digiti minimi, which is innervated by the C8,T1 nerve root.

50. E) The liver and gallbladder are located in the upper right quadrant of the abdomen.

Human Physiology

1. E) The top number of a blood pressure reading is the systolic number, and the bottom number is the diastolic number. The systolic pressure is representative of the blood pressure during ventricular contraction. The diastolic pressure represents the blood pressure during ventricular filling between cardiac contractions.

2. E) The hunting response is a reactive vasodilatation of local blood vessels after initial vasoconstriction. This occurs with the application of cryotherapy to a body part.

3. D) Acetylcholine is a chemical found at the endplate of a motor neuron, which plays a significant role in the transmission of nerve impulses at synapses and myoneural junctions.

4. A) The average level of desirable total cholesterol is less than or equal to 200 mg/100 dL.

5. A) The separation of electrically charged particles causing a transmembrane electrical potential difference is known as the resting membrane potential.

6. A) The two phases of an action potential are known as depolarization and repolarization.

7. B) The primary component of striated muscle is the muscle fiber.

8. C) A motor unit is made up of a motor neuron and the muscle fibers it innervates.

9. E) Type II or "fast twitch" muscle is more prevalent in the sprinter, as this type of activity is more anaerobic in nature.

10. B) Calcium (Ca++) is a mineral that is necessary for proper muscular contraction to occur. Ca++ is a necessary component in the activation of cross-bridging between actin and myosin to shorten the length of the sarcomere in the muscle myofibril.

11. C) During glycolysis, ATP is broken down to release energy. In addition to the release of energy, the byproducts ADP and PO_4 (phosphatase) are released.

12. A) The Krebs cycle is a complex series of chemical reactions in which there is oxidative metabolism of pyruvic acid, carbohydrates, proteins, and fats.

13. A) Sclerotomic pain is a deep, diffuse, aching pain that arises from deep somatic tissues and is transmitted by unmyelinated C fibers.

14. A) Fusiform muscle fibers are arranged in a cord-like shape, while the pennate muscle fibers are arranged in a feather shape.

15. B) Amenorrhea is defined as an absence of flow during menses.

16. A) Laxatives and enemas can lead to dehydration and electrolyte imbalance, which can endanger the athlete's health and impair performance.

17. E) Hemophilia is a disorder in which the plasma coagulation factor VIII is lacking, resulting in abnormal bleeding.

18. D) The rate of passive diffusion of oxygen from the alveoli depends on the partial pressure of oxygen, the thickness of the alveolar capillaries, and the amount of surface area available for diffusion to take place.

19. E) Vital capacity is the maximal amount of air that can be expired after maximal inspiration.

20. E) During the follicular phase of the menstrual cycle, which lasts from day 5 or 6 to day 13, the primary follicles grow. Toward the end of this phase, just prior to ovulation, one follicle reaches maturity and becomes a graafian follicle.

21. C) The two main phases of menstruation are the follicular or preovulatory phase and the luteal or postovulatory phase.

22. D) The pulp of a tooth is innervated, not the enamel.

23. D) By 4 weeks, a large laceration will heal by secondary healing. Areas of tissue loss are filled with scar tissue.

24. B) The stimulation of the periaqueductal gray area (PGA) of the midbrain and raphe nucleus of the pons and medulla during injury will cause analgesia. Endorphins and enkephalins are produced in these two areas of the brain.

25. B) It may take up to 1 year for a ligament to completely heal with scar maturation.

26. C) To avoid hypoglycemia and insulin shock from taking too much insulin and metabolizing significant

amounts of glycogen during exercise, the athlete should consume a snack of a complex carbohydrate and protein prior to exercise.

27. A) Cold therapy used in an acute injury will decrease the local metabolic rate.

28. B) If a scaphoid fracture is not properly immobilized, aseptic necrosis may occur and the fracture will not heal.

29. E) Hematuria means blood in the urine.

30. E) The scalene muscles are striated and have an arrangement of contractible proteins in a cross-striated pattern.

31. D) Valsalva's effect occurs when the athlete holds his or her breath during the contraction, which increases the intrathoracic pressure and causes a dramatic rise in blood pressure.

32. A) Ballistic stretching causes constant stimulation of the muscle spindles, which causes continuous resistance to further stretching. A muscle must be stretched a long enough time to stimulate the Golgi tendon organs.

33. B) The adrenal glands, which are part of the endocrine system, are responsible for secreting the hormones cortisol, epinephrine, aldosterone, estrogen, norepinephrine, and androgen.

34. B) The primary function of the testes is to produce spermatozoa and testosterone.

Exercise Physiology

1. A) The training effect during exercise is reflected by changes in cardiac output. Cardiac output in the trained athlete is a product of an increased stroke volume and a decreased heart rate.

2. A) Three sessions a week is how often (frequency) the athlete should exercise. Forty-five minutes is how long (duration) the exercise should continue, and 80% of VO_2 max is the intensity of exercise.

3. B) Total cholesterol is comprised of low-density lipoproteins (LDL), high-density lipoproteins (HDL), and very-low-density lipoproteins (VLDL).

4. B) The sternocleidomastoid and scalenes assist during inspiration by lifting the ribs to allow for the intake of greater volumes of air.

5. E) The hypothalamus stimulates the thyroid gland in very cold environments to generate internal heat.

6. C) Applying a static stretch to the muscle inhibits the muscle spindle and stimulates the inverse myotatic reflex, which originates in the Golgi tendon organs and causes relaxation of the muscle.

7. C) An athlete who is hypermobile/hyperflexible may be more susceptible to joint injuries, such as sprains and strains.

8. E) Interval training involves alternating intense, continuous periods of work with periods of active recovery. This type of training is very effective when conditioning athletes who participate in sports that involve short bursts of activity and are followed by a period of recovery.

9. A) The off-season period should be a time when the athlete is not training as frequently or as intensely as the in-season period, but he or she should participate in an activity that maintains a level of flexibility, strength, and endurance. The off-season can be broken down into the transition and preparatory periods, while the in-season may also be referred to as the competition period. In turn, these periods may be further divided into subphases.

10. C) The principles of overload, specificity of training, proper progression, and consistency must be adhered to in order to obtain optimal training effects.

11. B) Physiological adaptations to resistive exercise include increased ligament and tendon strength, increased mineral content of bone, and improved maximal oxygen intake.

12. A) When the muscle is in a position where there is maximum interaction of the cross-bridges between the actin and myosin myofilaments in a sarcomere, the tension within the muscle will be at its greatest point.

13. D) Heart rate and stroke volume determine the volume of blood that is pumped through the heart during a given period of time.

14. E) Target heart rate can be calculated with the following formula: 0.8 x (220 - age), or 0.8 x (220 - 20) = 160.

15. B) Contract-relax requires that the antagonist muscles contract isotonically just prior to the "relax" (stretch) phase of the exercise.

16. D) The triceps and pectoralis major must contract concentrically during the "lift" phase of a bench press.

17. C) Circuit training is one of the best means of improving muscle strength and flexibility because it includes weight training, flexibility, and calisthenics at various stages.

18. C) The hypothalamus is responsible for thermoregulation of the body.

19. B) Periodization includes the following phases: postseason, off-season, preseason, and in-season conditioning.

20. C) A proper cool down aids the return of blood to the heart and assists in decreasing lactic acid levels in the muscle.

21. E) Plyometric exercises emphasize a quick eccentric stretch prior to a forceful concentric contraction and are useful in building power.

22. E) The amount of testosterone present in the body has a significant impact on the amount of hypertrophy that will occur with weight training.
23. A) The greatest loss of heat from the body occurs at the head and neck. It is wise to keep these areas well-covered in cold weather.
24. D) Those individuals with blonde or light hair and fair complexions are much more susceptible to severe sunburn as a result of prolonged exposure to ultraviolet light. This type of athlete should use a sunscreen that has an SPF of 15 or greater.
25. C) The ozone levels are most diminished in the late afternoon because of the lower temperatures and decreased amount of traffic on the roads.
26. A) An athlete with the sickle-cell trait who trains in high altitudes is susceptible to an enlarged or ruptured spleen.
27. A) Because sweat contains a lower concentration of salt than the blood, there is a much greater loss of water when the athlete sweats. Therefore, fluids, especially water, should be unlimited.
28. C) Plyometric exercises include eccentric exercise, which is the most common cause of DOMS.
29. E) Milton's law states that the joint capsule, the muscles that move that joint, and the skin that covers that joint are supplied by the same nerve source.
30. D) A protein level of "trace" or +1 by urinalysis is not considered an abnormal finding in an adolescent.
31. A) Women have a lower strength:body weight ratio (due to a higher percent of body fat) than men.
32. D) There is increased mitochondrial density in the skeletal muscle with endurance exercise.
33. C) During a 400-meter sprint, which lasts approximately 45 seconds to 1 minute, the anaerobic glycolysis system is the predominant source of energy.
34. C) The diastolic blood pressure should remain close to resting levels during endurance exercises.
35. A) Hemolysis is the destruction of red blood cells caused by the repeated impact of the foot on the ground.

Biomechanics

1. D) A contraction that occurs as the muscle is shortening is known as a concentric contraction. An eccentric contraction occurs as the muscle lengthens against resistance.
2. A) The foot becomes a rigid lever in preparation for push-off during gait when the foot is supinated in midstance.
3. E) The knee has 2 degrees of freedom, allowing for flexion and extension in the sagittal plane and rotation in the horizontal plane.
4. E) During shoulder abduction, the humerus and scapula move simultaneously. This is known as scapulohumeral rhythm. For every 30 degrees of shoulder abduction, 20 degrees of motion occurs at the glenohumeral joint and 10 degrees occurs with the scapula rotating on the thorax. During shoulder abduction, the scapula contributes 60 degrees of movement, while the remaining 120 degrees occurs at the glenohumeral joint.
5. B) The agonistic muscle is the primary mover, while the antagonistic muscle is the muscle that causes the opposite action (ie, the quadriceps are the agonist muscle and the hamstrings are the antagonistic musculature during knee extension).
6. E) The most common lever system that exists in the body is the third lever system, where the point of attachment of the muscle causing the motion is closer to the joint axis than the resisting motion (ie, biceps flexing the forearm against gravity).
7. D) The movement arm of a force is always greatest when the angle of application is at 90 degrees to the lever being moved.
8. A) An anatomic pulley (such as the patella) can change the direction of the muscle force but not the magnitude of the force.
9. A) Muscular tension may be increased by increasing the frequency of the motor units firing or by increasing the number of motor units that are simulated.
10. C) Pronation of the foot is a complex movement. It is a combination of eversion, abduction, and dorsiflexion.
11. B) Plantar flexion of the ankle is an example of a second-class lever (ie, the resistance arm is shorter than the force arm).
12. C) Each lever has a force arm, which is the perpendicular distance from the line of force to the axis, and a resistance arm, which is the perpendicular distance from the resistance to the axis.
13. D) Running utilizes linear motion of the entire body and angular motion of the arms and legs.
14. B) Momentum = mass x velocity. Momentum is the force of motion that is acquired by a moving body as a result of its continued motion.
15. D) Potential energy is energy that is stored in a body when it is at rest. The amount of potential energy a body has depends on its position in space. Kinetic energy is the energy of a body in motion.
16. A) Cervical rotation occurs in the horizontal (transverse) plane around a vertical (longitudinal) axis of motion.
17. D) Applying an external force parallel to the tibia will result only in a distraction force.
18. E) An avulsion fracture of a bone is caused when tissue and bone are stretched and tension is produced

beyond its yield point. This is known as a stretching injury.

19. A) This situation results in an isometric contraction.

20. E) The carpometacarpal joint is a saddle joint. A saddle joint has one articulating surface that is concave and one articulating surface that is convex.

21. E) The maximum degrees of freedom (number of axes of movement) a joint can have is 3 degrees.

22. E) The elbow joint is a hinge, or ginglymus, joint and has 1 degree of freedom.

23. D) The frontal plane divides the body into anterior and posterior parts.

24. B) When performing a push-up, the distal end of the upper extremity is in a fixed position.

25. A) The tibia externally rotates on the femur during knee extension. This action is known as the screw-home mechanism.

26. A) With compressive loading, the articular surfaces are brought closer together.

27. E) Loading of a joint that is unstable as a result of ligament rupture produces abnormally high stresses on the joint cartilage.

28. C) Shoulder abduction occurs in the frontal plane around an anterior-posterior axis.

29. D) In the anatomic position, hip rotation occurs in the horizontal plane around a vertical axis.

30. B) A spiral fracture occurs when the foot is planted on the ground and the body is violently rotated. The bone breaks in an S-shaped line. The mechanism of injury is a torsion force.

31. B) Blisters may form in the epidermal layer of the skin as a result of continuous friction to the area.

Psychology

1. B) Progressive muscle relaxation is a relaxation technique by which the athlete learns to manage anxiety and control pain. This form of relaxation training incorporates systematically tensing and relaxing muscles in groups (such as the thighs and buttocks). This technique, when practiced routinely, allows the athlete to tune into his or her body reactions and gain more control of these reactions.

2. B) A passive-aggressive personality procrastinates, makes excuses for delays, and tends to criticize individuals on which he or she is dependent, but cannot separate from their company. These individuals also lack assertiveness and are indirect with their needs.

3. D) Signs of anabolic steroid abuse include mania and depression, bouts of anxiety and insomnia, changes in libido, and aggressive behavior.

4. B) The general adaptation syndrome is a stress response theory developed by Dr. Hans Selye in which there are three stages an organism may pass through: the alarm stage, resistance stage, and exhaustion stage. The alarm stage consists of the flight-or-fight response, which prepares the body to take action; the resistance stage is when the body directs the stress to a particular body site (such as to the stomach); and the exhaustion stage is when the body may become dysfunctional because of chronic stress.

5. E) An athlete who is "burned out" may display a variety of physical and emotional symptoms, including negative self-concept and attitudes regarding his or her sport and teammates, chronic fatigue, headaches, insomnia, and gastrointestinal problems.

6. D) The body passes through three distinct psycho-physiological phases in response to an injury: alarm, resistance, and exhaustion. The adrenal glands secrete adrenaline, which stimulates the flight-or-fight response during the alarm stage.

7. C) It has been shown that an abrupt cessation of exercise can lead to "sudden exercise abstinence syndrome," which is characterized by depression, sleep disorders, arrhythmias, eating disorders, and emotional problems.

8. E) In order for the athlete and athletic trainer to have a good relationship, it is crucial that the athlete trusts the individual who is providing his or her health care.

9. B) Having the athlete draw a mental picture of the healing process can have a positive impact on his or her recovery.

10. A) Two methods of cognitive restructuring are thought stopping and refuting irrational thoughts.

11. D) Obsessive-compulsiveness, mild feelings of denial, behavior that masks feelings of fear, providing self-worth, and taking extreme risks are factors that lead to overcompliant behavior.

12. A) Repeatedly rehearsing various plays in his mind while experiencing pain is a means of diverting his attention away from the pain.

13. E) Anger, loss of appetite, and chronic fatigue are signs of depression.

14. C) The athlete must be cooperative and take responsibility if he or she is to completely rehabilitate an injury.

15. A) "Purging" by self-induced vomiting or self-administered laxatives is a symptom of bulimia.

16. D) If the athlete is anxious, it is best to reassure him and not belittle his fear.

17. B) Staleness is characterized by an apathetic attitude, chronic fatigue, restlessness, and an increase in acute chronic injuries and infections.

18. C) Athletes between the ages of 15 to 24, those sustaining a serious injury with a long rehabilita-

tion process, and those with the prospect of losing their position to a teammate may become severely depressed.

19. A) Teaching the athlete about his or her injury and the healing process can significantly reduce the athlete's anxiety about rehabilitation.

20. E) This athlete is demonstrating denial of his condition.

21. C) Arranging the rehabilitation sessions around the athlete's daily routine will help the athlete to be more compliant.

22. D) Athletes who have little perceived control over their health care will tend to experience a greater amount of stress than those who feel they have some control over their environment.

23. A) A ritualistic cleaning of equipment is a sign of an obsessive-compulsive disorder.

24. B) Biofeedback is a technique that reflects the athlete's efforts to control a specific physiological response, such as muscular tension.

25. B) Individuals diagnosed with anorexia nervosa tend to be perfectionists and overachievers.

26. D) It is best for the athletic trainer to remain empathetic and calm and help the athlete to see the problem in proportion to the situation so she can deal effectively with the outcome.

27. B) An athlete who threatens suicide must be taken very seriously. It is important to be empathetic and listen to the athlete as he discusses what is troubling him. The team doctor should be immediately contacted so that a proper referral to a psychologist or psychiatrist may be made.

Nutrition

1. D) Vitamin A exists in two forms: provitamin A carotenoids, which are found in dark green and orange vegetables, and preformed vitamin A, which is found in liver, fish oils, fortified milk, and eggs.

2. C) Vitamin C is also known as ascorbic acid. Retinol is vitamin A, and thiamin and niacin are B vitamins.

3. B) Ultraviolet light in sunlight converts a form of cholesterol to vitamin D in the skin.

4. B) During glycolysis, glucose is broken down into pyruvate and ATP. Pyruvate is then broken down into CO_2 and water aerobically or into lactic acid during anaerobic exercise.

5. A) The best time for an athlete to consume carbohydrate-rich foods is within 2 hours after training, as glycogen synthesis is the greatest at this time.

6. C) Muscle cells primarily burn fat during low workloads (eg, a brisk walk) because the supply of ATP generated is able to handle that level of work.

Intense exercise that may not last more than 30 seconds uses phosphocreatine and some anaerobic glycolysis to replenish ATP.

7. E) Phosphorus can be found in milk and cheese products, eggs, legumes, nuts, whole grain cereals, meat, fish, and poultry.

8. B) Proteins are long chains of organic compounds called amino acids. There are 22 amino acids, which are used by the body to produce hormones and enzymes. Because the body cannot store excessive protein, some protein is converted into energy or fat.

9. E) Sodium and chloride are electrolytes, which are lost in the greatest amounts while sweating.

10. D) Do not wait for the athlete to complain of being thirsty before supplying fluids. Because the thirst mechanism does not function well when large amounts of fluids are lost by the body during activity, the athlete may need to be reminded to consume fluids frequently.

11. D) The six classes of nutrients include carbohydrates, proteins, water, fats, vitamins, and minerals.

12. C) Water is the most abundant nutrient in the body and must be present in an adequate supply for the body to function normally.

13. C) The new nutrient food label format is known as reference daily intakes (RDI).

14. A) Hydrostatic weighing, electrical impedance, and skin-fold thickness measurements are all means of measuring body composition.

15. B) When more calories are expended than consumed, a negative caloric balance exists and the individual will lose weight.

16. E) Triglyceride, which is a form of fat, is stored in adipose cells and released as the intensity and duration of exercise increases.

17. B) Increasing muscular exercise and dietary intake in appropriate amounts are necessary to increase muscle mass.

18. C) A female athlete who has been diagnosed with a combination of an eating disorder, amenorrhea, and osteoporosis has female triad syndrome.

19. E) Calcium supplements may be necessary to prevent osteoporosis in an athlete who is at high risk for this disease.

20. B) Lactovegetarians eat a diet consisting of plant foods and milk products, but exclude meat products, eggs, and fish. Iron and zinc may be deficient in this diet.

21. A) The body will begin to utilize protein in the event that the athlete's dietary carbohydrate supply is inadequate.

22. D) Athletes who lack the enzyme lactase have a difficult time digesting dairy products, which causes the

development of intestinal gas, diarrhea, and cramping.

23. D) If the body experiences significant electrolyte losses during exercise, the athlete may experience muscular cramping and become susceptible to heat illnesses.

24. A) The kidneys and brain are responsible for regulating water excretion from the body.

25. C) A diet that is significantly lacking in vitamin A will cause poor night vision.

Pharmacology

1. B) Lomotil is an antidiarrheal medication.

2. E) Prozac is a medication used to treat depression, obsessive-compulsive disorder, and bulimia nervosa.

3. E) Pepcid is a medication used to treat heartburn and acid indigestion. It has no stimulant effects.

4. D) Ibuprofen (ie, Advil, Motrin) is available in 200-mg, 400-mg, 600-mg, and 800-mg tablets.

5. B) Diclofenac is known by the brand name Voltaren.

6. A) The recommended dosage for Naprosyn is 250 to 500 mg twice a day.

7. B) An athlete who has overdosed on a stimulant will be agitated and excitable, demonstrate an increase in the respiratory and pulse rates with possible arrhythmias, exhibit tremors, and might become hyperthermic and have convulsions (cocaine affects central thermoregulation) if left untreated.

8. C) Because beta-blockers slow the heart rate, they are potentially performance enhancing during archery.

9. A) Caffeine consumed in moderate amounts will stimulate the cerebral cortex and the medulla, which will increase mental alertness.

10. E) Diarrhea is not a symptom of human growth hormone abuse.

Physics

1. C) The effective radiating area (ERA) is the area of the applicator that emits ultrasound waves to the surface tissue.

2. A) The frequency range of therapeutic ultrasound is between 1.0 to 3.0 MHz.

3. A) Archimedes' principle states that an object immersed in water experiences an upward force that is equal to the weight of the water displaced by the object.

4. B) TENS is a modality for pain relief that is based on the gate control theory.

5. A) A pulsed current during electric stimulation may be monophasic or biphasic.

6. B) The most common frequency used with shortwave diathermy is 27.33 MHz.

7. C) Microwave diathermy produces electromagnetic radiation with a frequency of 2450 megacycles per second and has a wavelength of less than 1 meter.

8. E) There is no "surge" setting on a TENS unit.

9. E) With iontophoresis, ionized medication, such as dexamethasone, is driven through the skin by a direct electrical current.

10. C) Work = force x distance.

11. E) Medication delivered by iontophoresis must be ionized.

12. A) According to Joule's law, heat produced by high frequency electrical currents is directly proportional to the square of the current strength, resistance of the conductor, and the time during which the current flows.

13. E) Ohm's law states that the strength of an electric current is equal to the electromotive force divided by the resistance, or $I = V/R$.

14. A) Heat transfers to the skin from a moist heat pack via conduction, which is the transfer of heat by direct contact.

15. C) An alternating current (AC) is an electrical current that reverses direction at a regular interval. A TENS unit utilizes AC current.

16. C) To change a temperature reading from Celsius to Fahrenheit, the following formula must be used: (temperature in Celsius x 9/5) + 32.

17. C) The impedance of a circuit is the resistance that exists within the circuit.

18. E) Moist heat applied during the acute phases of tendinitis will increase pain and enhance the inflammatory process.

19. C) Amperage is the strength of a current flow. It is expressed in amperes.

20. A) According to Poiseuille's law, the length and radius of a blood vessel are significant in determining resistance to blood flow.

21. A) Medium-intensity ultrasound is between 0.8 to 1.5 watts per square centimeter.

22. D) The transducer head should be kept between 0.5 to 1 inch from the skin surface during underwater treatment.

23. C) The anode is the positive pole of an electric source.

Answer Key— Written Simulation Sample Questions

Appendix C

Key

++ = Most appropriate

+ = Appropriate, but not first priority

0 = No relevance to the problem

- = Not a priority/harmful

-- = Detrimental

Problem I

Section A

The current situation: You know your athlete has injured his right lower leg during a dismount off the rings.

Your immediate responsibility: To perform your initial evaluation to determine the type and severity of the injury.

1. ++) Since this injury was not witnessed, information should be obtained from the athlete about what occurred as part of the "history" portion of the initial evaluation. (The athlete tells you he was not balanced and landed on his right side.)

2. ++) Because the opening scene has implied there is a significant lower extremity injury, the athletic trainer should ask the athlete if he heard/felt a "snap" or "pop," which may indicate a ligament injury or fracture. (The athlete definitely felt a "snap.")

3. ++) This will give the athletic trainer an idea of the athlete's willingness to move his leg. (The athlete won't move his leg because of pain.)

4. +) Observing for areas of swelling and/or bleeding is part of a secondary survey. (The distal lower extremity is swollen with deformity.)

5. +) Palpation of the injured area is part of the secondary survey. (The athlete has significant pain with palpation of the lower leg.)

6. ++) Because this appears to be a significant injury, it would be prudent for the athletic trainer to monitor the athlete's vital signs. (Blood pressure is 128/88 and his pulse is 88.)

7. ++) The pulses of the lower leg should be assessed to make sure there is adequate circulation to the affected limb. (The right popliteal pulse is palpable and strong.)

8. --) Heating the affected area is contraindicated during the acute phase of the injury. (The effusion becomes enormous.)

9. -) The injured leg should not be moved until your initial evaluation is complete. (The athlete screams in pain.)

10. +) It has been determined this injury is serious enough to warrant calling for an ambulance.

11. -) It has been determined that there is a significant injury to the right lower extremity. It is not necessary to spend a lot of time examining the athlete's entire body for injuries. (A lot of time has been wasted.)

12. +) If the area that is injured is not immediately accessible, it may be necessary to cut away the athlete's uniform. (You can clearly see where the injury is located.)

13. 0) Until the severity of the injury is established, immobilization of the limb may be a premature action.

Section B

The current situation: The athlete is complaining of severe right lower leg pain and the lower leg is swollen and obviously deformed. The athlete's vital signs are stable.

Your immediate responsibility: Continue your evaluation, then stabilize the leg and make the athlete comfortable.

14. --) If a fracture is suspected, the athletic trainer should never manipulate the injured area, as this will cause further injury. (The deformity is worsened.)

15. -) The athlete should not be moved until the immobilizer or splint is in place and secured on the affected limb. (The athlete screams in pain.)

16. 0) This action would only be necessary if a crowd is gathering and/or there is equipment that is in the way.

17. +) This action is appropriate to decrease pain and minimize effusion. (The athlete feels better with ice on his leg.)

18. ++) It is critical to check the pulses of the ankle and foot to determine if there is adequate circulation to the injured limb. (The right dorsalis pedis pulse is palpable, but weak.)

19. ++) If the leg appears hard and swollen, it may indicate the beginning of a Volkmann's contracture, which is a paralytic contracture that results from ischemia of muscles and nerves in an extremity. (The lower leg appears tight and swollen.)

20. 0) The competition should be stopped if the athlete is in harm's way or an entrance/exit to the gym area is blocked because of crowding.

21. --) Moving the athlete may cause further injury; initial immobilization should take place with the athlete in side-lying position. (The deformity is made worse by moving the leg.)

22. -) It has been determined by this time that the athlete has a significant lower leg injury. Evaluating the hip at this time is both unnecessary and inappropriate. (You wasted valuable time.)

23. +) Assuming the leg is immobilized at this point, short-term elevation may help retard swelling.

24. -) Checking for crepitus at this time is inappropriate. (The athlete screams in pain.)

25. ++) If a fracture of the lower extremity is suspected, immobilization is a priority in preventing further injury. (The leg is immobilized while the athlete is in side lying.)

26. --) Massaging the area of injury is inappropriate and will cause increased pain and swelling. (The athlete screams in pain.)

Section C

The current situation: You have determined the athlete has sustained a lower leg fracture. The athlete's leg is immobilized.

Your immediate responsibility: Prepare to transport the athlete to the hospital and monitor the athlete until the rescue squad arrives. Document the event and your actions.

27. +) This is an appropriate action to assess circulation and neurological function. (The athlete complains his foot feels numb.)

28. --) This action would be inappropriate. The athlete should be transported by a gurney to minimize movement of the lower body. (The athlete trips with the crutches.)

29. --) Issuing any medications to this athlete would not be an appropriate action at this point in time because it is unknown what other medications he will be given at the hospital. (The team physician finds out and is furious.)

30. -) It is not necessary for the coach to accompany this athlete to the hospital. It is the duty of the athletic trainer to follow up with this athlete after the meet is finished. (A parent substitutes for the coach and the team loses.)

31. --) It is unknown what the athlete will be given at the hospital (eg, medications, etc) or if he may need anesthesia. It is dangerous to allow the athlete to eat or drink as he wants until he is told it is okay by the medical staff at the hospital. (The athlete aspirates in the operating room and dies.)

32. -) It is unknown what this athlete's status is at this time, and the decision to return to play will be up to the team physician. (The coach wants to know if you spoke with the team physician.)

33. 0) If the trainer has a personal rapport with the emergency room staff, this is a nice touch, but not necessary. The rescue squad will alert the hospital of their arrival. (The emergency room nurse politely thanks you for your call.)

34. ++) Monitoring the athlete for symptoms of shock is always appropriate with a traumatic injury, and your findings should be passed along to the EMS team. (The athlete appears pale and his blood pressure has dropped to 90/60 with a pulse rate of 90.)

35. ++) It is important that the athletic trainer emotionally support the athlete. Realize he is in pain and scared and will need reassurance that he is in good hands. (The athlete is calm with your presence.)

36. 0) Fitting the athlete for a pair of crutches is unnecessary. (The hospital will handle it.)

37. +) If this athlete is a minor, his parents should be contacted and given information on what occurred, what actions were taken to care for the athlete, and to which hospital he was sent. (The parents leave for the hospital and are grateful you called.)

38. +) An injury report should be filled out to ensure the circumstances surrounding the injury and what steps were taken during his care are documented. (You avoid a potential malpractice lawsuit.)

PROBLEM II

Section A

The current situation: You know your athlete has sustained a traumatic injury to her eyes and/or face as a result of a blow by a hockey ball.

Your immediate responsibility: To perform your initial evaluation to determine the nature and severity of the injury.

1. 0) With the exception of the goalie, there is no head/face protective equipment in field hockey.

2. -) From the information provided by the opening scenario, you know the athlete has an eye and/or facial injury. Testing the athlete's fine motor skills is inappropriate. (There is no problem with the athlete's fine motor skills.)

3. -) It has been determined that this is an injury to the eye and/or face. Attempting to test this athlete's balance is inappropriate. (The athlete wonders why you want her to balance on one leg.)

4. --) The use of an ammonia capsule would be unnecessary and inappropriate. The athlete may jerk her head, possibly causing further injury. (The athlete sustains a retinal detachment.)

5. --) This athlete may have a potentially serious eye injury. The athlete should remain in a recumbent position until the initial injury assessment is complete. (The athlete complains of "throbbing" pain.)

6. +) This is an appropriate action but does not directly relate to your evaluation. (The athlete is more comfortable.)

7. 0) Asking the athlete who made the shot is an inappropriate question. (Who cares?)

8. +) This is an appropriate question during an injury assessment as part of the "subjective" information portion of the evaluation. (The athlete complains of pain above the right eye.)

9. 0) Although examining the shoulders will not harm the athlete, it has been determined the injury is to the eye. (The athlete has no shoulder pain.)

10. ++) It is important the athletic trainer perform a primary survey and thoroughly examine the head, face, or neck as indicated once the mechanism of injury has been determined. (It is determined this is not a life-threatening situation.)

11. ++) Gently palpating the orbital rim and nose for point tenderness, crepitus, or deformity is part of the initial assessment of an eye injury. (There is tenderness over the left eyebrow with a large hematoma. No crepitus is noted.)

12. ++) Because this was a traumatic injury involving a small high-velocity projectile, it is highly likely blood will be present. (Donning gloves is part of universal precautions.)

13. -) A "battle sign" is present when there is a basilar skull fracture. It is known from the opening scene that the athlete has suffered an eye/facial injury.

14. 0) Asking the athlete if she is a scholarship athlete is unnecessary and inappropriate. (The athlete asks why that matters.)

15. ++) Checking the area for bleeding is a fundamental component of your initial examination of this athlete. (There is a profuse amount of blood present.)

16. +) This is an appropriate question when assessing the severity of injury to the eye itself. (The athlete's vision is blurred.)

Section B

The current situation: You know the athlete has a deep laceration above the left eyebrow. It does not appear that the athlete has sustained any facial fractures.

Your immediate responsibility: To clean and dress the wound and treat the athlete for pain and swelling.

17. ++) It is important to check pupillary response for possible cerebral injury. (The pupillary response is normal.)

18. --) This would be contradicted in an acute injury to the eye. (The bleeding and swelling increase dramatically.)

19. +) Rinsing the wound with saline solution will help to remove any dirt or debris that may cause an infection.

20. 0) Because this is a deep laceration, the athlete will have to be referred to a physician for treatment. Application of an antiseptic or antibiotic to the area after a thorough cleansing will be done by the physician.

21. +) Both eyes should be covered during the athlete's transport to the hospital to minimize eye movement. (The athlete feels better with her eyes closed.)

22. 0) The mechanism of injury was determined by the opening scenario. (This is obvious.)

23. +) Because there is no apparent injury to the eye itself, an ice pack applied lightly to the surrounding area of the eye will help minimize swelling. (The pain and swelling are controlled.)

24. +) The application of Steri-Strips will help to minimize bleeding and approximate the wound until the physician sutures it. (You are able to close the wound.)

25. -) It is inappropriate to ignore the athlete. It is the job of the athletic trainer to answer her questions honestly and be reassuring to minimize her anxieties. (The athlete appears fearful.)

26. --) Only a physician can suture a wound; an athletic trainer is not qualified or licensed to do so. (You are sued for malpractice.)

27. +) If there is a suspected serious eye injury, the athlete should be transported to a hospital while lying in a recumbent position. (You act cautiously.)

28. --) The athlete should be kept calm and comfortable while waiting for the ambulance and should not be left alone. (The athlete passes out in the parking lot.)

29. -) In case of a serious eye injury, no direct pressure should be applied to the eye. (You find out later you might have made the injury worse.)

30. ++) A secondary evaluation is a detailed assessment that focuses on the nature and extent of the injury. (You know the athlete has a bad laceration and suspect a potentially serious eye injury.)

Section C

The current situation: The athlete has sustained a deep laceration over the left eyebrow with a potential eye injury.

Your immediate responsibility: Keep the athlete calm while waiting for the rescue squad and document the course of events.

31. +) The athletic trainer should be a source of reassurance. This is an appropriate action. (The athlete is grateful you are staying with her.)

32. -) The athlete's condition and playing status have not been determined. Announcing the athlete's condition is inappropriate. (You anger the coach and parents with this announcement.)

33. -) The student's insurance coverage should not be a deterrent for an emergency room visit. (You delay treatment.)

34. -) It is not the duty of the school nurse to accompany the athlete to the emergency room. (She reminds you that this is part of your job.)

35. --) Once the initial dressing is applied and the bleeding is controlled, it is inappropriate to change the bandage multiple times. (The Steri-Strips come off, and the cut bleeds again.)

36. +) The athlete may need reassurance from her coach that her position is not in jeopardy. (The coach tells the athlete there is no need to worry.)

37. -) Speaking with the press about the athlete's condition is not appropriate. (You are reprimanded by your athletic director.)

38. ++) Washing your hands thoroughly after handling a "blood-spill" is a fundamental universal precaution.

39. ++) Documenting the incident and treatment given is appropriate.

40. 0) Dispensing vitamins to the athlete is unnecessary and inappropriate.

41. +) Once the athlete is stable and not in any immediate danger, it is wise to inform the athlete's coach on the nature and severity of the injury and what is being done for her. (The coach thanks you for doing a thorough job.)

PROBLEM III

Section A

The current situation: You know your athlete has been injured after incorrectly landing on a crash mat. He is not moving.

Your immediate responsibility: To evaluate the injury to determine the type and nature of the injury.

1. -) This would be a premature action as you have not completed your initial evaluation of the injury.

2. +) This question should be asked as part of the "history" portion of the initial assessment. (The athlete complains of dull neck pain.)

3. ++) A primary survey is necessary to determine if there is a life-threatening injury. (The athlete is conscious and is breathing without difficulty. Blood pressure is 130/90 and pulse is 82.)

4. +) Noting the position of the athlete is important when deciding how the athlete is to be treated and transported. (The athlete is lying on his right side with his knees flexed.)

5. -) The athlete should not be moved unless the airway is blocked and there is additional help available. (The athlete is breathing without difficulty.)

6. +) This is a quick screen to assess motor function of the upper and lower extremities. (The athlete states he cannot move his fingers or toes.)

7. +) If the athlete is conscious and can answer questions, it is appropriate to ask this as part of the history portion of the evaluation. It helps in determining the mechanism of injury. (He reports he did not tuck his chin in and landed on his head, snapping his head forward.)

8. 0) Applying an ice pack to the athlete's neck is unnecessary and inappropriate.

9. 0) It is known from the opening scenario that the area of injury is not the lower extremity.

10. +) It is an appropriate action as part of the primary survey to assess the athlete for areas of significant bleeding. (The athlete's face in uninjured.)

11. 0) Until the initial evaluation of the injury is completed, this would be a premature and inappropriate action. (You waste valuable time.)

12. ++) Checking the athlete's level of consciousness is a necessary step during the primary survey. (The athlete is coherent and responds appropriately to questions.)

Section B

The current situation: The athlete is conscious and coherent and is breathing without difficulty. His vital signs are stable, but he is unable to move his extremities.

Your immediate responsibility: To continue your evaluation to determine the athlete's neuromuscular function, protect the athlete from further injury, and prepare him for transport to the hospital.

13. --) Moving the athlete at this time without securing him to a spine board may cause further injury. (The athlete sustains a complete spinal cord injury and is quadriplegic.)

14. --) Having the athlete move his head may be a potentially fatal or debilitating action. (The athlete sustains a vertebral fracture/dislocation and dies.)

15. ++) Determining sensation to the extremities is important in assessing the severity of the injury. (The athlete complains he cannot feel anything from his armpits down to his feet.)

16. ++) This is a fundamental action in preventing further injury to the athlete.

17. 0) This is an unnecessary action, as you have ruled out a head injury. (The athlete is conscious and alert.)

18. -) The findings of the primary survey do not indicate there is a head injury. (You waste time.)

19. ++) Log-rolling the athlete with assistance onto his back is necessary for stabilization and transport of the athlete. (You successfully position the athlete into supine.)

20. 0) Unless the athlete is in an area where he may be subjected to further injury, it is not necessary to stop the meet at this time. (You keep the area clear of spectators.)

21. ++) Securing the athlete to a spine board is an appropriate action. (You successfully secure the athlete onto a spine board with help.)

22. ++) While you stay with the athlete, an ambulance should be summoned to the field. (The ambulance is close by and arrives in 5 minutes.)

23. +) This is an appropriate action with a suspected neck injury. (You successfully apply a cervical collar.)

24. +) Monitoring the athlete's vital signs is a fundamental aspect of your care. (The athlete's vital signs remain stable.)

Section C

The current situation: You have evaluated the injury and suspect the athlete has sustained a serious cervical spinal injury. The athlete is transported to the hospital via ambulance.

Your immediate responsibility: To contact the team physician, parents, and other appropriate individuals with information regarding the accident. Document what occurred and who was involved.

25. +) Communicating with the team physician would be appropriate at this time. (Your athletic training student contacts the team doctor's office.)

26. +) It is important to document the incident. (You protect yourself against a malpractice lawsuit.)

27. 0) If another certified athletic trainer is available to cover the rest of the meet, it would be appropriate to go to the hospital. Otherwise, you should follow up with the athlete at the hospital after the meet.

28. 0) The athlete is coherent and able to provide this information to the EMS and hospital personnel.

29. 0) Whether or not the athlete is on a scholarship is not pertinent to the treatment of this athlete.

30. +) Contacting the parents of the injured athlete would be an appropriate step. (The parents go directly to the hospital.)

31. -) Leaving an athletic training student in charge of covering a state track meet without direct supervision of a certified athletic trainer is inappropriate. (You are reprimanded by your athletic director and are lucky no one else is hurt while you are gone.)

32. -) This is an inappropriate comment. (The athletic director suggests that you stick to your duties as an athletic trainer.)

PROBLEM IV

Section A

The current situation: An athlete comes to your office complaining of chronic left anterior knee pain. No specific mechanism of injury has been identified.

Your immediate responsibility: To perform your initial evaluation to determine the nature and severity of the condition.

1. 0) Applying an ice pack will not cause further injury, but may not help the athlete either because the problem has not been thoroughly evaluated at this time.

2. +) A postural assessment is part of the evaluation of anterior knee pain. (Both knees are in genu valgum.)

3. +) Palpation of the knee joint is a basic element of a knee evaluation. (The athlete complains of patellar tendon and medial knee pain.)

4. +) With subjective complaints of anterior knee pain, it is highly likely the athlete's iliotibial band will be tight. Both sides must be tested for comparison. (Ober's test is positive on the left lower extremity.)

5. +) This question should be asked while taking the athlete's history, as a "popping" sensation is often associated with patellofemoral pain syndrome. (The athlete reports it "pops" intermittently while running.)

6. -) It is known from the athlete's subjective complaints that this is a knee injury. (The athlete tells you her feet are fine.)

7. 0) Patrick's test is a special test of the hip that when positive is indicative of degenerative joint disease.

8. +) This is an appropriate question to ask when gathering information regarding the mechanism of injury. (The athlete has pain going down stairs and running downhill.)

9. ++) Because activity appears to increase the pain, it would be wise to advise the athlete to stop running when it hurts. (The athlete feels much better when she is not landing on it.)

10. -) Temporary orthotics may not be necessary or appropriate; the initial evaluation is not complete. (You waste time making them and the athlete reports no change in her pain.)

11. +) Observing the knee for swelling or deformity is a fundamental component of the initial evaluation. (No swelling is noted.)

12. +) Palpating the knee joint and surrounding soft tissue structures is a fundamental component of the initial evaluation. (The athlete complains of pain with palpation of the medial facet.)

13. -) A KT-1000 arthrometer is used to test for anterior cruciate laxity and would not be appropriate in this situation. (It is known from the opening scenario that this is not an acute injury, and injury to the anterior cruciate ligament is unlikely.)

Section B

The current situation: The athlete has pain running downhill, especially over the patellar tendon and medial aspect of the knee. She has pain over the same areas with palpation, although there is no swelling present. She also experiences a "popping" sensation with running. She stands in genu valgum and presents a tight iliotibial band on the left leg.

Your immediate responsibility: Make recommendations to the athlete to decrease her pain with activities and teach the athlete lower limb stretching and strengthening exercises to realign the patella.

14. +) A soft knee brace designed to help stabilize the patella may help decrease the athlete's pain during activity. (The athlete reports a decrease in pain and feeling of "popping" while wearing the knee sleeve.)

15. 0) Strengthening the hamstrings does not have a direct effect in stabilizing the patella.

16. +) Strengthening the vastus medialis obliques will help to improve the tracking of the patella in the femoral groove. (The athlete has fewer episodes of "popping.")

17. --) Repetitive deep squatting exercises cause high compressive loading on the patellofemoral joint and will aggravate the athlete's knee. (The athlete complains of significant anterior knee pain.)

18. +) Patella taping is a useful tool in evaluating and treating patellar misalignment problems. (There is reduction of pain with taping.)

19. ++) A tight iliotibial band will cause mistracking of the patella. (There are fewer episodes of "popping.")

20. ++) Tight hamstrings may cause mistracking of the patella in the femoral groove. (The athlete has bilateral hamstring tightness.)

21. -) Recommending an oral NSAID might be appropriate, but a certified athletic trainer is not qualified or licensed to dispense a prescription drug such as Voltaren. (The athlete has an adverse reaction to the medication and you are sued for malpractice.)

22. -) The athlete should avoid hard or hilly surfaces. (The athlete continues to complain of "popping" and knee pain with running.)

Section C

The current situation: You have determined from your evaluation that this athlete has a subluxing patella secondary to weak anteromedial thigh musculature and a tight iliotibial band and hamstrings.

Your immediate responsibility: Continue to work with the athlete to develop a structured rehabilitation program to encourage proper alignment of the patella, which will in turn eliminate the pain.

23. 0) A TENS unit is a modality that can be used temporarily for pain. A TENS unit will not contribute directly to the elimination of the origin of the problem. (The athlete has no pain when she is not running.)

24. -) The patella subluxes as a result of weak anterior and medial thigh musculature; PNF exercises that emphasize motions which encourage hip abduction with internal rotation facilitate strengthening of the lateral thigh musculature. (The athlete experiences an increase in episodes of patella subluxation.)

25. 0) Ultrasound treatments will not have a direct impact on the cause of the problem.

26. --) Because plyometric exercises employ ballistic movements, which generate high forces, the initiation of this type of exercise would not be appropriate. (The athlete now complains of anterior knee pain at rest.)

27. ++) Strengthening the quadriceps musculature in both open- and closed-chain positions is appropriate as long as the exercise is pain-free.

28. +) It may be beneficial to evaluate the athlete's running gait to assess what is occurring at the knee. (The athlete's feet severely pronate during midstance.)

29. ++) Strengthening the hip adductors will augment the strength of the vastus medialis oblique muscle.

30. +) The continual application of ice to the knee will help minimize any pain or inflammation from exercises. (The athlete is able to control postactivity soreness.)

PROBLEM V

Section A

The current situation: An athlete comes to you complaining of right shoulder pain that occurs after throwing. He is able to voluntarily sublux both his shoulders.

Your immediate responsibility: To perform an initial evaluation to determine the nature and severity of the problem.

1. ++) Asking the athlete how long the problem has existed is a fundamental question to ask during the history portion of the evaluation. This will give the athletic trainer an idea if this is an acute or chronic problem. (The athlete states it has hurt over the past 3 weeks.)

2. +) A more appropriate question might be to ask the athlete if the right shoulder had ever been injured in the past and when the injury occurred. (The athlete states he has not had a shoulder injury prior to this recent episode.)

3. +) This is an appropriate question to ask during the history portion of the evaluation. (The athlete states that he cannot specifically tell you what position[s] make the pain worse.)

4. 0) This would be an inappropriate question. Whether or not the athlete is consuming an adequate amount of protein has nothing to do with this problem.

5. ++) This would be an appropriate question given the information that has been provided in the opening scenario. (The fact that the athlete is able to voluntarily sublux his shoulder.)

6. 0) This question is unnecessary and inappropriate. The athlete has already provided you with information in the opening scenario relating to his joint laxity.

7. 0) This question is unnecessary and inappropriate. Whether or not the athlete is taking supplemental vitamins has no direct correlation to the present problem.

8. +) Asking the athlete about the intensity of his pain will provide the athletic trainer information regarding the severity of the condition. (The athlete reports his pain level is moderate, 5/10 after pitching.)

9. -) This is an inappropriate question. Whether or not his father played baseball is irrelevant and whether or not his father had injured his shoulder has no direct correlation to the present problem. (The athlete has no idea if his father ever had a shoulder problem.)

10. +) Asking the athlete about any medications he may be taking is appropriate during the history portion of the initial evaluation. (The athlete reports he has been taking aspirin for the pain with temporary relief.)

Section B

The current situation: The athlete has subacute right shoulder pain with joint laxity. He is able to voluntarily sublux both his shoulders. Aspirin provides minimal pain relief.

Your immediate responsibility: Perform special tests to identify the etiology of the athlete's pain.

11. -) This is an inappropriate test for this problem. Phalen's test is performed when carpal tunnel syndrome is suspected.

12. +) A clunk test is an appropriate test to perform if a glenoid labral tear is suspected. (The athlete has a negative clunk test.)

13. -) The pivot shift test is performed to evaluate the knee for anterolateral instability secondary to tearing the anterior cruciate ligament. This is an inappropriate test for this problem.

14. -) Patrick's test is performed to evaluate the hip for iliopsoas, sacroiliac, or joint pathology. This is an inappropriate test for this problem.

15. -) Thompson's test is performed when the possibility of an Achilles' tendon rupture exists. This is an inappropriate test for this problem.

16. +) The apprehension test (anterior and posterior) is an appropriate test to perform for this problem. A positive test may be indicative of either anterior or posterior glenohumeral instability. (The athlete has a positive apprehension sign.)

17. +) The Hawkins-Kennedy impingement test is used to test for pain and apprehension relating to shoulder impingement. This would be an appropriate test to perform for this problem. (The athlete has a positive test.)

18. +) Neer's sign is used to test for pain and apprehension relating to shoulder impingement, primarily of the biceps long head and supraspinatus tendons. (The athlete has a negative Neer's sign.)

19. +) The posterior drawer test of the shoulder is used when there is suspicion of posterior instability of the glenohumeral joint. This would be an appropriate test for this problem. (The athlete has a negative posterior drawer sign.)

20. -) Ober's test is used to determine iliotibial band/tensor fasciae latae tightness of the lower extremity. This is an inappropriate test for this problem.

21. -) Trendelenburg's test is used to determine if there is weakness of the gluteus medius muscle. This is not an appropriate test for this problem.

22. +) Testing for a sulcus sign is appropriate when assessing the athlete for multidirectional instability of the shoulder. This is an appropriate test for this problem. (The athlete has a positive sulcus sign.)

Section C

The current situation: The athlete has a positive impingement test, a positive sulcus sign, and a positive apprehension test.

Your immediate responsibility: Instruct and supervise an upper extremity strengthening program.

23. +) Shoulder shrugs strengthen the upper trapezius muscle, which helps to stabilize the scapula superiorly.

24. -) Although biceps curls are not inappropriate for general upper extremity strengthening, they will not contribute to strengthening the rotator cuff or scapula musculature.

25. +) Shoulder abduction strengthening exercises are appropriate, as they stabilize the scapula laterally and posteriorly.

26. -) Cervical isometric exercises are unnecessary and inappropriate for this particular problem, as they will not have a direct effect on stabilizing the scapula or strengthening the rotator cuff.

27. ++) Resistive exercises involving internal and external rotation of the shoulder directly strengthen the rotator cuff musculature.

28. +) Resistive exercises performed in the D2 extension pattern work the shoulder extensors, adductors, and internal rotators. This type of exercise would be appropriate for this problem.

29. -) Because the long head of the triceps brachii muscle arises from the infraglenoid tuberosity of the scapula, shoulder extension exercises would assist in scapular stabilization, but triceps curls (ie, elbow extension) would not have a direct effect on either the scapula or the rotator cuff.

30. +) Rowing exercises strengthen the rhomboids, triceps (long head), and latissimus dorsi, stabilizing the scapula medially and posteriorly.

31. +) Exercises involving resisted scapular protraction strengthen the serratus anterior muscle, stabilizing the scapula laterally.

32. -) Partial sit-ups strengthen the upper abdominals, which is unnecessary and inappropriate for this problem.

33. -) Prone trunk extensions strengthen the erector spinae musculature of the back, which is unnecessary and inappropriate for this problem.

34. -) Calf raises strengthen the triceps surae complex of the lower leg, which is unnecessary and inappropriate for this problem.

PROBLEM VI

Section A

The current situation: You know your athlete has sustained a left lower leg injury and the mechanism of injury was an indirect trauma.

Your immediate responsibility: To perform your initial evaluation of the injury to determine the type and extent of the injury.

1. -) It is obvious from the opening scenario that the athlete is breathing fine. (The athlete is howling in pain.)

2. -) It is obvious from the opening scenario that the athlete has a significant lower extremity injury; it is inappropriate to have the athlete attempt to walk until your initial evaluation is complete. (The athlete asks if you are an athletic training student.)

3. +) Asking the athlete what happened is an appropriate question that should be asked during the history portion of the initial evaluation. (He states he stopped suddenly and the left lower leg "gave out.")

4. -) It is obvious from the opening scenario that the athlete has not sustained a head injury. This would be an inappropriate action. (The athlete is very alert and in severe pain.)

5. +) Examining the athlete's leg for areas of external or internal bleeding (ecchymosis) is an appropriate action. (There are no obvious signs of bleeding at this time.)

6. ++) Asking the athlete where the pain is located is fundamental in determining what structures of the lower leg are involved. (The athlete points to the musculotendinous junction of the gastrocnemius and Achilles' tendon.)

7. ++) Observing the area of injury is an appropriate and necessary action as part of the initial assessment of an injury. (There is mild edema of the posterior lower extremity at the musculotendinous junction.)

8. ++) Asking the athlete whether or not he felt or heard a "pop" or "snap" provides the athletic trainer information regarding the nature and severity of the injury. (The athlete states he felt a "pop" with severe pain in the calf.)

9. 0) Applying ice at this point of your evaluation will not hurt the athlete but is premature, as your evaluation is not yet complete.

10. -) Asking the athlete if he has ever injured his uninvolved leg would be inappropriate at this time, as it is not a priority. (The athlete states his left lower extremity has never been hurt.)

11. --) It is obvious from the opening scenario that the left lower extremity has been significantly injured. Asking the athlete to stand and hop would be inappropriate and could cause further injury if attempted. (The athlete completely ruptures his gastrocnemius muscle.)

Section B

The current situation: You know from your evaluation that the athlete felt a "pop" accompanied by severe pain at the musculotendinous junction of the gastrocnemius and Achilles' tendon. There is mild edema present in the area.

Your immediate responsibility: To continue your evaluation to determine the severity of the injury.

12. ++) Palpating the injured extremity for swelling and deformity would be an appropriate action at this time. (There is now a moderate effusion of the lower extremity and a palpable defect at the musculotendinous junction.)

13. -) Performing a Lachman's test bilaterally would be an unnecessary and inappropriate action. The injury is to the left lower extremity, not the knee. (The athlete wonders why you are checking his knee.)

14. -) Performing a Thomas test bilaterally would be an unnecessary and inappropriate action. The Thomas test is performed to assess for tight hip flexors. (You have now wasted time examining the athlete's hip flexibility.)

15. +) Checking the active range of motion of both ankles is appropriate to assess the athlete's functional ability and willingness to move. (The athlete is unable to actively plantar flex his foot and has pain with the attempt.)

16. -) Checking the athlete's Q-angle is unnecessary and inappropriate. It is also known from the opening scenario that it is the left lower extremity, not the right, that is injured. (Be sure to carefully read through all the information provided.)

17. 0) Whether or not the athlete has bunions has nothing to do with this injury.

18. ++) Performing Thompson's test bilaterally would be an appropriate action to take during your assessment of this injury. (The test is positive on the left leg.)

19. -) Performing a Hawkin's test bilaterally would be unnecessary and inappropriate. The athlete's left lower extremity has been injured, not his shoulder. (The athlete wonders why you are examining his shoulder.)

20. -) Performing an anterior drawer test bilaterally on both ankles is unnecessary and inappropriate. The athlete's left lower leg has been injured, not his left ankle. (The athlete wonders why you are examining his ankles.)

21. 0) Palpating the femoral pulse is unnecessary and inappropriate for this problem. (The athlete's femoral pulses are fine.)

22. 0) Testing the patellar tendon reflexes bilaterally is an unnecessary and inappropriate action. (The athlete's patellar tendon reflexes are fine.)

23. +) Testing the strength of the ankle plantar flexors would be an appropriate action to take when initially assessing the severity of the injury. (The strength of the ankle plantar flexors is -2/5 and painful.)

Section C

The current situation: You suspect a torn left gastrocnemius muscle.

Your immediate responsibility: To begin treatment to control the pain and swelling and protect the athlete from further injury.

24. --) If the lower limb still has a significant amount of swelling, warm whirlpool treatments would be inappropriate. (The athlete's leg swells significantly during this treatment.)

25. ++) Applying ice to the injured area is an appropriate action to ease the pain and control the effusion. (The athlete is much more comfortable with the ice.)

26. ++) Applying a compression wrap to the injured area is an appropriate action to ease the pain and control the effusion. (The athlete is much more comfortable with the compression wrap.)

27. +) High-volt galvanic stimulation can be used to modulate pain and assist with edema reduction. (The athlete is much more comfortable after the treatment.)

28. ++) The application of a posterior leg splint is an appropriate action. This puts the lower extremity at rest and protects the area from further injury. (The athlete is much more comfortable with the lower leg immobilized.)

29. -) Attempting to use the BAPS board too early in the treatment may increase pain and swelling. This is an inappropriate action at this time. (The athlete complains of increased calf pain and is frustrated he is unable to move the board.)

30. --) Based on your initial assessment, this athlete has sustained a torn gastrocnemius muscle. This would be an inappropriate action if your assessment is correct. (The athlete howls in pain during the attempt to come up on his toes.)

31. +) This is an appropriate action, especially if the lower extremity is immobilized.

32. -) This is an inappropriate action. The defect is a result of a torn muscle, not an infection. (The athlete questions why you are smearing gel on him.)

33. 0) The athlete may or may not be able to perform hamstring curls early in the rehabilitation. (The athlete is able to lift light weights.)

34. --) Because this is an acute muscle tear, ultrasound treatments are contraindicated at this time. (The calf swells and becomes ecchymotic.)

35. -) While gentle range of motion exercises are appropriate, the injured limb is the left lower extremity, not the right. (The athlete reminds you that his right leg is fine.)

Section D

The current situation: Your athlete sustained a torn gastrocnemius muscle, which is now subacute in nature. The motion of his ankle and knee is normal, but he still has some strength deficits in plantar flexion.

Your immediate responsibility: Develop a strength and conditioning program designed to improve the athlete's left lower extremity strength and maintain his level of fitness.

36. ++) Stationary bicycling would be appropriate at this point of this athlete's rehabilitation. (The athlete is grateful to be aerobically active.)

37. --) Uphill jogging would be inappropriate. Based on the information provided, the athlete's strength in plantar flexion is still weak. This exercise is premature and may cause further injury. (The athlete retears the muscle.)

38. 0) Although push-ups will not harm the athlete, it is not a necessary exercise for this athlete's rehabilitation.

39. ++) Having the athlete performing progressive-resistive ankle exercises in all directions would be appropriate at this point of the athlete's rehabilitation. (The athlete has no pain or significant difficulty with resistive exercises.)

40. --) Knowing from the information given thus far that the athlete is weak in plantar flexion concentrically, plyometric exercises would be inappropriate and may cause further injury if initiated too soon. (The athlete retears the gastrocnemius.)

41. 0) Using the upper body ergometer during the athlete's rehabilitation would be appropriate to maintain aerobic fitness but is not directly related to rehabilitating a lower extremity injury.

42. +) Initiating exercises that enhance proprioception is a necessary and appropriate action to take in preparing the athlete to return to his sport. (The athlete demonstrates some difficulty in maintaining his balance on the injured leg.)

43. ++) Having the athlete perform exercises that directly work in strengthening the plantar flexors of the ankle is appropriate. (The athlete has no pain performing this exercise but still has difficulty performing unilateral calf raises.)

44. +) Partial squats with and without additional resistance is appropriate for lower extremity strengthening. (The athlete is able to do this without pain or difficulty.)

45. ++) Having the athlete perform resisted hamstring curls would be appropriate, as the gastrocnemius not only functions to plantar flex the ankle but is also a flexor of the knee.

46. +) It is important to make sure the rest of the leg is strengthened in addition to the specific area of injury, because the entire lower extremity loses strength during the initial phases treatment when the limb is immobilized. (The athlete has normal quadricep strength bilaterally.)

47. +) Making sure the athlete maintains his lower extremity flexibility is appropriate in preparing the athlete to return to his sport. (The athlete's flexibility is normal bilaterally.)

48. -) Focusing attention on upper extremity strengthening would not be necessary or appropriate during the rehabilitation of this injury.

49. -) Focusing attention on upper extremity strengthening would not be necessary or appropriate during the rehabilitation of this injury.

50. -) Until the strength of the athlete's plantar flexors on the injured limb is equal to the strength of the uninjured limb, initiating agility exercises would be inappropriate.

Section E

The current situation: This athlete has been performing a general lower extremity flexibility and strengthening exercise program as instructed without complaints of pain or difficulty. He is anxious to return to playing competitive tennis.

Your immediate responsibility: Reassess the athlete and have the athlete perform a series of functional exercises to determine if the athlete is ready to play.

51. +) Making sure the athlete can walk without a limp would be appropriate. (The athlete has no difficulty with this task.)

52. ++) The athlete should be completely pain-free at rest and during activity prior to returning to full-time competition. (The athlete is completely pain-free.)

53. ++) There should be no visible edema or ecchymosis at the site of injury. (There is no visible swelling or ecchymosis.)

54. +) The athlete should have no complaints of pain with deep palpation of the injured area. (The athlete reports he has no pain with palpation of the injured area.)

55. +) The athlete should have no complaints of pain with a resisted hamstring curl. (The athlete is pain-free with this motion.)

56. ++) The athlete should have full range of motion of both the ankle and knee before returning to full activity. (The range of motion of the injured ankle and knee is equal to the uninjured side.)

57. --) The athletic trainer should only return the athlete to competition when the athletic trainer and team physician determine the athlete is fully recovered. (The athlete returns too soon and is re-injured.)

58. +) The athlete should be able to hop on the injured lower extremity without pain before returning to full activity. (The athlete has no pain or difficulty pushing off or landing on the injured leg.)

59. +) The athlete should be able to jog a reasonable amount of time in a straight line before returning to full activity. (The athlete has no difficulty doing this.)

60. --) Although the athlete may not be as interested in his rehabilitation program as he is in his sport, the athlete's level of interest is not a credible parameter by which to determine whether or not he can return to full activity.

61. ++) The strength of the athlete's involved ankle should be equal to the strength of the uninvolved ankle before returning the athlete to full activity. (Both ankles are now graded as 5/5 during manual muscle testing.)

62. ++) It is prudent to have the team physician clear the athlete for return to full activity before the athlete participates in his sport. (The athlete is cleared for competition.)

63. 0) Whether or not the athlete can bench press 50 pounds or more has nothing to do with whether or not this athlete can compete in tennis. (The athlete can bench press 90 pounds.)

PROBLEM VII

Section A

The current situation: You know your athlete has sustained an indirect traumatic injury to his right knee. He is able to bear weight without assistance.

Your immediate responsibility: To perform your initial evaluation to determine the nature and severity of the injury.

1. ++) Having the athlete locate the area of pain is appropriate during the initial assessment of the injury. It is important in determining the nature of the injury. (The athlete reports he has pain along the medial side of the right knee.)

2. +) Observing for areas of swelling is appropriate during the initial assessment of the injury. (There is minimal edema noted along the medial side of the right knee.)

3. 0) Applying ice to the area prior to completing the initial exam is a premature action.

4. 0) Applying a knee immobilizer prior to completing the initial examination is a premature action.

5. 0) Issuing a cane to the athlete prior to completing the initial examination is a premature action. A cane may or may not be an appropriate assistive device for this injury.

6. ++) Palpation of the knee joint and the surrounding structures is a fundamental task of the initial evaluation. (The athlete reports he has a small amount of pain with palpation of the anteromedial joint line.)

7. -) Palpating the gluteus medius muscle is an inappropriate and unnecessary action. It is obvious from the opening scenario that this is a knee injury, not a hip injury. (The athlete asks why you are palpating his hip.)

8. -) Having the athlete perform multiple calf raises is not an appropriate action. It is known from the opening scenario that the athlete has pain in full weightbearing. (The athlete is unable to perform a calf raise because of knee pain and instability.)

9. ++) Evaluating the range of motion of both knees is appropriate during your initial evaluation of the injury. It assists the athletic trainer in determining the severity of the injury and the athlete's willingness to move. (The athlete has significant difficulty bending and completely straightening his knee because of pain.)

10. ++) Asking the athlete if he has injured his right knee before is an appropriate question during the history portion of the initial evaluation. (The athlete reports he had a minor knee injury 3 years ago but has been fine since that time.)

11. +) It is appropriate during the initial evaluation to assess the strength of the hip musculature bilaterally. (The strength of the hip flexors on the injured limb is +4/5.)

12. +) It is appropriate during the initial evaluation to assess the strength of the quadriceps musculature bilaterally. (The strength of the quadriceps musculature on the injured limb is -3/5.)

13. +) It is appropriate during the initial evaluation to assess the strength of the hamstring musculature bilaterally. (The strength of the hamstring musculature on the injured limb is -3/5.)

14. 0) Checking the athlete's pupillary reaction is an unnecessary and inappropriate action. (The athlete tells you to get the light out of his eyes.)

Section B

The current situation: You have determined from your evaluation that the athlete has pain along the medial aspect of the knee with palpation, there is minimal edema present, and the athlete has pain with movement into knee flexion and extension.

Your immediate responsibility: To continue your evaluation by performing special tests on the right knee.

15. ++) Performing a Lachman's test bilaterally would be appropriate to assess the integrity of the anterior cruciate ligament. (The Lachman's test is negative.)

16. --) The vertebral artery test is performed to test the patency of the vertebral arteries. This would be inappropriate. (The athlete does not trust you at this point of the exam.)

17. --) Tinel's test is performed when carpal tunnel syndrome is suspected. This would not be an appropriate test for this problem. (The athlete reminds you that it is his knee that is injured, not his wrist or hand.)

18. ++) The valgus stress test is performed to test the integrity of the medial collateral ligament. Performing this test bilaterally would be appropriate. (The athlete complains of medial knee joint pain and there is increased valgus movement on the injured side.)

19. ++) The varus stress test is performed to test the integrity of the lateral collateral ligament. Performing this test bilaterally would be an appropriate action. (There is no complaint of pain with this test and minimal/no varus movement on the injured knee joint.)

20. +) Performing a posterior drawer test bilaterally would be appropriate to test the integrity of the posterior cruciate ligament. (The posterior drawer test is negative.)

21. --) The empty can test is performed to assess for supraspinatus weakness and is an inappropriate test for this problem. This athlete has a knee injury, not a shoulder injury. (The athlete's shoulders are fine.)

22. --) The Finkelstein test is performed to assess for tenosynovitis of the abductor pollicis longus and extensor pollicis brevis tendons and is an inappropriate test for this problem. (The athlete asks you what this test has to do with his knees.)

23. -) Yergason's test is performed bilaterally when bicipital tendinitis is suspected. (The athlete asks you what this test has to do with his knees.)

24. ++) Performing a McMurray's test bilaterally would be appropriate to test the knee for a meniscal tear. (McMurray's test is inconclusive because of the limitation in range of motion.)

25. +) Performing an anterior drawer test bilaterally would be appropriate to test the knee for an anterior cruciate tear. (The anterior drawer test is negative.)

26. +) Performing a pivot shift test would be appropriate to test the knee for anterolateral rotary instability secondary to a torn anterior cruciate ligament and posterolateral capsule. (The pivot shift test is inconclusive because the athlete is guarding.)

27. +) Performing a patellar apprehension test bilaterally would be appropriate to test the knee for patellar subluxation or dislocation. (The patellar apprehension test is negative.)

Section C

The current situation: You suspect from the results of your evaluation that this athlete has a medial collateral ligament sprain with a possible meniscus tear of the right knee.

Your immediate responsibility: Begin a treatment program with emphasis on pain control and early motion.

28. --) The application of heat early in the rehabilitation when the knee is swollen would be inappropriate. (The knee swells severely after the heat is applied.)

29. -) Massaging the knee joint is unnecessary and inappropriate. (This causes great pain to the athlete, and he avoids you the following week.)

30. --) Having the athlete attempt to use a rowing machine would be inappropriate during the initial stages of rehabilitation. (The athlete has significant knee pain and is unable to move the knee enough to operate it.)

31. ++) Placing the athlete on crutches to protect the joint is an appropriate action during the initial phases of treatment. (The athlete is much more comfortable and mobile with crutches.)

32. +) Assessing the strength of the quadriceps is important in determining the starting point for a rehabilitation program. (The athlete is unable to fully extend his knee against gravity.)

33. -) Starting isotonic hamstring strengthening exercises would be an inappropriate action if the goal is to treat the athlete for pain and swelling. (The athlete is unable to fully flex his knee against gravity.)

34. ++) Applying ice to the injured joint is appropriate for pain management and reducing edema. (The athlete reports pain relief with the ice packs in place.)

35. ++) It is important to have the athlete move his knee as soon as possible to his tolerance to maintain joint mobility. (The athlete is able to actively flex and extend his leg to a limited degree while lying in a supine position.)

36. 0) This would not be an appropriate suggestion. It is the right knee that has sustained the injury, not the left knee. (Make sure you read through the scenario carefully.)

37. --) It is not within an athletic trainer's scope of practice to issue medication with codeine as an active ingredient. (You are sued for trying to practice medicine.)

38. ++) The use of high-volt galvanic stimulation is indicated for reducing pain and swelling. (The athlete has good results with this treatment.)

Section D

The current situation: The athlete's pain is controlled well with modalities and is moving his knee with greater ease.

Your immediate responsibility: To begin the athlete on a rehabilitation program with an emphasis on maintaining the athlete's aerobic conditioning and beginning functional exercises.

39. +) Functional activities should be introduced into the rehabilitation program as soon as possible; swimming is an appropriate activity to increase aerobic conditioning. (The athlete is able to swim with minimal discomfort.)

40. +) Having the athlete perform calf raises is an inappropriate activity as an early functional exercise.

41. -) Having the athlete attempt to run on a treadmill 1 week after sustaining a second-degree medial collateral tear of the knee would be inappropriate and may subject the athlete to further injury. (The athlete reinjures his knee while trying to run.)

42. +) Introducing closed-chain exercises, such as stair-climbing (eg, Stairmaster), into the rehabilitation program as early as possible is an appropriate action. (The athlete is able to perform stair-climbing activities.)

43. ++) Having the athlete use the upper body ergometer to maintain aerobic fitness is appropriate. (The athlete is able to get a vigorous workout on this machine.)

44. 0) Wall pulley exercises for the upper extremity will not harm the athlete but are unnecessary and inappropriate if the goal is to maintain the athlete's aerobic capability.

45. ++) Introducing closed-chain exercises, such as stationary bicycling, into the rehabilitation program as early as possible is appropriate. (The athlete has minimal/no difficulty using the stationary bike.)

46. --) Fartlek training involves a type of cross-country running, which is varied in speed and terrain. This would be an inappropriate activity for the athlete to attempt early in the rehabilitation. (The athlete is unable to run, much less perform long-distance running through varied terrain.)

47. --) Plyometric exercises would be inappropriate in the early stages of rehabilitation. (The athlete attempts to jump up onto a stool from the floor and reinjures his knee.)

48. --) Resisted rowing early in the rehabilitation would be inappropriate. The ballistic motion may cause further pain or injury. (The athlete complains of significant pain during this activity.)

PROBLEM VIII

Section A

The current situation: You know this athlete has sustained a significant abdominal injury after being kicked by an opponent.

Your immediate responsibility: To perform an initial evaluation to determine the nature and extent of the injury and assess if it is a life-threatening situation.

1. ++) Performing a primary survey would be an appropriate action. (The athlete is conscious, coherent, and in obvious pain.)

2. 0) Giving the athlete oxygen is unnecessary and inappropriate. (The athlete angrily pushes the oxygen mask away from his face.)

3. -) Auscultating the athlete's heart is an inappropriate and unnecessary action. (The athlete's heart is fine.)

4. ++) It is appropriate to gently palpate the athlete's abdomen to assess for areas of pain and firmness. (The athlete has significant pain with palpation of the lower right quadrant and a moderately sized hematoma over the injury site.)

5. ++) It is appropriate during the history portion of the initial assessment to ask the athlete where the pain is located. This will give the athletic trainer an idea regarding the nature of the injury. (The athlete reports his pain is located in the lower right quadrant of his abdominal area.)

6. --) Having the athlete attempt to stand and jog is a premature action. You have not yet completed your evaluation and may cause further injury by excessively moving the athlete. (This athlete cannot stand, much less jog, because of the pain.)

7. 0) Having the athlete count backward from 100 would be inappropriate and unnecessary. It is known from the opening scenario that a head injury has not been sustained.

8. 0) Having a stretcher brought out to the field is a premature action, as the initial evaluation has not been completed.

9. 0) Unless there is any evidence of bleeding, donning latex gloves is not necessary.

10. ++) Observing the abdominal area for signs of edema or ecchymosis is fundamental during the initial assessment of the injury. (There is a contusion over the lower right quadrant.)

11. ++) Asking the athlete whether the pain radiates anywhere is essential in determining if there are any possible internal injuries and assessing the severity of the injury. (The pain is local to the area of injury.)

Section B

The current situation: Your evaluation reveals a localized injury to the athlete's lower right abdominal area. The injury is not life threatening.

Your immediate responsibility: Monitor the athlete's vital signs as a precaution. Begin treatment to control pain and minimize effusion.

12. ++) Applying an ice pack to the injured area would be appropriate to minimize pain and local effusion. (The athlete is much more comfortable with the ice treatment.)

13. +) Applying a compression wrap as soon as possible after the injury is appropriate to minimize pain and local effusion. (The athlete reports he feels a little better with the compression wrap in place.)

14. -) Massaging the athlete's lumbar area would be unnecessary and inappropriate. (The athlete questions what "rubbing his back" will do for him.)

15. --) Massaging the contused area will be irritating and encourage further bleeding into the area. (The athlete winces in pain.)

16. +) It would be appropriate to assist the athlete off the field so he can be monitored. (The athlete is able to walk off the field unassisted.)

17. 0) The application of a rib belt would be inappropriate for this injury.

18. +) It is appropriate to place the athlete in a position in which he is most comfortable, preferably a position in which he is not placing pressure on the abdominals.

19. ++) It is important to monitor the athlete for any changes in pain location or intensity. This will alert the athletic trainer to any deterioration in the athlete's condition. (The athlete has no increase in pain 30 minutes after the injury.)

20. ++) Because of the possibility of internal injury, it is prudent to monitor the athlete's vital signs including his pulse and blood pressure. (The athlete's vital signs remain stable 1 hour after the incident.)

Section C

The current situation: You have determined the athlete has sustained a moderate contusion to his lower right abdominal area. The pain and effusion have been well-controlled with your initial treatment.

Your immediate responsibility: Continue to use modalities to control the pain, monitor any changes in the athlete's condition, and protect the athlete from further injury.

21. ++) As long as the athlete has any pain, swelling, or ecchymosis present, it is appropriate to continue to apply ice to the injured area. (The athlete reports his pain is much less with the ice pack applied.)

22. -) Because the athlete is still complaining of pain, the application of moist heat packs would not be appropriate. (The athlete has some increased pain and swelling over the area of injury after treatment.)

23. --) A contusion to the abdominals is very painful and disabling to the athlete. Manually muscle testing the abdominals during the early phases of treatment is inappropriate. (The athlete has a difficult time rising from a supine position secondary to abdominal pain.)

24. +) It would be appropriate to re-evaluate the injury in greater depth the next day when the athlete is not in acute pain and there is more time to do so. (Your findings generally remain the same.)

25. 0) Although it is always important to keep an athlete well-hydrated, drinking a glass of Gatorade will not have any significant impact on the recovery of this athlete. (The athlete states he is not thirsty, but thanks you for your offer.)

26. ++) Protecting the injured area from further harm is appropriate and will give the athlete a sense of security. (The athlete is less apprehensive with the pad in place.)

27. +) Because this can be an incapacitating injury, maintaining the athlete's aerobic conditioning is critical during his recovery. Utilizing an upper body ergometer would be appropriate as long as the activity does not cause any discomfort. (The athlete has no difficulty with this activity.)

PROBLEM IX

Section A

The current situation: You know that your athlete has been injured as a result of a collision with another soccer player.

Your immediate responsibility: To perform your initial evaluation to determine the type and severity of the injury.

1. +) If the athlete is coherent, it is important for him to identify where there is pain. This gives the athletic trainer an idea of the severity and nature of the injury. (The athlete is awake and complains of neck pain.)

2. --) The athlete should not be moved until a neck or back injury has been ruled out. (The athlete is now a quadriplegic.)

3. ++) This is a quick screen to assess for possible spinal injury. (The athlete can move his fingers and toes.)

4. +) Gathering as much information as possible from those who witnessed the injury is important in understanding how the injury occurred and what the nature of the injury may be. (Another player states he saw the athlete's head "snap" back.)

5. +) As part of a primary survey, it is important to note if there is any bleeding (from a cut or from an orifice). (There is no evidence of bleeding.)

6. 0) Calling an ambulance prior to evaluating this athlete's status would be premature. (The ambulance crew wastes a trip.)

7. ++) It is necessary to assess the athlete's level of consciousness during the primary survey to determine if there is a life-threatening problem. (The athlete is awake and alert.)

8. ++) The primary survey is an assessment of any life-threatening problems involving the athlete's airway/breathing, circulation, or severe bleeding. (The athlete's airway is fine and his pulse is 80.)

9. +) If the athlete is conscious and oriented, it is important to have basic knowledge concerning the athlete's prior injuries, especially of the head/neck or back, to prevent potential problems even though there may not be any immediate threat to life. (The athlete states he has never had a head injury.)

10. +) The athletic trainer should make a mental note of the athlete's body position in case the athlete must be moved to be treated or transported. (The athlete is lying in supine.)

11. --) Asking the athlete to get up and walk during an initial evaluation is not appropriate until the injury is completely assessed. (The athlete stands and collapses.)

12. +) Checking the pupillary reactions will give the athletic trainer information concerning a possible head injury. (Both pupils react normally.)

13. 0) This action would not be appropriate while performing your initial evaluation on the field. (The athlete wonders why you are placing ice on his shoulder.)

14. --) Unless the athlete is in harm's way while lying on the field, he should not be moved until a complete assessment of his injuries is conducted. (The athlete complains of dizziness and passes out.)

15. +) If the athlete can communicate what occurred, it is important to elicit this information to determine the mechanism and nature of his injury. (The athlete remembers colliding with the other player and felt his head "hit something hard.")

16. +) As part of your primary survey, it is imperative to monitor the athlete's vital signs to detect changes in status. (All vital signs remain stable.)

17. 0) Asking a member of your support team to get a spine board at this time may be a premature action. (The athlete feels okay, is moving, and asks if he is allowed to stand up.)

18. --) The athlete should not be moved until a head, neck, or back injury has been ruled out. (The athlete becomes dizzy.)

Section B

The current situation: You know that the athlete is conscious and coherent, his vital signs are stable, but he may have sustained a concussion and/or a neck injury.

Your immediate responsibility: Continue with a more in-depth evaluation of his neuromuscular function.

19. ++) Once the athlete is on the sidelines, an assessment of his injuries may be conducted in greater detail. (He is able to move his arms but is complaining of left arm "tingling" and a slight headache. There is a small hematoma on his forehead.)

20. ++) It is appropriate to assess the athlete's cognition if there is any evidence of a head injury. (The athlete knows who you are, the date, place, and event.)

21. --) Unless a significant head injury has been completely ruled out, the athlete should be kept awake in order to monitor any changes in level of consciousness. (The athlete becomes lethargic and difficult to arouse.)

22. --) Aspirin has anticoagulant properties; administration of aspirin is contraindicated with a possible head injury. (The athlete has an epidural hematoma and dies.)

23. +) It would be necessary to palpate the cervical area while evaluating the athlete for a possible neck or shoulder injury. (The athlete complains of left upper trapezius soreness.)

24. +) Palpating the trapezius and shoulder girdle musculature may elicit information regarding a musculoskeletal injury to the neck and shoulders. (The athlete is complaining of left-sided neck soreness.)

25. +) This action is a quick screen for the function of C7,T1. (The athlete's left grip strength is weak.)

26. +) The athlete should not return to the game until a secondary survey is complete and the team physician feels confident there are no significant injuries and clears the athlete to play. (A doctor has not examined the athlete yet.)

27. +) Observing the athlete's "body language" will give the athletic trainer an idea of where the injury may be located. (The athlete is holding his left arm.)

28. 0) Assessing the athlete's skin color is not a priority at this time unless the athlete is bleeding severely or the trainer suspects the athlete's circulation may be compromised. (The athlete's skin color is normal.)

29. -) This is not an appropriate action because it does not apply to this situation at this time. (The parents are insulted.)

30. -) The team physician would not need to be notified of the injury at this time unless there was a life-threatening/potentially disabling injury. (The team physician is surprised you do not have the ability to assess the athlete's condition.)

31. -) Calling the athlete's parents would be a premature action. (The parents panic.)

32. 0) This is not an appropriate action because it does not apply to this situation. (The athlete shows no sign of shock.)

33. -) If the athlete can ambulate under his own power without difficulty, he will not need crutches. (There is no evidence of a lower extremity injury.)

Section C

The current situation: The athlete's vital signs remain stable, and he appears alert and oriented. You suspect the athlete may have sustained a concussion and an upper quarter injury.

Your immediate responsibility: Continue with a detailed examination of the athlete to determine the severity of the injury.

34. 0) Unless there is evidence of a significant problem at this time, monitoring vital signs as frequently as every 10 minutes may or may not be necessary. (The athlete's blood pressure is 120/80 and pulse is 74 and stable.)

35. +) Manually muscle testing the upper trapezius muscle would be appropriate during your evaluation of this injury. (The athlete can shrug but complains that the left side hurts.)

36. -) Adson's test is performed when thoracic outlet syndrome is suspected; this athlete has an acute injury. (Review this test and its indications.)

37. +) Manually muscle testing the deltoids would be appropriate during your evaluation of this injury. (The athlete has some difficulty abducting his left arm. Grade = 3/5.)

38. +) Manually muscle testing the rotator cuff musculature would be appropriate during your evaluation of this injury. (The athlete has some difficulty with external rotation of his left arm. Grade = +3/5.)

39. -) If the athlete has potentially injured his neck or back, this may make the injury worse. If the athlete was feeling lightheaded, it would be better to position him in supine with both legs elevated. (The athlete now has a headache.)

40. -) You have already determined from your sideline evaluation that there is no significant lower extremity injury. A functional movement test is not appropriate at this time. (The athlete is steady while standing and walking.)

41. 0) You have already determined from your sideline evaluation that the athlete is oriented. (The athlete counts backward by increments of seven without difficulty.)

42. +) As part of an upper quarter screen, it may be necessary to check upper extremity deep tendon reflexes. (The left triceps deep tendon reflex [DTR] is a little sluggish.)

43. -) The athlete is not in any respiratory distress. (The athlete refuses the mask.)

44. ++) If the physician is available at this time, it would be important for him or her to evaluate the athlete and determine his status for play. (The team physician will arrive in 10 minutes.)

45. --) With a suspected head injury, it would be poor judgment on the athletic trainer's part to allow the athlete to drive. (The athlete gets dizzy and hits a parked car in the parking lot.)

46. +) Checking the sensation of the upper extremities should be included in a detailed evaluation of the athlete in the athletic training room. (There is hypersensitivity in the C7,8 dermatomes.)

47. +) Checking the range of motion of the athlete's neck should be included in a detailed examination of the athlete. (The athlete has full cervical active range of motion.)

48. -) A positive Tinel's sign is indicative of carpal tunnel syndrome and would be inappropriate, as this was a known traumatic event. (No information is gained from this test.)

49. 0) Palpation of the lateral epicondyle would not provide any helpful information in the evaluation of this athlete. (The athlete states his elbow feels fine.)

50. +) Manually muscle testing the biceps would be appropriate during your evaluation of this injury. (The athlete has some difficulty with resisted elbow flexion. Grade = +3/5.)

51. +) Manually muscle testing the triceps would be appropriate. (The athlete has significant difficulty extending his elbow against resistance. Grade = 3/5.)

Section D

The current situation: You know that your athlete has sustained a first-degree concussion and a left-sided "burner."

Your immediate responsibility: Monitor the athlete for any changes in his condition and protect the athlete from further harm until he is cleared by the team physician to play.

52. 0) A "burner" is an injury to the nerves of the brachial plexus. An ice pack applied to the upper arm would be ineffective.

53. ++) Persistent sensory changes of the upper extremity would be significant in determining the extent of nerve involvement. (The athlete states his sensation is returning to normal.)

54. -) The athlete has to be cleared by the team doctor in order to return to play. (The athlete returns the next day and is reinjured.)

55. 0) This action would be at the discretion of the physician, not the athletic trainer. (You are reprimanded by your athletic director and team physician.)

56. --) Shoulder strengthening exercises are not indicated with an acute nerve injury. (This action causes further injury to the left upper extremity.)

57. --) This exercise would be contraindicated for an acute upper extremity nerve injury. (The athlete complains of increased pain.)

58. ++) It is prudent to monitor the athlete for a few days after a mild concussion to be sure there is no change in his status. (The athlete's condition returns to normal the next day.)

59. ++) It is imperative that the physician clear the athlete before he returns to full-time activity. (The athlete is cleared to play the second day after the injury.)

60. 0) Giving the athlete a soft neck collar will not cause further injury, but it may not help the athlete either. (The athlete receives a lot of attention from his teammates.)

PROBLEM X

Section A

The current situation: You know the athlete has sustained a direct blow to the nose causing recurrent nose bleeds.

Your immediate responsibility: Evaluate the athlete for a possible nasal/facial fracture. Stop the bleeding.

1. +) This question is important to ask as part of the history and in understanding the severity of the problem. (The athlete states he saw "stars.")

2. +) Asking whether or not there has been a similar problem in the past is a question that should always be asked when taking a history. (He has had one episode of recurrent nosebleeds 2 years ago from a blow to the nose.)

3. 0) Whether or not the athlete's parents are aware of his nosebleed is irrelevant at this time.

4. 0) Whether or not the athlete has any allergies is insignificant information. (He tells you he is allergic to cats.)

5. -) This action may increase the flow of bleeding. (The bleeding becomes copious.)

6. +) The athlete should be seated in case he becomes faint from the bleeding or pain. (The athlete has no complaints of dizziness.)

7. 0) This action is not necessary in this situation.

8. 0) A noseguard should not be necessary. (This should not be a chronic problem.)

9. --) This action is inappropriate, as heating the area will cause further bleeding. (You have difficulty stopping the bleeding.)

10. 0) It is known from the opening scenario that the origin of this nosebleed was from a blow to the nose, not from chronic high blood pressure.

11. -) Pressure should be applied to the affected nostril, not to the cheek. (This action does nothing to slow the bleeding.)

12. ++) The trainer should palpate the athlete's nose and surrounding areas to be sure no other areas were injured as a result of the earlier trauma (eg, nasal fracture). (The athlete reports tenderness over the bridge of his nose, but there is no crepitus with palpation or deformity.)

13. ++) Swelling with or without deformity may be indicative of a possible nasal fracture. (A small hematoma is noted over the bridge of the nose.)

14. 0) An ice pack placed behind the athlete's neck will be ineffective—it should be placed over the nasal area.

15. --) Under no circumstances should the athlete blow his nose, as this will increase the bleeding. (The bleeding becomes heavy.)

16. ++) Placing a cotton plug under the athlete's top lip will assist in stopping the bleeding. (The bleeding slows down considerably.)

Section B

The current situation: The athlete has a nosebleed. There is no evidence of a nasal or facial fracture.

Your immediate responsibility: Stop the bleeding.

17. -) This is an unnecessary step at this time. (It is obvious that this is not a life-threatening problem.)

18. -) This is an inappropriate step at this time. (The athlete shows no signs of shock.)

19. ++) Having the athlete maintain pressure on the affected nostril will help completely stop the bleeding. (The bleeding stops.)

20. +) It is a prudent step to take, since you will not be following this athlete on a long-term basis. (The coach appreciates your assistance.)

21. -) Most nosebleeds are a minor problem and relatively easy to control. Unless the bleeding cannot be stopped within a 5-minute period, the athlete should be able to return to the competition. (The athlete is furious with you for not allowing him to compete.)

22. 0) This is only necessary if it is determined that this athlete has fractured his nose. (So far there is no indication of a fracture.)

23. -) The athlete should sit upright with his head in a neutral position. (The athlete becomes nauseated from the taste of blood.)

24. -) Calling the visiting team's athletic trainer during your initial treatment is not an appropriate action. (The other athletic trainer wonders why you are calling him during your treatment.)

25. ++) A cotton nose plug soaked with epinephrine hydrochloride will enhance clotting. (The bleeding stops.)

26. --) Aspirin should never be given during active bleeding, as it is an anticoagulant. (The bleeding increases again.)

27. ++) Checking to see that no blood is present on the athlete, his clothing, the mat, and floor are appropriate steps in following universal precautions. (You do a thorough job making sure the blood is cleaned up.)

Section C

The current situation: The athlete has sustained a nosebleed secondary to a traumatic blow to the nose, which is beginning to resolve.

Your immediate responsibility: Stop the bleeding and return the athlete to competition.

28. -) As long as the nosebleed has been brought under control, it is not necessary to call your team doctor. (The doctor is upset you wasted time calling him.)

29. --) It is not your place to call the visiting team's doctor regarding a minor nosebleed. (The physician thinks you are incompetent.)

30. 0) This action may only serve to unnecessarily alarm the athlete and his parents and should only be initiated if the nose needs to be cauterized by a doctor. (You panic the parents.)

31. -) There is no reason to restrict this athlete's fluid intake. (The athlete becomes dehydrated.)

32. ++) As long as the bleeding has completely stopped, the athlete can return to competition. (He wins his match.)

33. -) This is an unnecessary action if no swelling or deformity of the nose is evident, as the bleeding has stopped. (The team physician is upset that you suggested this.)

34. ++) It would be a responsible step to contact the athlete's home athletic trainer to report the incident and what treatment was administered. (The athletic trainer appreciates your information.)

35. --) Sit-ups temporarily increase blood pressure and capillary pressure, which may produce another spontaneous nosebleed. (The athlete's nose begins bleeding again.)

36. ++) Biohazard bags should be used as a universal precaution. (The athletic director appreciates you following protocol.)

37. +) The athlete should be monitored during the competition for any further problems. (The athlete has no further episodes of bleeding.)

38. +) The athlete should keep an ice pack on his nose while he is not competing to minimize pain and encourage clotting. (He reports the pain and swelling have decreased.)

PROBLEM XI

Section A

The current situation: You know your athlete has injured his left ankle.

Your immediate responsibility: To perform your initial evaluation to determine the nature and severity of the injury.

1. -) You witnessed the injury. It is obvious that his left ankle is involved, not his back. Evaluating this athlete's low back is unnecessary. (The athlete thinks you are incompetent.)

2. -) It is obvious from the information given in the opening scenario that the athlete is able to bear weight on the ankle without assistance. Getting a wheelchair is inappropriate. (The athlete wonders for whom you are getting a wheelchair.)

3. 0) This is an unnecessary action. It has been determined that the athlete has injured his left ankle. (Now the athlete definitely does not trust you.)

4. +) It is important to make a bilateral comparison of both ankles when observing for swelling, ecchymosis, or deformity during the initial evaluation. (The left ankle is swollen on the lateral side.)

5. --) This is an inappropriate action and may cause further injury. (The athlete reinjures his ankle.)

6. --) This is an unnecessary and inappropriate action that may cause further injury. (The pain and swelling increase.)

7. -) Lachman's test is not a special test for the ankle. (The athlete's knees are fine.)

8. +) An anterior drawer test should be performed bilaterally to determine if there is any ankle joint instability. (There is a positive result on the left ankle.)

9. ++) Palpation is an integral portion of the initial evaluation. (There is tenderness over the anterior talofibular [ATF] and calcaneofibular [CF] ligaments.)

10. ++) Checking the athlete's willingness to move is an integral segment of the initial evaluation. Comparing the active range of motion of the involved joint to the uninvolved side is a necessary step in an orthopedic assessment. (The athlete complains of pain with active movement into dorsiflexion and eversion.)

Section B

The current situation: The athlete has a grade II inversion sprain of the left ankle with injury to the ATF and CF ligament.

Your immediate responsibility: To begin treating the injury to reduce the pain and swelling.

11. ++) During the acute stages of treatment, the athlete should be kept in nonweightbearing or partial weightbearing to minimize pain and swelling. (There is less pain in nonweightbearing.)

12. -) Although aspirin is an anti-inflammatory with analgesic properties, it would be contraindicated at this time because it may cause further bleeding into the joint. (The swelling increases.)

13. ++) Rest, ice, compression, and elevation are primary components of the initial treatment of an acute musculoskeletal injury. (The pain and swelling decrease.)

14. 0) Calling the team doctor at this time is unnecessary and inappropriate. (The doctor wonders why you don't know how to treat an acute ankle sprain.)

15. --) Ultrasound is a deep-heating modality. This is a definite "no-no" during the acute stage of treatment. (The pain and swelling increase significantly.)

16. --) As with ultrasound, a warm or hot whirlpool will only make the pain and swelling worse. (The ankle is very swollen.)

17. +) Keeping the athlete in nonweightbearing at this time is proper protocol in the immediate care of an acute injury. (The athlete is able to ambulate comfortably with crutches.)

18. 0) Unless you suspect a more significant injury at this point, this action is inappropriate. (The athlete has not seen a doctor.)

19. 0) The immediate care of an acute ankle sprain does not include upper body reconditioning.

20. +) It is the athletic trainer's duty to keep the athlete's coach well-informed about the athlete's injury and treatment. (He appreciates your report.)

21. -) Resistive ankle strengthening exercises would be inappropriate at this time. (The ankle is too weak and the pain is increased with resistance.)

Section C

The current situation: You have determined the athlete has sustained a grade II inversion sprain with injury to the ATF ligament and CF ligament. Treatment has been initiated to reduce the pain and swelling.

Your immediate responsibility: To ensure the athlete knows how to care for his injury at home.

22. -) Although going to the emergency room would not hurt the athlete, it may not be necessary either. (The athlete spends 3 hours in the emergency room to be diagnosed with a sprain.)

23. 0) It is courteous to contact the parents if the athlete is a minor, but this may be an unnecessary step. (The athlete is able to follow your instructions overnight.)

24. --) Closed-chain exercises would be contraindicated with such an acute ankle injury. (The ankle pain increases.)

25. ++) This is a fundamental component of treatment of an acute musculoskeletal injury. (The pain and swelling are controlled.)

26. +) This is a fundamental component of treatment of an acute musculoskeletal injury. (The swelling is controlled.)

27. 0) Wearing high-top sneakers will not change the athlete's condition. (Although they look "cool.")

28. --) Attempting to hop on an acutely injured ankle is inappropriate and will cause further injury to an already traumatized joint. (The athlete falls and sprains his ankle again.)

PROBLEM XII

Section A

The current situation: You have been made aware of an athlete who may have a serious eating disorder.

Your immediate responsibility: Educate and advise the coach not to encourage her current behavior, but to emphasize the importance of proper nutritional habits and to keep the athletic training staff informed of her behavior.

1. --) Because anorexia nervosa is an eating disorder that is characterized by a distorted body image and is caused by a deep-seated and complex interaction of psychological and sociocultural factors, the athlete must be gently confronted and not attacked. Unless the athlete is in immediate danger, threatening the athlete is inappropriate. (The athlete is so upset, she quits the team.)

2. +) Continual fixation on the athlete's weight changes in relation to her athletic performance may encourage destructive behavior.

3. 0) Keeping a diary of the time or place the athlete eats is unnecessary. Treatment should be implemented by those qualified to do so, such as a psychologist or physician. (The coach wastes a lot of paper.)

4. +) Emphasizing the importance of good nutritional habits in optimizing athletic performance is an appropriate action. (The athlete seems to respond in a positive manner and begins eating a small, but regular breakfast.)

5. ++) Any behavior(s) associated with eating disorders that become prominent must be relayed to the athletic training staff so the athlete can be immediately referred for professional help. (You are able to provide the team physician with valuable information.)

Section B

The current situation: You have identified an athlete who has an eating disorder and you have advised the coach how to properly handle the situation.

Your immediate responsibility: Continue to monitor the athlete's behavior and educate and support the athlete.

6. +) Providing constructive advice is an appropriate action. (The athlete agrees to try to reach the set goals.)

7. -) Using an approach that threatens the athlete in any fashion is not appropriate. (The athlete feels challenged and continues to abuse laxatives anyway.)

8. +) Encouraging the athlete to express her feelings is an important and necessary step in her recovery. (She states she feels her parents won't love her if she is not the best gymnast on the team.)

9. 0) Addressing the issue with the athletic director is not necessary. (He tells you to discuss the matter with the team doctor.)

10. -) To make the assumption that the athlete will be removed from the team is premature and is ultimately a decision that will be made by the coach. (The athlete panics.)

11. --) It is not wise to make promises that you may not be able to keep. If this athlete is seriously ill, the coach may cut her from the team. (The coach is debating what to do.)

12. -) This athlete will need the support of the coaching and athletic training staff to actively seek professional counseling. (The athlete does not have the self-esteem to initiate counseling on her own.)

13. ++) The athlete needs to be gently confronted with specific behaviors that the coach and athletic trainer have observed to move the athlete toward recovery. (The athlete admits she has a problem.)

Section C

The current situation: You have identified an athlete with a significant eating disorder. The athlete acknowledges she has a problem.

Your immediate responsibility: Make sure the athlete is referred to a psychologist for treatment.

14. ++) The team physician needs to be aware of the problem to arrange for psychological or psychiatric treatment. (The team doctor tells you he will make a referral to a psychiatrist.)

15. 0) This is an appropriate action but should occur in conjunction with the team physician.

16. -) Anorexia nervosa and bulimia are primarily psychological disorders. Placing the athlete on a diet intended to encourage weight gain will not be enough to solve this problem. (She follows the diet for 2 days.)

17. 0) Weighing the athlete will not have an impact on changing her behavior at this time.

18. --) The athletic trainer is not qualified to arrange for this type of intervention. (The team doctor is very upset with your actions.)

19. -) This would be an inappropriate referral for this athlete. (The sports nutritionist reminds you she does not have a degree in psychology.)

20. 0) Although having the athlete eat these foods would not hurt her, she is not likely to comply. She needs professional psychological treatment, so this action would not be appropriate. (This athlete is a vegetarian and hates bananas.)

Problem XIII

Section A

The current situation: Your athlete presents to you with abdominal cramping and diarrhea of unknown origin, which has lasted 2 days.

Your immediate responsibility: To try to identify the etiology of the problem and perform an initial evaluation to determine the extent of the problem.

1. ++) It is important to evaluate what types of food and drink the athlete has consumed because certain foods (such as spicy foods) may lead to dyspepsia or diarrhea. (The athlete states he has not eaten any spicy foods.)

2. +) Anxiety can contribute to gastrointestinal upset. This is an appropriate question to ask the athlete during the history portion of your initial assessment. (The athlete admits he is nervous.)

3. ++) This is an appropriate question to ask during the history portion of the initial evaluation because it will help to identify if the athlete has an underlying gastrointestinal problem. (The athlete states this frequently happens at the beginning of the season.)

4. 0) This action would be appropriate if you suspect the athlete is dehydrated. (The athlete complains his lips feel dry, but he is not excessively thirsty. Blood pressure is 115/70.)

5. +) This is an appropriate action because the athlete might have a fever secondary to an infection. (The athlete's oral temperature is within normal limits.)

6. 0) This is an inappropriate action. It does not directly relate to the athlete's condition.

7. 0) This is an unnecessary and inappropriate action. (The athlete complains of "gas pain" with palpation of his abdomen.)

8. --) Running or increased activity will only contribute to gastrointestinal upset and is an inappropriate action at this point. It will not provide any information regarding the cause of the problem. (The athlete has a severe episode of diarrhea after running).

Section B

The current situation: You have determined that the athlete has developed gastrointestinal upset because of precompetition anxiety.

Your immediate responsibility: Treat for abdominal cramping, diarrhea, and prevent dehydration.

9. +) If the athlete is very uncomfortable and is feeling "weak," this would be an appropriate action to take. (The athlete feels better at rest.)

10. ++) This would be an appropriate action to monitor the athlete for degree of dehydration. (The athlete loses 3 pounds after a strenuous workout.)

11. ++) An over-the-counter antimotility medication, such as Imodium or Pepto-Bismol, may reduce the cramping and diarrhea. (The athlete responds well to this and the diarrhea stops.)

12. -) Certain vegetables may cause intestinal gas formation and would be inappropriate to add to the athlete's diet at this time.

13. --) It would be best to give the athlete clear fluids. Milk may cause nausea and increased flatulence; soda and tea contain caffeine, which has a diuretic effect. (The athlete becomes significantly dehydrated.)

14. 0) This would be an inappropriate action. Only one of your athletes is complaining of gastrointestinal distress. (The hotel management finds out what you are doing and is outraged.)

15. 0) Although this is not necessary, drinking bottled water will not be harmful to the athlete.

Problem XIV

Section A

The current situation: You know your athlete has injured his right knee while playing soccer, and he is only able to partially bear weight on the involved limb.

Your immediate responsibility: To perform your initial evaluation to determine the type and severity of the injury.

1. +) Palpating the joint and the surrounding soft tissue structures is an appropriate action during the initial evaluation of the injury. (The athlete is significantly tender over the anteromedial joint line and the medial retinaculum.)

2. --) Performing a functional movement such as a deep squat is inappropriate during the initial assessment. (The athlete refuses to do this.)

3. ++) Since you were not present during the actual injury, you must rely on the athlete's account of what occurred to determine the mechanism of injury. (The athlete reports feeling a "pop" and sharp knee pain after planting his right leg to kick the ball with his left leg.)

4. +) It is an appropriate action to check the circulation of the injured limb distal to the injury site. (The circulation is fine.)

5. +) This is an appropriate question to ask during the history portion of the evaluation. (The athlete has told you he felt a "pop.")

6. -) This is an inappropriate test for a knee injury. Speed's test is used to assess for the presence of bicipital tendinitis.

7. ++) Based on information given in the opening scenario and the mechanism of injury, this would be an appropriate special test to perform. (Lachman's test is positive on the right knee.)

8. 0) Although this was a traumatic incident, there was no direct insult. Crepitus would be present with a possible fracture or a chronic problem, such as patellofemoral joint disease.

9. ++) Asking the athlete if he ever sustained a prior knee injury is an appropriate question during the history portion of the initial evaluation. (The athlete states he had a partial anterior cruciate tear of the right knee a year ago.)

10. +) Assessing the range of motion of the knee joint would be appropriate at this time. This demonstrates the athlete's willingness to move and assists in determining the level of disability. (The athlete has difficulty fully flexing and extending the knee.)

11. 0) Testing the strength of the athlete's hip abductors will not provide any information that will lead to determining the nature and extent of the knee injury.

12. 0) It is obvious from the opening scenario that this is a knee injury; having the athlete attempt toe raises would be unnecessary and inappropriate. (The athlete has difficulty doing this.)

13. ++) From the information given at the opening scenario and the mechanism of injury, performing a pivot shift test would be appropriate and should be performed bilaterally for comparison to the uninvolved extremity. (The test is inconclusive because the athlete is so guarded.)

Section B

The current situation: The athlete is complaining of pain along the anteromedial joint line and medial retinaculum. The athlete felt a "pop" and has significant edema of the right knee. He has difficulty flexing and extending the knee and has a positive Lachman's test on the right knee.

Your immediate responsibility: Protect the knee from further injury and control the pain and swelling.

14. +) Issuing crutches with a toe-touch weightbearing status would be an appropriate action. (The athlete is more comfortable ambulating with crutches.)

15. ++) Applying ice and elevating the injured extremity are appropriate actions during the initial phases of treatment. (The pain and swelling are controlled.)

16. ++) The team physician should be contacted to evaluate the athlete. (The team physician has athletic training room hours that afternoon.)

17. 0) At this point, you realize this is not a patellofemoral joint problem. McConnell taping would be unnecessary and inappropriate. (The athlete questions why you are taping his kneecap.)

18. --) Applying heat to a swollen joint is contraindicated in the initial treatment of this injury. (The pain and swelling increase significantly.)

19. 0) Ordering a functional knee brace at this phase of treatment would be premature.

20. -) The application of pulsed ultrasound would be an inappropriate action. (The pain and swelling increase.)

Section C

The current situation: The team physician has examined the athlete and agrees with your suspicions. The MRI results are pending.

Your immediate responsibility: Instruct the athlete in a home program emphasizing pain and edema reduction, early joint mobilization/range of motion, and isometric strengthening.

21. +) It is important to restore normal joint range of motion as soon as possible. This would be an appropriate action. (The athlete's range of motion improves 50% over the following week.)

22. ++) Applying ice on a routine basis during the initial stages of recovery is critical. (The pain and swelling decrease significantly.)

23. -) The athlete should remain on the crutches to protect the injured limb until the diagnosis is confirmed. (The athlete's knee buckles while walking with a cane and he falls.)

24. 0) Working on the proprioception of the unaffected limb is unnecessary. (The athlete's balance is fine.)

25. ++) Instructing the athlete to perform early isometric exercises is an appropriate step in preventing atrophy of the musculature around the knee joint. (The athlete is compliant.)

26. 0) The pain is controlled well with ice; a TENS unit is not contraindicated but is not necessary.

27. --) The athlete should be restricted from activities that may cause further injury until the diagnosis is confirmed and the athlete is cleared by the doctor. (The athlete reinjures his knee.)

PROBLEM XV

Section A

The current situation: An athlete has requested assistance in developing a lower body strength and general conditioning program. He is currently in preseason.

Your immediate responsibility: Educate the athlete about the goals of preseason training and in proper methods to develop good habits to develop lower extremity flexibility strength. Assist the athlete in progressing his program and in preparing for his sport.

1. --) An athletic trainer is not qualified to administer steroids. This is an inappropriate action. (The athletic director finds out and you lose your job.)

2. +) A good flexibility program is a fundamental aspect of a general conditioning program. (The athlete's flexibility improves.)

3. --) Having the athlete participate in such a vigorous activity is inappropriate. (The athlete develops heat exhaustion.)

4. 0) There is nothing in the opening scene to indicate the athlete has a respiratory problem. This is an unnecessary action.

5. +) Adequate warm-up and cool-down periods are fundamental elements of a comprehensive fitness program. (The athlete had spent little time warming up prior to your recommendations.)

6. ++) Optimal results occur from training when the athlete mimics movement patterns and speeds that are similar to the activities in which he participates (eg, training a soccer player by performing short, high intensity sprints).

7. -) Having the athlete participate in another sport during the preseason may not be wise because of the increased risk of injury just before the season begins. (The athlete sprains his ankle and cannot participate for the first 2 weeks of the season.)

8. ++) Having the athlete work on the strength of his lower extremities would be appropriate.

9. -) The athlete should be assisted in maintaining a well-balanced nutritional diet. Limiting the athlete to one or two food groups is not appropriate. (The athlete complains of feeling lethargic.)

10. --) A regular training schedule should be maintained during the preseason period to allow for a progressive program. (Because of the many changes in the schedule during the preseason, the athlete is not in an acceptable state of fitness by the beginning of the season.)

11. --) Keeping the training schedule intense is acceptable, but often coaches prolong the workout, increasing the quantity rather than the quality of the session. (The athlete becomes overly fatigued and pulls a hamstring.)

12. ++) Progressing the conditioning program gradually is an appropriate action. (The athlete is at his physical peak going into the season.)

13. +) Making sure the athlete has acclimated to the heat prior to the season is appropriate. (The athlete avoids episodes of heat cramps or heat exhaustion.)

Section B

The current situation: The athlete has started a preseason conditioning program as per your instructions to improve his lower body strength and general conditioning. He is now in-season.

Your immediate responsibility: Continue to supervise his program to maintain a proper level of fitness that is tailored for his sport and position, and add variety to prevent staleness.

14. +) Establishing a regular aerobic exercise routine while in-season is an appropriate action. (The athlete maintains a good aerobic conditioning level.)

15. ++) Maintaining a regular strength training program throughout the season is appropriate. (The athlete maintains a good strength level for his lower extremities.)

16. --) Rest is important, but too much time off while in-season is counterproductive. (The athlete starts to show signs of deconditioning.)

17. 0) This action is unnecessary unless the athlete has a known or suspected cardiovascular problem.

18. +) This is an appropriate action depending on the athlete's position. (The athlete is a running back.)

19. ++) Establishing a maintenance program for training while in season is necessary and appropriate. (The athlete maintains a good level of aerobic and strength conditioning.)

20. -) Putting the athlete on a clear diet is inappropriate. (The athlete begins to show signs of fatigue and malnutrition.)

21. +) Cross-training during the season may serve to maintain a good fitness level and prevent staleness during training. (The athlete swims one to two times per week.)

22. 0) Although this action is not harmful, it is not sport specific and is not a necessary activity.

23. --) This action is not necessary and is inappropriate. (The athlete is thrown during a competition and is injured.)

Section C

The current situation: It is now postseason. The athlete has done well thus far with the conditioning program you have designed.

Your immediate responsibility: Continue to educate the athlete regarding proper flexibility and strengthening techniques. Adjust the workload so that the athlete will avoid boredom and maintain a good level of fitness at a lower intensity.

24. ++) Maintaining a good flexibility program year-round is appropriate. (The athlete remains injury-free during the off-season.)

25. ++) Cross-training is appropriate during the entire year but is especially effective during the off-season period to maintain proper fitness levels and prevent boredom with training. (The athlete uses a rowing machine during the off-season.)

26. --) The off-season is a period of detraining in which there is a gradual decrease of the workload. Jogging 4 to 5 days a week would be inappropriate. (The athlete shows signs of overtraining and quits the team.)

27. --) Along with a decrease in activity intensity during the off-season, there should be a decrease in the calorie intake by the athlete. Having the athlete consume a high-calorie diet during the off-season is inappropriate. (The athlete reports to preseason practice 10 pounds overweight.)

28. 0) Having the athlete learn the skill of visual imagery may enhance performance techniques but is not a necessary activity in maintaining fitness during the off-season.

29. --) Having the athlete become completely sedentary during the off-season period is inappropriate. (The athlete gains 20 pounds during this time and becomes aerobically unfit).

30. +) Allowing the athlete time off from training will prevent burnout. (The athlete appreciates the much-needed break.)

31. +) Participating in another sport during the off-season will help the athlete maintain a proper level of fitness. (The athlete plays basketball during the off-season.)

PROBLEM XVI

Section A

The current situation: You know your athlete has suffered a serious traumatic injury after colliding with the boards.

Your immediate responsibility: To perform your initial evaluation to determine the nature and severity of the injury and assess if it is a life-threatening situation.

1. -) Performing a secondary survey prior to doing a primary survey would be premature and inappropriate. (The athlete is in respiratory distress and you have wasted valuable time.)

2. ++) If the athlete is lying prone and it has been determined he is not breathing, this would be an appropriate action. (The athlete is unconscious and not breathing.)

3. --) This is an inappropriate action. The helmet should not be removed until a neck or spinal injury has been ruled out. (The athlete has sustained a spinal cord injury and is now a quadriplegic.)

4. ++) Determining responsiveness and the ABCs is the immediate priority. This is an appropriate action. (The athlete is unconscious and not breathing.)

5. ++) This is an appropriate action. Determining level of consciousness is part of the primary survey.

6. --) Chest compressions should not be started unless it has been established that the athlete has no pulse. (The athlete has a weak carotid pulse.)

7. 0) This would be an inappropriate action. It is apparent from the opening scenario that the primary site of injury is not an extremity.

8. -) This is an unnecessary action. It is known from the opening scenario that the athlete hit the boards with his head. (You spend too much time asking questions instead of evaluating the athlete.)

9. --) This is an inappropriate action. The athlete should not be moved until a neck or back injury has been ruled out.

Section B

The current situation: The athlete has been carefully placed into supine and is unconscious and not breathing. He has a weak pulse.

Your immediate responsibility: Establish an airway and ventilate the athlete. Activate the EMS system.

10. -) The immediate priority is establishing an airway. Performing a secondary survey is inappropriate at this time. (The athlete has now been without oxygen for 1.5 minutes.)

11. +) This would be an appropriate action, as a true emergency has been determined. (The ambulance arrives within 5 minutes of the call.)

12. --) This is an inappropriate action and may cause further injury to the athlete.

13. 0) Although this action is appropriate, it is not a priority at this time.

14. ++) Cutting the face mask off the helmet is a necessary step to allow for CPR and artificial respiration. (You are now able to ventilate the athlete.)

15. -) This is an unnecessary and inappropriate action.

16. -) This is an unnecessary and inappropriate action. (Romberg's sign is a test used to assess balance.)

17. --) This is an inappropriate action. (The athlete vomits, aspirates, and dies.)

18. ++) This is an appropriate action; opening the airway and ventilating the athlete is a priority. (You are able to open the airway and administer mouth-to-mouth respiration.)

19. 0) This action is unnecessary as it has already been determined the athlete has a pulse.

20. +) Removing the mouthguard is necessary to clear the airway. This is an appropriate action.

21. +) Using a jaw-thrust to open the airway is an appropriate action. (You suspect a possible spinal cord injury.)

Section C

The current situation: The athlete responds to your resuscitation efforts, becomes conscious, and is able to respond to questions. He reports feelings of gross anesthesia.

Your immediate responsibility: Assess and monitor the athlete's vital signs, assess the extent of loss of sensation and motor control, and document what occurred and who was involved. Prepare to transport the athlete to the hospital via ambulance.

22. ++) Once the athlete is conscious and breathing independently, it is a priority to perform a secondary survey. (Respiratory rate is 14 breaths per minute, blood pressure is 110/70, and pulse is 88. Gross sensation is absent from the armpits caudally, and no significant bleeding or deformities are noted.)

23. +) Monitoring the athlete's vital signs is appropriate. (You are able to give the EMS team vital information.)

24. -) This is an inappropriate action. (You do not have enough information regarding the athlete's permanent outcome.)

25. +) This is an appropriate action. (The athlete is ready to be transferred to the hospital.)

26. 0) This would be an inappropriate action at this time. (This would not be helpful at this time.)

27. +) Checking the pupillary response is an appropriate action to determine if the athlete has sustained a head injury. (Both pupils respond normally.)

28. -) This is an inappropriate action. (The policy on helmet removal should be established before a catastrophic injury occurs.)

29. -) This is an inappropriate action. Once the athlete is transferred into the care of the emergency medical team, you are still responsible for the remaining athletes. (You leave the practice area and a second athlete gets injured.)

30. +) This would be an appropriate action. (You avoid a malpractice suit.)

Section D

The current situation: Your athlete has suffered a serious spinal cord injury and has been transported by the rescue squad to the hospital.

Your immediate responsibility: Provide emotional support to the athlete and his teammates. Provide accurate information of what occurred to the team physician and provide support for the athlete's parents.

31. ++) This would be an appropriate action. (The athlete is very scared and is grateful you came.)

32. +) This is an appropriate action. (The team doctor documents what occurred.)

33. +) This is an appropriate action. (The parents meet you at the emergency room.)

34. --) This is an inappropriate action. An athletic trainer is not qualified to determine the athlete's prognosis. (You have given the athlete false hope, and he becomes severely depressed.)

35. 0) This is an unnecessary action. (It is too late to change this now.)

36. --) This is an inappropriate action. (You are reprimanded by the school administration.)

37. +) This is an appropriate action. (The coach appreciates the information.)

38. +) This is an appropriate action. (The rest of the hockey team expresses how they are feeling.)

39. -) This is an inappropriate action. (The physician never makes the phone call and the athletic director finds out about the accident the following day from a coach.)

PROBLEM XVII

Section A

The current situation: You know from this athlete's complaints that his low back pain is chronic in nature and localized to the lumbar area.

Your immediate responsibility: To perform an initial evaluation to determine the etiology of his pain.

1. ++) When assessing a low back injury, it is appropriate to observe the athlete's posture in standing and sitting. (The athlete stands with a forward head and rounded shoulder posture and slouches when he sits. The athlete also has a slight scoliotic curve.)

2. +) Having the athlete describe his pain is appropriate, as it gives the athletic trainer information about the nature of the injury. (The athlete reports the pain is a "dull ache.")

3. 0) Checking the range of motion of the athlete's knees would not contribute any helpful information. This athlete has a low back problem, not a knee injury.

4. -) A Scour test of the hip is performed when the possibility of hip arthritis exists. This test would be unnecessary and inappropriate. The athlete is not complaining of any hip pain.

5. ++) Palpating the lumbar erector spinae is an appropriate action and is a fundamental component of the initial assessment. (The athlete reports mild muscle discomfort.)

6. +) Although it is not likely that muscular wasting will be observed, it is appropriate to visualize the area of injury for any unusual changes, such as atrophy, swelling, or deformity. (There is no evidence of muscular atrophy.)

7. +) Palpation of the entire lumbar and sacral regions is appropriate during the initial evaluation to check for any areas of point tenderness. (The athlete is pain-free with palpation of both posterior superior iliac spine [PSIS] and sacroiliac [SI] joints.)

8. 0) Genu varum is a "bow-legged" deformity of the lower extremities and has no correlation to the athlete's low back pain.

9. ++) Assessing the athlete for a leg-length discrepancy is appropriate. Even a subtle leg-length discrepancy can cause chronic low back pain. (The athlete's legs are of equal length.)

10. 0) Having the athlete perform a partial squat is unnecessary and inappropriate during the initial evaluation. Whether or not the athlete can perform this action will not provide the athletic trainer with significant information concerning the nature of the problem.

11. ++) Evaluating the range of motion of the lumbar spine will help the athletic trainer assess the athlete's willingness to move and provide information concerning the nature and severity of the problem. (The athlete complains of pain with lumbar flexion, right side-bending, and right rotation.)

12. -) Evaluating the athlete's hip abduction with a goniometer is not appropriate. This athlete does not have a hip injury.

13. +) It would be appropriate to check the flexibility of the muscles around the hip because tight hip flexors or hamstrings can contribute to chronic low back pain. (The athlete has tight hamstrings bilaterally.)

Section B

The current situation: You have determined from your initial evaluation that the athlete's pain is muscular in origin and he has tight bilateral hamstrings.

Your immediate responsibility: To provide immediate pain relief during rest and activity.

14. -) Friction massage is a deep, local massage technique that is most commonly performed around joints and over thin tissue areas that are hypomobile because of scarring or local spasms. This type of massage is inappropriate for this problem. (The athlete complains of significant pain during treatment.)

15. ++) The application of ice in the form of ice packs can break the pain-muscle spasm-pain cycle, allowing the athlete to move more comfortably, and is an appropriate modality to use. (The athlete reports pain relief during treatment.)

16. +) Because the injury is chronic in nature and the athlete is not in severe pain, moist heat in the form of a whirlpool may be useful in helping the athlete relax and will reduce discomfort. (The athlete reports pain relief with the heat treatments.)

17. ++) Because this is a chronic problem, ultrasound would be an appropriate modality choice. Deep heat improves circulation, which enhances healing.

18. -) Iontophoresis is a technique in which ions of a chemical substance are delivered through the skin through use of an electrical current. The most common application is the delivery of a steroid to reduce a local inflammatory response

(eg, tendinitis). Iontophoresis would not be an appropriate modality choice for this problem. (The athlete complains of irritation under the active electrode.)

19. 0) Although an ice massage would not harm the athlete, it would not be the optimal choice for decreasing chronic, diffuse low back pain. The application of ice massage would be more appropriate for decreasing pain in areas of point tenderness. (The athlete is not pleased with you rubbing ice all over his lower back.)

20. -) Sending the athlete for chiropractic treatments would not be appropriate. It is within the athletic trainer's scope of practice to be able to comprehensively manage this athlete's problem. (The chiropractor sends you a thank you note.)

21. +) TENS therapy would be an appropriate choice of modality in managing the athlete's pain. (The athlete reports pain relief when the unit is used.)

22. ++) The application of moist heat packs (especially prior to exercise) would be appropriate to enhance relaxation and reduce pain. (The athlete reports pain relief with moist heat treatments.)

23. +) Short-wave diathermy would be an appropriate modality choice for treatment of chronic low back pain. Short-wave diathermy is a deep heater, which improves local circulation and enhances healing. (The athlete reports feeling better after treatment.)

24. 0) Although stationary bicycling would be appropriate for aerobic conditioning, it has no direct effect regarding pain reduction of the low back or improving lumbar movement.

25. --) Functional electric stimulation is not an appropriate modality choice in the treatment of chronic low back pain. It is primarily used for neuromuscular re-education. (The athlete has more pain because of the muscular stimulation.)

26. --) Cervical traction would not be an appropriate modality for this problem. This athlete has a low back problem, not a neck injury. (Please read the opening scenario.)

27. --) Paraffin bath would not be an appropriate modality choice for this problem. Paraffin treatments are most commonly used for hand and foot conditions. (The athlete is very upset that you are pouring a very warm, waxy substance on his back.)

28. ++) Effleurage would be an appropriate action to take. This massage technique can be very effective in relaxing the athlete and in encouraging improved venous and lymphatic drainage. (The athlete reports significant relief of his muscular discomfort after your treatment.)

29. +) A neoprene lumbar support would be an appropriate item to recommend to the athlete to use during activity. It provides warmth and a sense of support that is effective in reducing pain with movement. (The athlete reports he is able to move easier during practice.)

Section C

The current situation: The athlete's low back pain is beginning to reduce with the treatment he has been receiving.

Your immediate responsibility: To instruct the athlete in a series of exercises to improve his lumbar mobility and strength.

30. -) Active trunk extensions against gravity would be inappropriate in the initial stages of rehabilitation, especially while the athlete is still complaining of lumbar pain with active movement. This may aggravate his lumbar pain. (The athlete is fine extending his back while standing but reports increased pain attempting this in prone.)

31. +) Gentle active-assisted low back flexibility exercises, such as knee-to-chest exercises, are useful in the initial phases of rehabilitation to restore lumbar movement. (The athlete has minimal discomfort with these exercises.)

32. 0) Resisted knee extensions will not cause further injury to the athlete but are not necessary in the initial treatment of chronic low back pain. (The athlete has strong hip flexors and quadriceps.)

33. ++) Stretching the hamstrings would be an appropriate action to take. Tight hamstrings can contribute to chronic low back pain. (The athlete has bilateral tight hamstrings.)

34. ++) Having the athlete perform active posterior pelvic tilts would be an appropriate exercise to initiate during the early phases of rehabilitation. (The athlete has no difficulty or pain with this exercise.)

35. +) Stretching the hip flexors would be appropriate if it is found during the initial evaluation that the muscles were tight. If the hip flexors are too tight, it can place a strain on the low back area. (The athlete's hip flexors flexibility is within normal limits bilaterally.)

36. +) Strengthening the muscles around the hip is important because these muscles also serve to support the pelvis and lumbar areas. This would be an appropriate exercise only if it does not cause the athlete further discomfort.

37. +) Lower trunk rotations in supine are useful in the initial phases of rehabilitation to restore lumbar movement. (The athlete has no discomfort with these exercises.)

Section D

The current situation: The athlete now has no complaints of low back pain during rest or activity.

Your immediate responsibility: Progress the athlete's program with an emphasis on lumbar stabilization to prevent a reoccurrence of low back pain.

38. ++) PNF exercises for the trunk would be appropriate as long as the chosen exercises cause the athlete no discomfort. (The athlete fatigues easily.)

39. ++) Resistive abdominal strengthening would be appropriate exercises to initiate during the later stages of rehabilitation as long as the exercises cause the athlete no discomfort. (The athlete fatigues easily.)

40. 0) Resistive cervical strengthening would be unnecessary and inappropriate for this problem.

41. +) Resisted prone hip extension requires activation of the lumbar musculature. This would be an appropriate exercise to perform for lumbar stabilization. (The athlete has no discomfort with this but fatigues easily.)

42. -) Achilles' stretching exercises are unnecessary and not appropriate for this problem. (The athlete questions why stretching his calves is important.)

43. -) Groin stretching exercises are unnecessary and not appropriate for this problem. (The athlete's groin musculature is not tight.)

44. --) Shoulder press exercises are unnecessary and inappropriate during the rehabilitation of this problem. Loading the spine with overhead exercises could cause further harm. (The athlete complains this exercise bothers his back.)

45. 0) Jogging would be appropriate to maintain aerobic conditioning but would not be the optimal choice of exercise for an athlete with a low back injury. Swimming would be a safer choice if a pool is available. (The athlete complains of mild lumbar discomfort with this activity but is able to jog short distances.)

46. ++) Swimming would be the optimal exercise for aerobic conditioning. (The athlete has no lumbar discomfort while swimming.)

47. ++) Resisted bridging exercises are an effective exercise for lumbar stabilization and an appropriate exercise choice. (The athlete has no pain with this exercise.)

48. ++) In the late stages of rehabilitation, trunk extensions against gravity are appropriate to strengthening the erector spinae. (The athlete now has no complaints of lumbar discomfort but continues to fatigue easily with this exercise.)

PROBLEM XVIII

Section A

The current situation: This athlete is complaining of ear pain and itching. You suspect the athlete has an ear infection.

Your immediate responsibility: Protect the athlete's ear to prevent the infection from getting worse and refer the athlete to a physician for treatment.

1. --) Dispensing antibiotics is a medical task, not an athletic training task. It is illegal for an athletic trainer to dispense antibiotics. (You are brought up on charges for practicing medicine.)

2. -) Cleaning the athlete's ear with epinephrine is an inappropriate action. Inserting any foreign object into the ear canal should be avoided. Epinephrine is a vasoconstrictor and is an inappropriate chemical for the treatment of external otitis. (The athlete hollers in pain during your attempt to "clean" his ear.)

3. +) It is important that the athlete is referred to the team physician as soon as possible so the athlete can begin treatment. (The athlete is placed on antibiotics by the team doctor.)

4. -) Protecting the ear that has an ear infection is best accomplished by plugging it with lamb's wool that is soaked with lanolin. (The athlete complains that the gauze pad is "not doing anything" and he removes it.)

5. +) It is best to avoid having the infected ear exposed to cold wind. Wearing a hood or hat that covers the ears will help protect the ear and reduce pain. (The athlete is much more comfortable when wearing a hood outside.)

6. --) The use of a TENS unit would not be appropriate in this situation. (Even the athlete knows this is wrong!)

7. -) Because swimmer's ear is caused by an infection as a result of fluid trapped in the ear canal, the application of a moist heat pack would not be an appropriate action. (The infection gets worse.)

8. +) It is appropriate to allow the athlete to continue swimming as long as the athlete habitually dries the affected ear with a soft towel and uses ear drops containing a 3% boric acid and alcohol solution before and after swimming.

Section B

The current situation: The athlete has begun treatment by a physician.

Your immediate responsibility: Instruct the athlete in methods to prevent the infection from getting worse.

9. ++) Using ear plugs while swimming to protect the infected ear is appropriate to reduce the amount of water entering the ear canal.

10. 0) Having the athlete utilize a bathing cap may help decrease the amount of water entering the ear while swimming but may not be totally effective in doing so if ear plugs are not used.

11. -) If properly managed, the athlete should be able to return to swimming on a regular basis.

12. 0) Wearing goggles is unnecessary and inappropriate regarding treatment of this problem.

13. ++) Having the athlete refrain from inserting any foreign objects into the ears is appropriate in protecting the athlete from further injury or additional infection.

PROBLEM XIX

Section A

The current situation: You know this athlete has suffered a traumatic mouth/facial injury resulting from a blow by a hockey stick.

Your immediate responsibility: To perform an initial evaluation to determine the type and extent of the injury.

1. ++) Having the athlete clear the mouth with water and cleansing the face with water will allow the athletic trainer better visualization of the injured area.

2. -) Cleaning the athlete's mouth out with a paper towel is inappropriate. (The athlete is not pleased with pieces of paper sticking to her teeth and the roof of her mouth.)

3. ++) Anytime there is blood present during an injury, universal precautions must be observed.

4. -) The athlete has just received a significant blow to the mouth; wouldn't you be crying? (The athlete is upset with your insensitivity.)

5. +) It would be appropriate to check to see if the athlete was wearing a mouthguard. If she was wearing it, the fit must be checked. (She states she forgot it today and was not wearing it.)

6. -) Reviewing the school's liability insurance policy would be inappropriate. (It does not matter at this time.)

7. +) It would be an appropriate action to observe the mouth and surrounding areas for lacerations or abrasions. (There is an abrasion on the inside of the upper lip.)

8. +) Palpating the mouth and surrounding structures for deformity would be appropriate to check the athlete for a possible facial or jaw fracture. (Although edema is present, no gross deformity is palpable.)

9. -) Placing the athlete in a cervical collar would be unnecessary and inappropriate.

10. +) Having the athlete open and close her mouth will provide the athletic trainer some information concerning the extent of the injury. (The athlete is able to open and close her mouth, although it is painful.)

Section B

The current situation: Your findings indicate that the athlete's inner upper lip has been abrased and there is some swelling present with a moderate amount of bleeding. There is no gross deformity of the face/jaw, and the athlete is able to open and close her mouth. One of the athlete's front teeth is missing.

Your immediate responsibility: Recover the tooth, if possible, and try to reposition it, if possible. Refer the athlete to a dentist as soon as possible.

11. -) Asking the officials to stop the game would be unnecessary and inappropriate. (The officials deny your request.)

12. 0) Having a athletic training student bring the athlete to the school nurse would be unnecessary and inappropriate. (There is nothing the school nurse could do that you could not do.)

13. +) Speaking with the athlete's parents would be appropriate, especially since the athlete is a minor. (The parents are grateful you filled them in on the situation.)

14. -) Calling the team physician would not be appropriate. (He wonders why you need his assistance.)

15. +) Applying ice to the injured area would be appropriate to control the athlete's pain and reduce the bleeding. (Although the athlete still has pain, she is more comfortable.)

16. +) Applying a cotton plug between the lip and injured gum will help control the bleeding and decrease the swelling. (The bleeding begins to stop.)

17. ++) Placing the displaced tooth in a container of sterile saline solution would be appropriate and is an important step toward saving the tooth if it is not possible to reposition the tooth in its socket.

18. +) The displaced tooth should be rinsed off with water to clean it of any dirt or debris.

19. ++) Sending the athlete and the tooth to a dentist within 30 minutes is critical if the tooth is to be saved. (The parents immediately leave with the athlete.)

20. --) Discarding the tooth is inappropriate unless it is a known fact that the tooth is no longer alive. (The parents threaten to sue you when they find out the tooth could have been saved.)

21. 0) Having the athlete lie down in a side-lying position has no bearing on this situation.

PROBLEM XX

Section A

The current situation: You have been asked by an athlete to assist him in losing weight during his off-season period.

Your immediate responsibility: Assist the athlete in developing a nutritionally balanced diet and proper eating habits. Assess the athlete's current condition.

1. --) Having the athlete consume a protein drink daily with one of his regular meals will not encourage weight loss and should not be used in lieu of a regular meal. (The athlete gains another 7 pounds in 2 weeks.)

2. +) Using calipers to measure the athlete's percent body fat would be appropriate to obtain a baseline measurement. (The athlete's body fat is 12%.)

3. --) It is unrealistic to give the athlete a cookbook and expect him to lose weight as a result of that one action. This would be an inappropriate action. (The athlete admits he never even opened the book.)

4. --) Sending the athlete to an acupuncturist for this problem is not appropriate. (The athlete refuses to go.)

5. ++) Having the athlete record his food and drink intake in a personal log will assist the athletic trainer in adjusting the athlete's diet to ensure he is eating a nutritionally sound diet. (The athlete's current diet is high in fatty food and fluids high in sugar.)

6. ++) Monitoring the athlete's weight once a week will help the athletic trainer modify the athlete's diet accordingly and ensure the athlete is losing weight at a safe pace. (The athlete begins to lose weight after 3 days from initiating the new diet.)

7. --) Having the athlete fast is an inappropriate and potentially dangerous action. Fluids in particular should not be restricted. (The athlete becomes significantly dehydrated and ends up at the hospital.)

8. +) It is important that the athlete consume plenty of water while losing weight to avoid dehydration. (The athlete is compliant with this recommendation.)

9. ++) Weighing the athlete prior to beginning his program will provide the athletic trainer with a baseline weight so weight reduction can be tracked. (The athlete is overweight by 10 pounds.)

10. --) Having the athlete sit in a sauna is an inappropriate and potentially dangerous suggestion. (The athlete sits in a sauna for an extended period of time and becomes significantly dehydrated.)

11. ++) Monitoring the athlete's exercise program is essential in providing a comprehensive weight loss program.

12. ++) Sitting down with the athlete to put together a balanced diet that he will adhere to is appropriate. Having the athlete be an active participant in his own care will help to maintain compliance. (The athlete is satisfied with the diet that is developed.)

13. --) Wearing a rubber suit during activity to encourage rapid dehydration is an inappropriate and very dangerous practice. (The athlete becomes severely dehydrated during a workout and collapses.)

14. 0) Although having the athlete perform progressive-resistive exercises for his lower extremities certainly will cause no harm to the athlete, it will serve no specific purpose in decreasing this athlete's weight. (In fact, the athlete's weight might increase with the increased muscle bulk.)

Section B

The current situation: You have concluded from your assessment of this athlete that he is somewhat overweight and is eating a diet that is high in fat and sugar. He is compliant with your program and is beginning to show signs of success.

Your immediate responsibility: Continue to encourage the athlete in maintaining good eating habits and monitor the athlete on a regular basis to track his progression.

15. +) It would be appropriate to have the athlete keep a diet log so he can continue to keep track of what he eats and drinks. This will make it easier to make adjustments in his diet as necessary. (The athlete thinks this is a good idea.)

16. -) Having the coach monitor the athlete's food intake is inappropriate and not practical. (The coach has enough to do just coaching the team.)

17. ++) Having the athlete maintain a good level of hydration is always important. (This poses no problem.)

18. -) Increasing the level of physical activity does not necessarily require the athlete to exercise twice as long as his current exercise program requires. How the intensity and duration of the exercise program is modified will depend on the athlete's current level of activity. (The athlete becomes chronically fatigued.)

19. --) The use of laxatives to lose weight is inappropriate and potentially dangerous because of their dehydrating effects. (The athlete overdoses and collapses from dehydration and an electrolyte imbalance.)

20. 0) Involving a sports nutritionist is not necessary unless complicating conditions exist, such as medical problems (eg, diabetes, ulcerative colitis, etc) or the athlete desires to seek help from a professional nutritionist.

21. ++) To discourage binge eating, encouraging the athlete to eat numerous small meals throughout the day would be an appropriate suggestion. (The athlete nibbles on fruit, crackers, and small amounts of cheese during the day.)

22. 0) Although having the athlete perform progressive-resistive exercises for his upper extremities will cause him no harm, it serves no specific purpose in decreasing this athlete's weight. (The athlete sees no change in his weight since beginning an upper extremity strength program.)

PROBLEM XXI

Section A

The current situation: You know this athlete has sustained a traumatic lower extremity injury from a hard landing.

Your immediate responsibility: To perform an initial evaluation to determine the type and extent of the injury

1. --) Manipulation of the limb is premature until the severity of the injury is established.

2. ++) Blood pressure is 110/78, and the pulse is 90.

3. 0) This is unnecessary at this point.

4. -) You can see the primary deformity has occurred at the hip. Performing a Lachman's test is a premature action.

5. 0) The athlete is breathing without difficulty.

6. ++) The athlete tells you his right hip is "killing him."

7. -) You have caused disruption of the blood supply to the head of the femur and injury to the sciatic nerve.

8. +) Both extremities are grossly intact to light touch.

9. -) Moving the athlete at this time is inappropriate; you have not established the nature/severity of the injury or stabilized the athlete for transport.

10. --) The athlete screams in pain.

11. +) This would be an appropriate action.

12. +) You rule out injuries to the neck, upper body, and left lower extremity.

13. +) The athlete states "I don't know; I got whacked on my right side."

14. ++) You prevent additional injury to the right lower extremity.

15. +) You do not find any areas of deformity or pain with palpation of the right knee or ankle.

Section B

The current situation: You realize from your initial findings that the athlete's right hip is grossly malaligned and that there is no injury to the right knee or ankle.

Your immediate responsibility: Monitor (and treat as necessary) the athlete for shock, minimize pain, and prevent further injury.

16. 0) This is not a priority at this time.

17. ++) The athlete's respiratory rate is 16 breaths per second; blood pressure is 100/70, pulse rate is 94 and thready.

18. -) Competition was stopped at the time of the injury, and the athlete has not yet been removed from the field.

19. +) You have the room you need to work without obstruction, and the athlete feels less anxious without his teammates watching him.

20. -) You have just caused a sciatic nerve injury as a result of moving the athlete.

21. -) The athlete screams in pain as you try to straighten his knee.

22. +) The pain is minimized with the application of an ice pack.

23. -) The aspirin causes increased internal bleeding at the site of the injury.

24. -) The athlete screams in pain.

25. -) The athlete tells you that he cannot move his right leg.

26. ++) The popliteal and dorsalis pedis pulses are palpable but weak.

27. +) This helps to prevent additional injury.

Section C

The current situation: You have stabilized the athlete in anticipation of the EMS team's arrival.

Your immediate responsibility: Assist the EMS team with the transfer of the athlete onto a spine board, ensure the athlete's family and your athletic director are informed of the athlete's status, and properly document the incident.

28. 0) The EMTs have taken care of this.

29. -) The athlete should not eat or drink anything prior to arriving at the hospital.

30. 0) The coach is needed at the venue to keep his team together. You go to the hospital after the game.

31. +) The athlete tells you he is scared and thanks you for staying with him.

32. 0) The athlete has already done this.

33. ++) You assist the EMTs with the transfer and stabilization of the athlete onto a spine board successfully.

34. +) You protect yourself from a possible malpractice suit.

35. +) The parents thank you for your care and proceed to the hospital.

36. +) Your athletic director appreciates being kept informed.

Problem XXII

Section A

The current situation: The referee presents with a quick onset of nausea and chest discomfort with associated diaphoresis. His past medical history is unknown.

Your immediate responsibility: To perform an initial evaluation to determine the type and origin of his condition.

1. ++) He states he was jogging up the court and suddenly has "pressure in his chest" and "just felt bad."

2. -) There is no such thing as an ACE.

3. --) You ignore obvious signs of physiologic distress and are eventually sued for negligence.

4. 0) This is an inappropriate action at this time.

5. +) It would not be wise to continue the game while you are attending to an ill referee.

6. ++) The referee's blood pressure is 130/80, and his pulse is 100 and regular.

7. +) The referee tells you he takes nitroglycerin for angina pectoris, Claritin for allergies, and naprosyn for knee arthritis.

8. --) You lose your certification, state license, and are sued for practicing medicine without a license.

9. -) The referee states he is dizzy and unable to stand at this time.

10. ++) The referee tells you he had a "mild heart attack" ten years ago.

11. +) The referee states, "I've been trying to quit…."

12. +) The referee tells you he definitely has pain in his right shoulder area.

Section B

The current situation: You determine from your initial evaluation that the referee has a past medical history of cardiac issues and he is a smoker. Although his vital signs are stable, he is exhibiting signs/symptoms of a myocardial infarction.

Your immediate responsibility: Monitor vital signs and escalating symptoms, keep the referee calm, and activate EMS.

13. 0) The team doctor is not immediately available for assistance.

14. ++) This is an appropriate action based on your assessment of the situation.

15. -) The referee tells you lying on his back "makes it hard to breathe."

16. --) The referee panics and his symptoms exacerbate.

17. --) This is an inappropriate action.

18. 0) Placing ice on the back of the referees' neck is an inappropriate action.

19. 0) Why? Having the referee cough has no purpose.

20. +) The referee tells you that he is having a hard time "catching his breath."

21. 0) Poor capillary refill of the digits is a sign of peripheral vascular problems and is not a symptom of a myocardial infarction.

22. +) The referee may experience anxiety and a feeling of "impending doom," so it is important to keep him calm and be supportive.

23. ++) This should be obvious; you are informed that an ambulance has been dispatched.

Section C

The current situation: The referee suddenly collapses.

Your immediate responsibility: To confirm that he is unresponsive and begin the sequence for CPR and the application of the AED.

24. ++) This is the first step in CPR.

25. --) The referee dies as you waste time in the stands looking for assistance.

26. ++) The referee is breathing and you palpate a carotid pulse.

27. -) This is an inappropriate action.

28. -) You do not need a spine board right now. CPR can be performed on the court.

29. 0) A facial droop is a sign of a stroke, not of a myocardial infarction.

30. ++) This action could save the referee's life.

31. -) This action is inappropriate for this situation.

32. ++) This action could save the referee's life.

33. 0) This will not make the referee's condition better or worse, but it will impede your ability to perform CPR.

Section D

The current situation: The paramedics have stabilized and transported the referee to the hospital.

Your immediate responsibility: Document the incident and give a verbal report to your athletic director.

34. --) You are severely reprimanded by your athletic director and the superintendent for giving confidential information to the media.

35. ++) It is important to document how the incident occurred and what actions you took to ensure the victim's care.

36. +) The athletic director appreciates you keeping him updated and commends you on a job well done.

37. -) Play resumes without you present and one of your athletes gets injured. You are reprimanded by the athletic director for leaving the game unattended.

38. +) The rest of the game is uneventful and you check on the referee's condition the next day.

PROBLEM XXIII

Section A

The current situation: Your athlete presents to you with dyspnea and chest discomfort.

Your immediate responsibility: To perform an initial evaluation to determine the etiology of his condition.

1. -) Shortness of breath is not a symptom of diabetes. The athlete denies that he is a diabetic.

2. +) The athlete tells you he is asthmatic.

3. 0) Imodium is a drug used to slow peristalisis. The athlete denies having any symptoms of diarrhea.

4. -) The athlete experiences increased difficulty in breathing.

5. ++) The athlete acknowledges he owns an inhaler.)

6. +) You are able to keep the athletes respiratory rate at 14 breaths per second.

7. --) This is a premature action. You have not determined the nature/severity of the problem.

Section B

The current situation: The athlete reveals he is an asthmatic and owns an inhaler.

Your immediate responsibility: Make the process of breathing easier by instructing the athlete to breathe through his nose and slow down his pace of activity. Monitor the athlete for further symptoms at least four hours after his episode of EIB.

8. ++) Breathing through the nose warms and humidifies the air.

9. 0) The athlete's pulse rate is 74 and regular.

10. -) The athlete is not hyperventilating.

11. -) A short-acting inhaler works best as a pre-treatment after a warm-up routine to prevent an attack for 2 to 6 hours.

12. ++) A 10 to 30 minute cool-down after vigorous activity will help to avoid thermal changes in the airways.

13. 0) The athlete thanks you for the offer, but hot tea or chocolate will not help him breathe.

14. 0) The athlete states he feels better if he "just walks around".

15. +) Taking the athlete out of the game is an appropriate action.

16. ++) It is important to monitor the athlete after the symptoms decrease or subside because the athlete may develop another bout of bronchospasm 4 to 12 hours after exercise. He has no symptoms after 5 hours of observation.

PROBLEM XXIV

Section A

The current situation: Your athlete presents to you with low back pain and radiating symptoms down his right leg after a weight-lifting session.

Your immediate responsibility: To perform an initial evaluation to determine the type and severity of the injury.

1. -) There is no reason to use iontophoresis when the nature/severity of the injury has yet to be determined.

2. -) The initial evaluation should be completed before any modality is used.

3. ++) Palpation of the injured area is a vital step in the evaluative process. The athlete tells you the right side of his lower back and right sacroiliac joint are sore.

4. ++) A right lateral shift is observed.

5. 0) The athlete tells you his knees feel fine.

6. ++) The athlete has a positive Slump test.

7. +) The athlete states that he has pain down the back of his right leg to just below the knee joint.

8. +) The athlete states he has had similar pain two years ago after helping a friend move into his apartment.

9. 0) The athlete reports the massage feels great but it has not changed his leg pain.

10. -) The athlete replies he now feels sharp pain in his right calf.

Section B

The current situation: The pain is significantly increased with forward flexion and his pain is radiating to the L5-S1 dermatome.

Your immediate responsibility: Decrease the radicular pain with prone press-ups and pain modalities.

11. ++) The athlete reports his pain is now out of his calf and thigh and is concentrated in his right buttock.

12. -) The athlete reports his pain has intensified to the back of his right knee.

13. 0) The athlete reports the tape has not changed his pain level.

14. --) Administration of a medication without the direction of a physician is beyond the scope of practice for an athletic trainer.

15. --) It is the physician's decision whether or not a MRI is ordered.

16. -) The athlete loses confidence in your skills to evaluate his condition.

17. ++) The athlete reports the pain has moved from his leg to his right buttock.

18. +) The athlete reports good relief of low back pain with the ice.

Section C

The current situation: The athlete is responding favorably to the prone press-ups and pain modalities.

Your immediate responsibility: Instruct the athlete in proper body mechanics while lifting and make sure the athlete continues to perform lumbar extension exercises

to counteract any forward flexion he performs during the day (i.e., sitting or lifting).

19. 0) The athlete is able to side bend with greater ease, but it does not affect his pain intensity or location.

20. +) The athlete agrees not to lift any heavy objects at this time.

21. ++) You observe the athlete bending at the knees as he picks up his sweatshirt off the floor.

22. +) The athlete has decreased spasm of the lumbar area as he moves.

23. -) NSAIDS may ease the immediate discomfort but does not eliminate the underlying problem involving the intervertebral disc.

24. --) The athlete bends over to tie his sneakers and winces in pain.

25. -) The athlete experiences peripheralization of his pain.

26. +) The athlete's low back pain is reduced.

Problem XXV

Section A

The current situation: An athlete presents to you with changes in cognition, skin temperature, texture, and color after running for a prolonged period of time.

Your immediate responsibility: To perform your initial evaluation to determine the etiology of his condition.

1. --) You are sued for practicing medicine without a license.

2. +) The athlete replies "nothing."

3. ++) The athlete's core temperature is 102°F.

4. ++) The athlete's blood pressure is 90/60, and his pulse rate is 122.

5. 0) The athlete has no cranial nerve dysfunction.

6. 0) The athlete does not have a deep vein thrombosis.

7. 0) The athlete's capillary refill is fine.

8. +) The athlete is oriented to self, time, and place.

Section B

The current situation: You determine from your evaluation that the athlete is suffering from symptoms of heat exhaustion.

Your immediate responsibility: Monitor and treat for shock, reduce the athlete's core temperature as soon as possible, rehydrate him, and instruct him on the signs and prevention of heat illness.

9. -) The athlete has no symptoms of hyperventilation.

10. ++) It is imperative to get the athlete's core body temperature reduced as soon as possible.

11. ++) You are able to prevent symptoms of shock.

12. 0) The athlete is indifferent to your attempt to relax him.

13. --) The athlete becomes completely disoriented, his temperature rises, and his blood pressure falls.

14. +) The athlete's vital signs begin to stabilize as his core temperature returns to normal and he is rehydrated.

15. --) There is no decrease in the athlete's core temperature.

16. ++) The athlete's core temperature returns to normal.

17. +) The athlete thanks you and follows your recommendations.

Problem XXVI

Section A

The current situation: You know this athlete has sustained a blunt trauma injury to the right side of her chest.

Your immediate responsibility: To perform an initial evaluation to determine the severity of the injury.

1. +) The athlete's skin color/lips appear normal

2. --) The athlete loses consciousness

3. 0) The athlete is obviously able to move her extremities.

4. --) The athlete experiences respiratory distress.

5. ++) The athlete is breathing, and the pulse rate is 90 BPS.

6. --) The athlete screams in pain as she tries to elevate her right arm.

7. -) You have determined there is no neck injury.

8. +) You notice the athlete coughing up small amounts of frank blood.

9. ++) The athlete winces from pain as you palpate the right lower ribs, and you feel some crepitus.

Section B

The current situation: You find the athlete's vital signs are stable, but you suspect a rib injury with a possible lung injury as a result of blunt chest trauma.

Your immediate responsibility: Monitor vital signs, splint the chest area to make inspiration easier, keep the athlete calm, and activate EMS. Follow-up with the team physician and document the incident.

10. ++) The athlete's respiratory rate is 18 breaths per minute and is shallow.

11. ++) The athlete's vital signs remain stable.

12. --) The bandage is too constrictive and limits the athlete's ability to breathe freely.

13. 0) The athlete asks you what that "cold stuff" is.

14. ++) The athlete reports she feels much more comfortable.

15. +) You notice an indentation over the eighth rib.

16. --) The athlete screams in pain.

17. 0) The athlete does not have thoracic outlet syndrome.

18. 0) The athlete does not have carpal tunnel syndrome.

19. +) An ambulance has been dispatched.

20. ++) The athlete is able to breathe easier.

21. ++) You contact the team physician as soon as the game is over.

Problem XXVII

Section A

The current situation: Your athlete presents with a change in level of cognition (LOC) and you are aware his is diabetic.

Your immediate responsibility: Perform an initial evaluation to determine the extent of his condition.

1. 0) The athlete is breathing with difficulty.

2. +) The athlete is profusely diaphoretic.

3. +) The athletes pulse rate is 74 BPS.

4. ++) The athlete tells you he injected himself with regular insulin at 7:00 AM this morning right after breakfast.

5. 0) The athlete's face appears to be fine.

6. 0) There are no signs of cranial nerve involvement.

7. 0) The Romberg's test is not indicated for this problem.

8. --) The athlete is highly insulted by your suggestion of drug abuse, and you miss signs of the athlete's problem.

9. +) The athlete does not have fruity smelling breath.

Section B

The current situation: Based on your initial findings, you determine the athlete has become hypoglycemic secondary to increased activity.

Your immediate responsibility: Monitor vital signs and administer a mixture of sugar and juice to increase the blood glucose levels.

10. --) The athlete goes into a coma and dies.

11. 0) Lack of protein is not this athlete's problem.

12. 0) There is no change in the athlete's condition.

13. +) The athlete's vital signs are stable.

14. ++) The athlete responds quickly and feels much better. He is alert and asks, "What happened?"

15. 0) There is no change in the athlete's status.

16. 0) The athlete recovers minimally.

Section C

The current situation: The athlete has fully recovered from the hypoglycemic event.

Your immediate responsibility: Instruct the athlete in the prevention of hypoglycemia during exercise.

17. ++) The athlete reports he "forgot" to eat some fruit and crackers before coming to the athletic training room.

18. --) The athlete goes into insulin shock as a result of injecting himself prior to his rehabilitation session.

19. +) The athlete has no problem during his events.

20. +) The athlete tells you he has hard candy in his duffle bag.

21. 0) Do they have diabetic support groups?

HELPFUL WEBSITES

GENERAL

American Academy of Kinesiology and Physical Education
www.aakpe.org/newsletr/currpres.htm

American Academy of Orthopedic Surgeons
orthoinfo.aaos.org

American Academy of Physician Assistants
www.aapa.org

American Academy of Podiatric Sports Medicine
www.aapsm.org

American Alliance for Health, Physical Education, Recreation, and Dance
www.aahperd.org

American College of Sports Medicine
www.acsm.org

American Medical Association
www.ama-assn.org

American Occupational Therapy Association
www.aota.org

American Orthopedic Society for Sports Medicine
www.sportsmed.org

American Physical Therapy Association
www.apta.org

American Red Cross
www.redcross.org

American Society of Exercise Physiologists
www.asep.org

Association of American Medical Colleges
www.aamc.org

Canadian Athletic Therapists Association
www.athletictherapy.org

College Athletic Trainers' Society (CATS)
www.collegeatc.org

International Federation of Sports Medicine
www.fims.org

International Society of Biomechanics
www.isbweb.org

Japanese Athletic Trainers' Organization
www.jato-trainer.org

Joint Review Committee on Educational Athletic Training Programs
www.jrc-at.org

National Academy of Sports Medicine
www.nasm.org

National Athletic Trainers' Association (NATA)
www.nata.org

NATA Board of Certification
www.bocatc.org

NATA Education Council
www.nataec.org

National Association of Emergency Medical Technicians
www.naemt.org

National Collegiate Athletic Association
www.ncaa.org

National Operating Committee on Standards for Athletic Equipment
www.nocsae.org

National Registry of Emergency Medical Technicians
www.nremt.org

National Safety Council
www.nsc.org

National Strength & Conditioning Association
www.nsca-lift.org

Professional Baseball Athletic Trainers Society
www.pbats.com/malt/rangers.htm

Professional Football Athletic Trainers Society
www.pfats.com/

United States Olympic Committee
www.usoc.org

World Federation of Athletic Training & Therapy
www.wfatt.org

PUBLICATIONS

Athletic Therapy Today
www.mylitsearch.org/pub/100673337

BioMechanics
www.biomech.com

First Aider
www.cramersportsmed.com/first_aider.jsp

Gatorade Sports Science Exchange
www.gssiweb.com/sportssciencecenter/topic.cfm?id=96

Hughston Health Alert (newsletter)
www.hughston.com/hha/hha.htm

Journal of Applied Biomechanics
www.humankinetics.com/JAB/index.cfm

Journal of Athletic Training
www.nata.org/jat/

Journal of the American Medical Association
jama.ama-assn.org

Medicine & Science in Sports & Exercise
www.ms-se.org

Orthopedics Today
www.orthosupersite.com

Penn State Sports Medicine Newsletter
www.psu.edu/ur/news.html

EDUCATIONAL PROGRAMS

Please note that this list is representative of educational programs offering a degree in athletic training.

Alabama

Huntingdon College
www.huntingdon.edu/academic_programs/athletic_training

Samford University
www.samford.edu

Troy University
www.troy.edu

University of Alabama
www.ches.ua.edu/atep

University of Mobile
www.umobile.edu/acad/ed/athlettrain.asp

University of West Alabama
at.uwa.edu

Arizona

Grand Canyon University
www.gcu.net/campus/programs/bachelor-of-science-in-athletic-training.php

Northern Arizona University
www.nau.edu/hp/dept/exs

Arkansas

Arkansas State University
www.clt.astate.edu/hpess/AthleticTrainingProgram/athome.html

Ouachita Baptist University
www.obu.edu/atep/

University of Arkansas
www.uark.edu/depts/atepweb/

University of Central Arkansas
www.uca.edu/divisions/academic/kped/Admission.html

California

Azusa Pacific University
www.apu.edu/educabs/undergraduate/physicaleducation/bachelors/training

California Lutheran University
www.clunet.edu/Academic_Programs/Departments/Exercise_Science/ESSM/ATEP.html

California State University-Fresno
www.csufresno.edu/kines/ATEP/default.html

California State University-Fullerton
hdcs.fullerton.edu/at/

California State University-Northridge
www.csun.edu

California State University-Sacramento
www.hhs.csus.edu/khs

Chapman University
www.chapman.edu/educ/atep/

Humboldt State University
www.humboldt.edu/~hpe/atep.htm

Point Loma Nazarene University
www.ptloma.edu/Kinesiology/athletic/

San Diego State University
www.rohan.sdsu.edu/dept/athletic/athletictraining/ATPPINFO.htm

San José State University
www.sjsu.edu/depts/hup/gradath/ugath.html

University of La Verne
www.ulv.edu/athletictraining

Vanguard University
www.vanguard.edu/athletics/training

Colorado

Colorado State-Pueblo
ceeps.colostate-pueblo.edu/exhpr/athletic_training.htm

Fort Lewis College
www.fortlewis.edu/academics/school_education/exersci/athtrain/athtrain/athtrain.html

Mesa State College
www.mesastate.edu/schools/sbps/hpw/athletictraining-home.htm

Metropolitan State College of Denver
www.mscd.edu/~hpslweb/program/ath_train.shtml

Connecticut

Quinnipac University
www.quinnipiac.edu/x1002.xml

Sacred Heart University
www.sacredheart.edu/academics/catalogs/undergraduate/cat2000ehpat.html#ehp3

Delaware

University of Delaware
www.udel.edu/catalog/cat2001/hns/hesc/athtr.html

Florida

Barry University
www.barry.edu/hpls/BS/athleticTraining/default.htm

Florida State University
www.chs.fsu.edu/nfes/undergraduate_athletic_training.php

Florida Southern College
www.flsouthern.edu

Palm Beach Atlantic University
www.pba.edu/academic/ATEP/

The University of Tampa
www.ut.edu/academics/liberalarts/departments/exercs-ports/training.html

University of Florida
www.hhp.ufl.edu/about

University of Central Florida
www.cohpa.ucf.edu/health.pro/athletic

University of North Florida
www.unf.edu/coh/cohatweb.htm

University of Miami
www.education.miami.edu/AthleticTraining/index.html

University of South Florida
pe.usf.edu/ath_trng/04atspecs.php

University of West Florida
cops.uwf.edu/hles/Athletic_Training.cfm

Georgia

Georgia Southern University
www.georgiasouthern.edu/

The University of Georgia
www.coe.uga.edu/departments/academic.html

Hawaii

University of Hawaii Manoa
www.hawaii.edu/kls/atsm/

Idaho

Boise State University
kinesiology.boisestate.edu/atep/

University of Idaho
coe2.ed.uidaho.edu/index.cfm?SiteID=9

Illinois

Eastern Illinois University
www.eiu.edu/~athtrain

Illinois State University
www.cast.ilstu.edu/isuatep/

Lewis University
www.lewisu.edu/academics/athtrain/

Millikin University
www.millikin.edu/athletictraining/

Northern Illinois University
www.niu.edu/knpe/at/index.htm

North Park University
www.northpark.edu/acad/athletic_training/

Southern Illinois University
www.siu.edu/~athtrain

Trinity International University
www.tiu.edu/athletictraining/

Western Illinois University
www.wiu.edu/Kinesiology/atrain.shtml

University of Illinois
www.kines.uiuc.edu/atcentral

Indiana

Anderson University
www.anderson.edu/athletics/ausm

Franklin College
www.franklincollege.edu/athweb/training/

Manchester College
www.manchester.edu/Academics/Departments/HPE/AthleticTraining/

University of Evansville
hkss.evansville.edu/at.html

University of Indianapolis
athtrg.uindy.edu/

Iowa

Buena Vista University
www.bvu.edu/academics/education/athletictraining/atep.asp

Central College
www.central.edu/athletics/training.html

Graceland University
www.graceland.edu/show.cfm?durki=481

Iowa State University
www.hhp.hs.iastate.edu/athletic-training.php

Northwestern College
www.nwciowa.edu/athletictraining/

Simpson College
www.simpson.edu/physed/programs/atadmission.html

University of Iowa
www.uiowa.edu/~exsci

University of Northern Iowa
www.uni.edu/athtrn

Kansas

Benedictine College
www.benedictine.edu

Bethel College
www.bethelks.edu/academics/atep/

Emporia State University
www.emporia.edu/athletics/athletictraining/athltrain/
atwebpg.htm

Fort Hays State University
www.fhsu.edu/hhp/athletictraining/training.shtml

Kansas State University
www.ksu.edu/kines

Kansas Wesleyan University
www.kwu.edu/atep/

MidAmerica Nazarene University
www.mnu.edu/academics/education/ath_training/

Southwestern College
www.sckans.edu/athletictraining/index.php?page_ID=590

Tabor College
www.tabor.edu/academics/undergrad_dept.php?id=17

University of Kansas
www.soe.ku.edu/depts/hses/undergraduate/athletic_training/

Washburn University of Topeka
www.washburn.edu

Kentucky

Eastern Kentucky University
www.physed.eku.edu

Louisiana

Louisiana College
www.lacollege.edu/academics/atep/index.html

Louisiana State University
appl003.lsu.edu/educ/kines.nsf/$Content/Athletic+Training+Concentration?OpenDocument

Nicholls State University
www.nicholls.edu/ahs/health/athletic/admission.htm

Southeastern Louisiana University
www.selu.edu/atep

University of Louisiana at Lafayette
kinesiology.louisiana.edu/Programs/ATEP/

Maine

University of Maine at Presque Isle
www.umpi.maine.edu/programs/pgms/phedbs.htm

University of New England
www.une.edu/cas/esp/

University of Southern Maine
www.usm.maine.edu/sportsmed/athletictraining.html

Maryland

Frostburg State University
www.frostburg.edu/admin/athletics/

Salisbury University
www.salisbury.edu/academic/checklists/03_05/ATTR.pdf

Towson University
wwwnew.towson.edu/kinesiology/athletictraining.htm

Massachusetts

Bridgewater State College
www.bridgewater.edu/~bhlong/

Endicott College
www.endicott.edu/servlet/RetrievePage?site=endicott&page=SSFAthTrain

Lasell College
www.lasell.edu/academics/alliedhealth_sportscience.asp

Merrimack College
secure.merrimack.edu/athletictraining

Northeastern University
www.bouve.neu.edu/department/at/at.html

Sargent College
www.bu.edu/sargent/programs/undergraduate/athletic_training/index.html

Springfield College
www.spfldcol.edu

Westfield State College
www.wsc.ma.edu/dept/mssls

Michigan

Albion College
www.albion.edu/athletic_training/

Aquinas College
www.aquinas.edu/health/ath_training.html

Central Michigan University
www.chp.cmich.edu/atep

Eastern Michigan University
www.emich.edu/hphp/athletic_training.htm

Grand Valley State University
www.gvsu.edu/move-sci/index.cfm?id=37891252-0A8D-F791-38DE857239694C85

Hope College
www.hope.edu/academic/kinesiology/athtrain

Lake Superior State University
www.lssu.edu/recstudies/at/

Michigan State University
athletictraining.msu.edu/

Northern Michigan University
www.nmu.edu/hper/athletic_training/

Saginaw Valley State University
www.svsu.edu/catalog/undergraduate/Education/physical_and_health_education.htm#athtraining

Minnesota

Bethel College and Seminary
www.bethel.edu/career-services/career-planning/career-links/athletic-training

Gustavus Adolphus College
www.gustavus.edu/oncampus/athletics/atr/

Minnesota State University
https://www.mnstate.edu/athtrng/

Winona State University
www.winona.edu/athletictraining/

Mississippi

University of Southern Mississippi
www.usm.edu/athletictraining

Missouri

Central Methodist College
www.centralmethodist.edu/athtr/index.asp

Culver-Stockton College
www.culver.edu/academics/divisions/education/athletic-training/

Lindenwood University
www.lindenwood.edu/

Missouri State University
www.missouristate.edu/sportsmed

Park University
www.park.edu

Southeast Missouri State University
www.semo.edu/study/athletictraining/index.htm

Truman State University
hes.truman.edu

William Woods University
www.williamwoods.edu/2005catalog/2005FallSchedule/majorcourses.asp?SCMajorID=48

Montana

University of Montana
www.soe.umt.edu/hhp/athletic_training/default.shtm

Nebraska

Creighton University
www.creighton.edu/athletictraining/root_folder/at_homepage/at_homepage.htm

Nebraska Wesleyan University
www.nebrwesleyan.edu/depts/ateducation/

University of Nebraska –Lincoln
cehs.unl.edu/nhs/undergrad/athlTrain.shtml

University of Nebraska at Kearney
aaunk.unk.edu/catalogs/current/dptpe.htm

University of Nebraska-Omaha
www.unocoe.unomaha.edu/hper/athletictraining/

New Hampshire

Colby-Sawyer College
www.colby-sawyer.edu/academic/ess/athletictraining/
index.html

Keene State College
www.keene.edu/programs/pe

University of New Hampshire
www.unh.edu/athletic-training

New Jersey

Kean University of New Jersey
www.kean.edu/~gball

Montclair State University
www.montclair.edu/pages/athletics/training/training.html

Rowan State University
www.rowan.edu/mars/exersci

Seton Hall University
artsci.shu.edu/biology/at.htm

William Paterson University of New Jersey
www.wpunj.edu/cos/ex-movsci/atep.htm

New Mexico

New Mexico State University
education.nmsu.edu/perd

University of New Mexico
www.unm.edu/~lobotrng/

New York

Alfred University
las.alfred.edu/~ath/html/

Canisius College
www.canisius.edu/sportsmed

Dominican College of Blauvelt
www.dc.edu/profess/athletic.html

Hofstra University
www.hofstra.edu/academics/SOEAHS/PESP/pesp_at.cfm

Ithaca College
www.ithaca.edu/admission/hshp/program_at_es.htm

Long Island University-Brooklyn Campus
www.brooklyn.liu.edu/health/bsathra.html

Marist College
www.marist.edu/science/athtrain/

State University of New York-Brockport
www.brockport.edu/pes/undergrad/atrain/index.htmll

State University of New York-Buffalo
sphhp.buffalo.edu/ens/at/

State University of New York-Cortland
www.cortland.edu/esss/majors/training2.htm

SUNY Health Science Center at Stony Brook
www.hsc.stonybrook.edu/shtm/at_index.cfm

North Carolina

Appalachian State University
www.hles.appstate.edu/areas/athletic_training/index.htm

Barton College
www.barton.edu/SchoolofArts&Sciences/ATEP/HOME.
htm

Campbell University
www.campbell.edu/coas/exercise/index.html

East Carolina University
www.ecu.edu/hlth/athletictr/athletetr.cfm

Elon University
www.elon.edu/athletictraining/index.html

Gardner-Webb University
aux.gardner-webb.edu//

Greensboro College
www.gborocollege.edu/athletics/sports/athletictraining.
htm

High Point University
www.highpoint.edu/academics/ess/athletictraining

Lees-McRae College
www2.lmc.edu/Sites/Academics/Divisions/
ScienceMathCS/AthleticTraining/athletic_training.htm

Lenoir-Rhyne College
www.lrc.edu/

Mars Hill College
www.athletictraining.mhc.edu

Methodist College
www.methodist.edu/athtraining

North Carolina Central University
www.nccu.edu/artsci/pe/AthleticTraining.html

University of North Carolina-Charlotte
www.uncc.edu

University of North Carolina-Wilmington
www.uncw.edu

Wingate University
www.wingate.edu/academics/sport_sciences/
athletic_training

North Dakota

North Dakota State University
www.ndsu.edu/ndsu/academic/factsheets/hde/athltrn.
shtml

University of Mary
www.umary.edu/AcadInfo/HPSDiv/athleticTraining.asp

University of North Dakota
www.med.und.nodak.edu/depts/fammed/SportsMed/

Ohio

Ashland University
www3.ashland.edu/academics/education/sportsci/ath-
training/

Baldwin-Wallace College
www.bw.edu/academics/hpe/programs/at/adreq/index.
html

Bowling Green State University
bgsufalcons.collegesports.com/school-bio/bgu-athletic-
training.html

Capital University
www.capital.edu/acad/as/hss/page2.html

Cedarville University
www.cedarville.edu/academics/athletictraining/

College of Mount St. Joseph
www.msj.edu/academics/courses/coursecat/undg0506/
dept/health/at/index.asp

Defiance College
www.defiance.edu/pages/edu_AT_detailed.html

Denison University
www.denison.edu/phed/ATindex.html

Heidelberg College
www.heidelberg.edu/offices/registrar/catalog/courses-g-
l.html#hpe

Kent State University
dept.kent.edu/athletictraining/

Marietta College
mcnet.marietta.edu/~spmd

Miami University
www.units.muohio.edu/eap/phs/Pages/athletictraining.
html

Mount Union College
raider.muc.edu/pe/athletic%20training/index.htm

Ohio Northern University
www.onu.edu/a+s/hpss/at

Ohio State University
amp.osu.edu/at/

Ohio University
www.ohiou.edu/~rspsdept/ohioated

Otterbein College
www.otterbein.edu/dept/HPE/

University of Cinncinnati
www.uc.edu/programs/viewprog.asp?progid=948

University of Toledo
www.undergradadmission.utoledo.edu

Urbana University
www.urbana.edu/athletic_training.htm

Wilmington College Of Ohio
www.wilmington.edu/wchome.htm

Wright State University
www.wright.edu/majors/atr_more.html

Xavier University
www.xu.edu/athletic_training/

Oklahoma

East Central University
www.ecok.edu/academics/schools/edu_psych/hper/athletic_train/atEducProg/sports_training_atep_welcome.asp

Oklahoma State University
www.okstate.edu/education/sahep/athletic_training/

Southern Nazarene
www.snu.edu

Southwestern Oklahoma State University
www.swosu.edu/atep/

University of Tulsa
www.cba.utulsa.edu/depts/athletic

Oregon

George Fox University
www.georgefox.edu/academics/undergrad/departments/ath_tr/

Linfield College
www.linfield.edu/hhpa/at/index.php

Oregon State University
oregonstate.edu/athletics/training

Pennsylvania

Alvernia College
www.alvernia.edu/academics/at

California University of Pennsylvania
www.cup.edu/education/hsss

Duquesne University
www.healthsciences.duq.edu/at/athome.html

East Stroudsburg University
www3.esu.edu/academics/05.06/unofficial/at.asp

Indiana University of Pennsylvania
www.hhs.iup.edu/hped

King's College
www.kings.edu/Academics/FactSheets/AthlTraining05.pdf

Lock Haven University
www.lhup.edu/training/index.htm

Mercyhurst College
www.mercyhurst.edu/

Messiah College
www.messiah.edu/departments/hhp/programs/athletic_training.html

Pennsylvania State University
www.hhdev.psu.edu/kines/undergrad/athletic_tr.html

Slippery Rock University
www.sru.edu/depts/hes/ers/at/att.htm

Temple University
www.temple.edu

University of Pittsburgh
www.upb.pitt.edu/academics/programs/athletic_training_major/index.htm

Waynesburg College
www.waynesburg.edu/~sportmed

West Chester University
health-sciences.wcupa.edu/sportsmed/sportsmed-new/sportsmed.htm

South Carolina

College of Charleston
www.cofc.edu/~rozzis/at.html

Erskine College
www.erskine.edu/academics/athletictraining

Lander University
www.lander.edu/pees/athletic_training.htm

Limestone College
www.limestone.edu/sfs/acad/profess/at/rc.htm

University of South Carolina
www.usca.edu/exercise

Winthrop University
coe.winthrop.edu/COE/health-pe/hpe_athletic_training.htm

South Dakota

Augustana College
www.augie.edu/dept/athtr/pages/education.html

Dakota Wesleyan University
www.dwu.edu/catalog/courses/athletic_training.htm

National American University
www.national.edu/Athletic%20Training/athletic_training.htm

Si Tanka University
www.sioux.org/sitankauniv.html

South Dakota State University
www3.sdstate.edu/Academics/CollegeOfArtsAndScience/
HealthPhysicalEducationandRecreation/Majors/
AthleticTraining/Index.cfm

Tennessee

Bryan College
www.bryan.edu/714.html

Carson-Newman College
www.cn.edu/CN.htm

Lincoln Memorial University
www.lmunet.edu/academics/undergrad/hpeat/

Lipscomb University
www.lipscomb.edu/page.asp?SID=4&Page=32

Middle Tennessee State University
www.mtsu.edu/~athtrain/index.htm

Tusculum College
www.tusculum.edu/academics/programs/athletic_training/
.

Union University
www.uu.edu/programs/atep/

University of Tennessee at Chattanooga
www.utc.edu/Academic/GraduateAthleticTraining/entry.
php#descr

University of Tennessee at Martin
www.utm.edu/departments/cebs/hhp/AthleticTraining.
php

Texas

Angelo State University
www.angelo.edu/org/sportmed/

Baylor University
www.baylor.edu/soe/HHPR/index.php?id=11856

East Texas Baptist University
www.etbu.edu

Hardin Simmons University
www.hsutx.edu/academics/sportsmed/index.htm

Southwestern University
www.southwestern.edu/athletics/ath_training.html

Southwest Texas State University
excet.hper.txstate.edu/Athletic%20Training/ATMission.
html

Texas A&M University-Commerce
www.tamu-commerce.edu/vpaa/MyPlan/coehs/Health_
Human_Performance/BS_Athletic_Training.htm

Texas Christian University
www.train.tcu.edu

Texas Lutheran University
www.tlu.edu/academics/athletic_training/

Texas Tech University Health Sciences Center
www.ttuhsc.edu/sah/mat/

The University of the Incarnate Word
www.uiw.edu/snhp/athtrain.html

University of Texas at Arlington
www.uta.edu/coed/kinesiology/atep/

Utah

Brigham Young University
ar.byu.edu/dept_academ_advise/gemajor/OO/dc/
663421DC.html

Southern Utah University
www.suu.edu/ed/pe/bs-athtrain.html

University of Utah
www.health.utah.edu/ess/athletic-trng

Weber State University
www.weber.edu/

Vermont

Castleton State College
www.csc.vsc.edu/athletictraining

Norwich University
www.norwich.edu/academics/mathematics/athletictraining.html

University of Vermont
www.uvm.edu/~dosa/chw/?Page=athletic.html

Virginia

Averett University
www.averett.edu/academics/physical-education/athletic-training/

Bridgewater College
www.bridgewater.edu/Sports/Athletic_Training/

Emory & Henry College
www.ehc.edu/cgi-bin/MySQLdb?FILE=/index1.html

George Mason University
www.gmu.edu/catalog/courses/atep.html
www.gmu.edu/departments/advising/majors/athl.doc

James Madison University
www.jmu.edu/healthsci/at/

Jefferson College of Health Sciences
www.jchs.edu/

Liberty University
www.liberty.edu/academics/education/sport/index.cfm?PID=85

Longwood University
www.longwood.edu/hrk/athletic_training/index.htm

Lynchburg College
www.lynchburg.edu/academic/athletictraining/

Radford University
www.radford.edu/~atep/AT%20Program/Athletic%20Training%20Program.htm

Roanoke College
www.roanoke.edu/education/athletic-training.htm

Shenandoah University
www.su.edu/academic.cfm?program=Athletic%20Training

Virginia Commonwealth University School of Medicine
www.medschool.vcu.edu/

Washington

Washington State University
education.wsu.edu/ELCP/programs/BA_AthleticTrng.html

Whitworth College
www.whitworth.edu/Academic/Department/Kinesiology&Athletics/Index.asp

West Virginia

Concord University
www.concord.edu/

Marshall University
www.marshall.edu/coehs/essr/athletic.training/

University of Charleston
www.ucwv.edu/

West Virginia University
www.wvu.edu/~physed/attrain/wvattr-1.htm

West Virginia Wesleyan College
www.wvwc.edu/aca/ped/dept/

Wisconsin

Carroll College
www.cc.edu/academics/academics_area_athletictrain.html

Carthage College
www2.carthage.edu/departments/athtraining/

Concordia University
www.cuw.edu/Academics/programs/athletic_training/

Marquette University
www.marquette.edu

University of Wisconsin-Eau Claire
www.uwec.edu/kin/majors/AT/atcourselist0304.pdf

University of Wisconsin-LaCrosse
www.uwlax.edu/AthleticTraining/undergraduate.htm

University of Wisconsin-Madison
www.education.wisc.edu/kinesiology/ugrad/at1.htm

University of Wisconsin-Milwaukee
www.uwm.edu/ugbulletin/SC/D_HS_K.html#ath_t_p

University of Wisconsin Stevens Point
www.uwsp.edu/hesa/athtraining/

Wyoming

University of Wyoming
uwadmnweb.uwyo.edu/ATHTRN/

BIBLIOGRAPHY

Albohm MJ, Campbell D, Konin JG. *Reimbursement for Athletic Trainers.* Thorofare, NJ: SLACK Incorporated; 2001.

American Academy of Orthopedic Surgeons. *Athletic Training and Sports Medicine.* 4th ed. Chicago, Ill: Author; 2004.

American College of Sports Medicine. *ACSM's Guidelines for Exercise Testing and Prescription.* 6th ed. New York, NY: Lippincott Williams and Wilkins; 2000.

Anderson M, Hall S, Martin, M. *Foundations of Athletic Training.* 3rd ed. New York, NY: Lippincott Williams and Wilkins; 2005.

Baechle TR, Earle RW. *Essentials of Strength Training and Conditioning.* 2nd ed. Champaign, Ill: Human Kinetics; 2000.

BOC. *Certification Update.* Omaha, NE: NATA; 2005.

BOC. Online Registration for Reg X. Available at: http://www.bocatc.org/becomeatc/regx/login/. Accessed September 1, 2005.

BOC. *Role Delineation Study.* 5th ed. Raleigh, NC: Columbia Assessment Services; 2005.

Cantu RC. *Neurological Athletic Head and Spine Injuries.* St. Louis, Mo: Mosby-Year Book; 2000.

Cartwright L. *Preparing for the Athletic Trainer's Certification Examination.* Champaign, Ill: Human Kinetics; 2002-2004.

Clarkson HM. *Musculoskeletal Assessment.* 2nd ed. New York, NY: Lippincott Williams and Wilkins; 2000.

Crouch JE. *Functional Human Anatomy.* 4th ed. Philadelphia, Pa: Lea and Febiger; 1985.

Denegar CR. *Therapeutic Modalities for Athletic Injuries.* Champaign, Ill: Human Kinetics; 2000.

Epler M, Wainwright S. *Manual Muscle Testing.* Thorofare, NJ: SLACK Incorporated; 1999.

Gall MD, Gall JP, Jacobsen DR, Bullock TL. *Tools for Learning: A Guide to Teaching Study Skills.* Alexandria, Va: Association for Supervision and Curriculum Development; 1990.

Gallaspy JB, May JD. *Signs and Symptoms of Athletic Injuries.* St. Louis, Mo: Mosby-Year Book; 1996.

Henry ML, Stapleton ER. *EMT Prehospital Care.* Philadelphia, Pa: WB Saunders; 1992.

Heyward VH. *Advanced Fitness Assessment and Exercise Prescription.* 3rd ed. Champaign, Ill: Human Kinetics; 1998.

Hoppenfeld S. *Physical Examination of the Spine and Extremities.* Norwalk, Conn: Appleton and Lange; 1976.

Hoppenfeld S, Zeide MS. *Orthopaedic Dictionary.* Philadelphia, Pa: JB Lippincott; 1994.

Houglum J, Harrelson G, Leaver-Dunn D. *Principles of Pharmacology for Athletic Trainers.* Thorofare, NJ; SLACK Incorporated; 2005.

Houglum PA. *Therapeutic Exercise for Athletic Injuries.* 2nd ed. Champaign, Ill: Human Kinetics; 2005.

Kleiner DM, Almquist JL, Bailes J, et al. *Prehospital Care of the Spine-Injured Athlete: A Document From the Inter-Association Task Force for Appropriate Care of the Spine-Injured Athlete.* Dallas, Tex: NATA; 2001.

Konin JG. *Clinical Athletic Training.* Thorofare, NJ: SLACK Incorporated; 1997.

Konin JG, Wiksten DL, Isear J, Brader H. *Special Tests for Orthopedic Examination.* 2nd ed. Thorofare, NJ: SLACK Incorporated; 2002.

Magee DJ. *Orthopaedic Physical Assessment.* 5th ed. Philadelphia, Pa: WB Saunders; 2004.

McFarlane P, Hodson S. *Studying Effectively and Efficiently: An Integrated System*. Toronto, Ontario, Canada: Governing Council of University of Toronto; 1983.

McMinn RMH, Hutchings RT. *A Colour Atlas of Human Anatomy*. London, England: Wolfe Medical Publications Ltd; 1998.

Mellion MB. *Sports Medicine Secrets*. Philadelphia, Pa: Hanley and Belfus; 1993.

Mellion MB, Walsh WM, Shelton GL. *The Team Physician's Handbook*. Philadelphia, Pa: Hanley and Belfus; 1990.

Michlovitz SL. *Thermal Agents in Rehabilitation*. 2nd ed. Philadelphia, Pa: FA Davis; 1990.

NATA. Education. Available at: http://www.nata.org/education/education1.html. Accessed August 27, 2005.

NATABOC. *Study Guide for the Entry-Level Athletic Trainer Certification Examination*. 2nd ed. Philadelphia, Pa: FA Davis; 1993.

Norkin C, Levangie P. *Joint Structure and Function: A Comprehensive Analysis*. 2nd ed. Philadelphia, Pa: FA Davis; 1992.

Norkin CC, White DJ. *Measurement of Joint Motion*. 2nd ed. Philadelphia, Pa: FA Davis; 1995.

O'Conner DP. *Clinical Pathology for Athletic Trainers: Recognizing Systemic Disease*. Thorofare, NJ: SLACK Incorporated; 2001.

Prentice WE. *Principles of Athletic Training*. 13th ed. New York, NY: McGraw-Hill; 2005.

Prentice WE. *Rehabilitation Techniques in Sports Medicine*. 4th ed. New York, NY: McGraw-Hill; 2003.

Prentice WE. *Therapeutic Modalities in Sports Medicine*. 5th ed. New York, NY: McGraw-Hill; 2002.

Prentice WE, Voight MI. *Techniques in Musculoskeletal Rehabilitation*. New York, NY: McGraw-Hill; 2001.

Ray R. *Management Strategies in Athletic Training*. 2nd ed. Champaign, Ill: Human Kinetics; 2005.

Rothstein JM, Roy SH, Wolf SL. *The Rehabilitation Specialist's Handbook*. Philadelphia, Pa: FA Davis; 1991.

Sladyk K, McGeary S, Sladyk L, Tufano R. *OTR Exam Review Manual*. 3rd ed. Thorofare, NJ: SLACK Incorporated; 2001.

Starkey C. *Therapeutic Modalities*. 3rd ed. Philadelphia, Pa: FA Davis; 2004.

Stedman's Concise Medical Dictionary for the Health Professions. 4th ed. Baltimore, Md: Williams & Wilkins; 2001.

Van De Graaff K. *Human Anatomy*. 5th ed. New York, NY: McGraw-Hill; 2000.

Van Ost L. *Goniometry*. Thorofare, NJ: SLACK Incorporated; 1999.

Vander A, Sherman J, Luciano D. *Human Physiology*. 8th ed. New York, NY: McGraw-Hill; 2001.

Voss DE, Ionta MK, Myers BJ. *Proprioceptive Neuromuscular Facilitation*. 3rd ed. Philadelphia, Pa: Harper and Row; 1985.

Wardlaw GM, Insel PM. *Perspectives in Nutrition*. 2nd ed. St. Louis, Mo: Mosby-Year Book; 1993.

WAIT
...There's More!

SLACK Incorporated's Health Care Books and Journals offers a wide selection of products in the field of Athletic Training. We are dedicated to providing important works that educate, inform and improve the knowledge of our customers. Don't miss out on our other informative titles that will enhance your collection.

Clinical Skills Documentation Guide for Athletic Training, Second Edition

Herb Amato, DA, ATC; Christy Hawkins, MS, ATC; and Steven L. Cole, MEd, ATC, CSCS

464 pp., Soft Cover, 2006, ISBN 1-55642-758-1, Order# 47581, **$34.95**

The esteemed Practical Exam Preparation Guide of Clinical Skills for Athletic Training has been updated, revised, and renamed to accurately reflect the material presented throughout the text that is necessary for athletic training students to master clinical skill sets as tested on throughout their educational career. With new chapters reflecting the progressing field of athletic training, a re-organization of the information presented, and the addition of 110 new clinical skill sets, this Second Edition is the critical first step necessary in developing clinical skill set mastery for athletic training students.

Special Tests for Orthopedic Examination, Third Edition

Jeff G. Konin, PhD, ATC, PT; Denise L. Wiksten, PhD, ATC; Jerome A. Isear, Jr. MS, PT, ATC-L; and Holly Brader, MPH, RN, BSN, ATC

400 pp., Soft Cover, 2006, ISBN 1-55642-741-7, Order# 47417, **$38.95**

Special Tests for Orthopedic Examination has been used for 10 years by thousands of students, clinicians, and rehab professionals and is now available in a revised and updated Third Edition. Concise and pocket-sized, this handbook is an invaluable guide filled with the most current and practical clinical exam techniques used during an orthopedic examination. This Third Edition takes a user-friendly approach to visualizing and explaining more than 150 commonly used orthopedic special tests, including 11 new and modern tests.

Athletic Training Exam Review: A Student Guide to Success, Third Edition

Lynn Van Ost, RN, PT, ATC, MEd; Karen Manfre, ATR, MA; and Karen Lew, MEd, ATC, LAT

272 pp., Soft Cover, 2006, ISBN 1-55642-764-6, Order# 47646, **$42.95**

Quick Reference Dictionary for Athletic Training, Second Edition

Julie N. Bernier, EdD, ATC

416 pp., Soft Cover, 2005, ISBN 1-55642-666-6, Order# 46666, **$28.95**

Athletic Training Student Primer: A Foundation for Success

Andrew P. Winterstein, PhD, ATC

256 pp., Soft Cover, 2003, ISBN 1-55642-570-8, Order# 45708, **$38.95**

Clinical Pathology for Athletic Trainers: Recognizing Systemic Disease

Dan O'Connor, PhD, AT

288 pp., Soft Cover, 2001, ISBN 1-55642-469-8, Order# 44698, **$40.95**

Goniometry: An Interactive Tutorial

Lynn Van Ost, RN, PT, ATC, MEd

CD-ROM, 1999, ISBN 1-55642-721-2, Order# 47212, **$49.95**

Athletic Training in Occupational Settings

Susan Finkam, MS, ATC, LAT, CEA

168 pp., Soft Cover, 2004, ISBN 1-55642-632-1, Order# 46321, **$39.95**

The Athletic Trainer's Guide to Psychosocial Intervention and Referral

James Mensch, PhD, ATC and Gary M. Miller, PhD

350 pp., Hard Cover, Due Early 2007, ISBN 1-55642-733-6, Order# 47336, **$44.95**